Glutamine and Glutamate in Mammals

Volume I

Editor

Elling Kvamme, M.D., Dr. med.

Professor of Neurochemistry
Neurochemical Laboratory
University of Oslo
Oslo, Norway

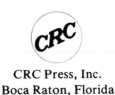

CRC Press, Inc.
Boca Raton, Florida

Library of Congress Cataloging-in-Publication Data

Glutamine and glutamate in mammals.

   Includes bibliographies and indexes.
   1. Glutamine--Metabolism.   2. Glutamic acid--
Metabolism.   3. Mammals--Physiology. I. Kvamme,
Elling, 1918-
QP562.G55G57   1988   599'.019'245   87-21788
ISBN 0-8493-6856-1 (v. 1)
ISBN 0-8493-6857-X (v. 2)

   Direct all inquiries to CRC Press, Inc., 2000 Corporate Blvd., N.W., Boca Raton, Florida, 33431.

© 1988 by CRC Press, Inc.
International Standard Book Number 0-8493-6856-1 (v. 1)
International Standard Book Number 0-8493-6857-X (v. 2)

Library of Congress Number 87-21788
Printed in the United States

PREFACE

The present comprehensive volume, which is based on the joint effort of a great many top scientists and covering most aspects of the metabolism and function of glutamine and glutamate in mammals, is a result of what we felt was a specific demand. Thus, the majority of previous books and review articles on glutamine and glutamate are confined to limited areas (e.g., energy metabolism, nervous transmission, etc.) or organs (e.g., brain, kidney, liver, etc.). This is not surprising in view of the vast amount of recent publications in each field, but it contributes to some sort of compartmentalization — to use a popular word — that creates barriers and subspecialization. The present volumes intend to act as a carrier between the various compartments. Similar to biological carriers, this one must be selective, since every discovery claimed to be done cannot be and does not deserve to be conveyed. However, what should be included will always be a matter of different opinion. Anyway, to communicate essential information from the many interrelated subfields appears to be necessary, since quite a few recent publications reflect the lack of knowledge of relevant findings in neighboring fields.

In addition to breaking down artificial barriers between subjects and fields, this volume also serves another purpose, namely to transmit different views on controversial matters. For that reason each author has been allowed to speak with his own voice and present his personal opinion on problems under debate. The careful reader will therefore discover that in spite of considerable overlapping in problems to be discussed, the flavor of the discussions may be different. Furthermore, although the reader may feel that he knows what is worth knowing about a subject after having read the relevant chapter, he may change his mind following the study of other chapters touching upon the same subject. However, the present volumes do not pretend to give the final answer to the many problems presented, but it intends to give a cross-section of a process under continuous development, and I wish to convey my sincere thanks to the authors who have all contributed to approach this goal.

Elling Kvamme

THE EDITOR

Dr. Elling Kvamme is professor of neurochemistry at the Oslo University and Head of the Neurochemical Laboratory.

In 1947, Dr. Kvamme received an M.D. at the Oslo University. Thereafter, he studied organic and physical chemistry, and in 1959 he received the scientific degree, Dr. med., at the Oslo University. After 3 years of service at Dikemark Hospital, Asker, and a 1-year internship (internal medicine and surgery) at the Ullevål Hospital, Oslo, he received a Fulbright/Smith Mundt Fellowship and worked as a Research Fellow at the Sloan-Kettering Institute for Cancer Research in New York from 1952 to 1954, and at the Public Health Research Institute of the City of New York, Department of Biochemistry, from 1954 to 1955. From 1955 to 1962, Dr. Kvamme was appointed Assistant Head of the Central Laboratory, Ullevål Hospital. Thereafter, he was appointed Head of the newly formed Neurochemical Laboratory at the Oslo University Psychiatric Clinic and, in 1966, appointed professor of Neurochemistry at the Oslo University. He is currently teaching neurochemistry to medical students and organizing postgraduate courses.

In 1962, Dr. Kvamme spent 6 months as a Technical Assistant Expert at the National Institute of Cancer, Rio de Janeiro, being appointed by the International Atomic Energy Agency, Vienna.

Dr. Kvamme has presented numerous papers at international meetings, as well as guest lectures at various universities and institutes in Europe and the U.S. He has also taken an active part in organizing many national and international meetings. Dr. Kvamme has served as the President of the Norwegian Biochemical Society from 1976 to 1978, the Treasurer of the International Society for Neurochemistry (ISN) from 1977 to 1981, the Chairman of ISN from 1981 to 1983, and the Chairman of the Policy Advisory Committee of ISN from 1985 to 1987.

Dr. Kvamme's main interest includes the metabolism and function of amino acids, in particular with regard to glutamine and glutamate. He has published a great number of scientific articles in international journals, in addition to several review articles in handbooks and scientific journals.

CONTRIBUTORS

Arthur J. L. Cooper
Associate Professor
Departments of Neurology and
  Biochemistry
Cornell University Medical College
New York, New York

Ivan Couée
Department of Biochemistry
Trinity College
Dublin, Ireland

A. M. Pujaras Crane
Department of Immunology
Baylor College of Medicine
Houston, Texas

Larry A. Denner
Department of Cell Biology
Baylor College of Medicine
Houston, Texas

Alan J. Garber
Professor of Medicine, Biochemistry, and
  Cell Biology
Baylor College of Medicine
and
Chief
Diabetes Metabolism Unit
The Methodist Hospital
Houston, Texas

Peter J. Hanson
Division of Biology, Molecular Sciences
University of Aston
Birmingham, England

Nils-Erik Huseby
Department of Clinical Chemistry
Institute of Medical Biology
University of Tromso
Tromso, Norway

Bang Hwang
Indiana University
Terre Haute Center for Medical Education
Terre Haute, Indiana

Elling Kvamme
Professor
Neurochemical Laboratory
University of Oslo
Oslo, Norway

Chin-Tarng Lin
Department of Pathology
National Taiwan University
Taipei, Taiwan

C. M. Maillet
Department of Biochemistry
University of Texas Health Science
  Center
Houston, Texas

J. D. McGivan
Department of Biochemistry
University of Bristol
Bristol, England

William J. Nicklas
Professor
Department of Neurology
Robert Wood Johnson Medical School
University of Medicine and Dentistry of
  New Jersey
Piscataway, New Jersey

Dennis S. Parsons
Department of Physiology
Oxford University
Oxford, England

David P. Simpson
Professor
Department of Medicine
University of Wisconsin
Madison, Wisconsin

Gerd Svenneby
Neurochemical Laboratory
University of Oslo
Oslo, Norway

J. Tyson Tildon
Professor
Department of Pediatrics
Department of Biological Chemistry
University of Maryland
Baltimore, Maryland

Keith F. Tipton
Department of Biochemistry
Trinity College
Dublin, Ireland

Ingeborg Aasland Torgner
Neurochemical Laboratory
University of Oslo
Oslo, Norway

Jang-Yen Wu
Professor
Department of Physiology
Milton S. Hershey Medical Center
Pennsylvania State University
Hershey, Pennsylvania

H. Ronald Zielke
Associate Professor
Department of Pediatrics
University of Maryland
Baltimore, Maryland

TABLE OF CONTENTS

Volume I

Volume II

GLUTAMINE AND GLUTAMATE IN THE CENTRAL NERVOUS SYSTEM

PATHOLOGY OF GLUTAMINE AND GLUTAMATE

Chapter 1

GLUTAMATE AND GLUTAMINE IN MAMMALS: AN OVERVIEW

William J. Nicklas

Glutamate and glutamine are key amino acids in mammalian intermediary metabolism, intimately associated with aerobic metabolism via the tricarboxylic acid cycle and with ammonia metabolism. In addition they are involved in the synthetic pathways of numerous biologically important compounds.[1] Research in various aspects of the metabolism and function of these amino acids has been continuous since the earliest days of modern biochemical studies.[2] The various contributions to this monograph attest to the vitality and conceptual depth of current research efforts. The direction of these studies has traced a path through the traditional biochemical methodologies and now encompasses other powerful techniques such as immunohistochemistry and molecular biology.

What is emerging from these multidisciplinary studies on different organ systems is a pattern of greater complexity and heterogeneity than previous work might have suggested. Not only does one find the expected intracellular and interorgan diversity, but intercellular heterogeneity is becoming a more commonly accepted phenomenon. Nowhere is this complexity and heterogeneity more apparent, nor has it been more intensely studied, than in the nervous system.[3-5] In the central nervous system (CNS), glutamate and its decarboxylation product, 4-aminobutyrate (GABA), may well function as important neurotransmitter substances.[6] Thus superimposed on the "normal" role of glutamate and glutamine in cellular metabolism with its accompanying transport systems and enzymes is the further complication of specific membrane-associated receptor proteins and the associated ion-channel systems. Furthermore, glutamate and related neuroexcitatory substances are also potentially neurotoxic. The pharmacological and toxicological consequences of multiple receptor types for excitatory dicarboxylic amino acids are only now being understood and exploited.[7,8] It is clear from this that exquisite regulatory mechanisms must be present to separate these various functions of ubiquitously distributed amino acids such as glutamate and glutamine. The homeostatic regulation of the neuroactive amino acids is associated with a heterogeneity of enzyme distribution among the neurons and glial cells that make up the nervous system.[9] Most current evidence would suggest that transmitter pools of glutamate are formed in glutamatergic synaptic endings from glutamine via the activity of phosphate-activated glutaminase [EC 3.5.1.2], which catalyzes the hydrolytic cleavage of glutamine to glutamate and ammonia. It is doubtful that this enzyme is localized principally in such neurons but there may be some relative enrichment. Regulation probably occurs via product inhibition and presence of other effectors, such as Ca^{2+}.[10,11] Glutamine synthesis in the brain appears to be principally associated with the activity of glutamine synthetase [EC 6.3.1.2] which catalyzes the ATP-dependent amidation of glutamate.[12] This also serves to remove ammonia from the circulation since the urea cycle is inoperative in brain. Early experiments in which animals were injected with radioactive precursors suggested that glutamine synthesis in the brain was compartmented. For example, when rats were injected intracisternally (thus avoiding problems with the blood-brain barrier) with ^{14}C-glutamate and the total pools of brain glutamate and glutamine acid-extracted, it was found that within minutes the radiospecific activity of the total glutamine was severalfold higher than that of the total brain glutamate.[13] This indicated that the radioactive extracellular glutamate was metabolized in a biochemical compartment in which glutamine was synthesized before the radioactive glutamate could mix with the bulk of tissue glutamate. Based on a great deal of similar in vivo and in vitro data, Balazs et al.[14] suggested the "compartment" in which glutamine was actively syn-

thesized was the astroglial cells of the brain. The subsequent immunohistochemical localization of glutamine synthetase in astrocytes in the brain[15] has definitively shown this
interpretation based on biochemical studies to be correct. These findings immediately suggest
problems of regulation of transport and metabolism which would not be so obvious in a less
complex model. However, this complexity also allows for the separate regulation of the role
of these amino acids in "normal" metabolism and their possible role in neurotransmission.

From these studies emerged a concept of a "glutamine cycle" between glia and nerve
endings.[9,16] In this hypothesis, glutamate and GABA levels within their respective nerve
terminals are maintained by glutamine derived from the extracellular space which in turn
can be replenished by synthesis in the glia via glutamine synthetase. In a series of studies
we attempted to answer the question as to whether this really occurred.[9] One consistent
finding that emerged from the many earlier studies done with radioactive precursors of
glutamate/glutamine was that radioactive acetate (either [14]C- or ^{3}H-labeled) is preferentially
metabolized in the glutamine-synthesizing compartment of the brain, i.e., the astrocyte,
whereas radioactively labeled glucose is metabolized in all compartments.[16] Numerous studies have shown that when various CNS preparations are allowed to metabolize labeled glucose
and/or acetate and then efflux of synaptic contents initiated by depolarization stimuli, there
is a preferential efflux of glucose-labeled glutamate.[9,17,18] In a series of experiments,[9] tissue
slice preparations from rat brains were incubated with a mixture of ^{14}C-glucose and [3]H-
acetate to label endogenous pools of amino acids. The alkaloid veratridine was used to cause
the efflux of synaptic glutamate and GABA. The proposed flow pathway from glutamine
synthesis in glia to glutamine utilization in the nerve endings was blocked by using 6-diazo-
5-oxo-L-norleucine (DON), an inhibitor of glutaminase, or L-methionine sulfoximine, an
inhibitor of glutamine synthetase. These treatments decreased the veratridine-induced release
of acetate-labeled glutamate and GABA preferentially. Therefore, glutamate and GABA
labeled from radioactive acetate metabolism (i.e., from glial metabolism) did indeed enter
transmitter pools of these amino acids via glutamine.[9] Moreover, the contribution of glutamine metabolism to the maintenance of transmitter amino acid levels seemed to be quantitatively important. The above studies were performed with in vitro preparations. Rothstein
and Tabakoff[19] have come to a similar conclusion after in vivo inhibition of glutamine
synthetase. Methionine sulfoximine was administered to rats intraventricularly and the glutamergic system of the striatum was studied. Striatal glutamine synthetase activity and
glutamine levels were decreased substantially for days with no change in total glutamate
levels. In addition, the Ca^{2+}-dependent, K^+-stimulated release of glutamate from striatal
slices of treated animals was diminished by 50%. When glutamine was present in the
perfusion medium in which release was measured, there was no difference in glutamate
efflux between slices from control or treated animals. The same authors had previously
reported that treatment of rats with intraventricular methionine sulfoximine decreased the
activity of dopaminergic terminals in the striatum.[20] This is of physiological interest because
it has been suggested that corticostriatal glutamergic inputs presynaptically facilitate the
release of dopamine from nigrostriatal nerve endings. At the present time, there is every
reason to conclude that the "glutamine cycle" is operative in the CNS and is of quantitative
and qualitative importance in the regulation of glutamate homeostasis.

When the first studies on amino acid metabolism in the brain were reported 2 decades
ago, there was a good deal of skepticism in the traditional biochemical community. Some
of this attitude was probably due to the perception of a relative homogeneity of amino acid
metabolism in other organs, for example, in the liver which was the benchmark for comparison. Another important reason, perhaps, was a lack of awareness of how to properly
interpret studies with tracer-radioactive precursors and the role played by high affinity active
transport systems for substances such as glutamate when tracer amounts are utilized in such
studies. In any case, doubts were slowly buried under an ever-increasing amount of data

culminating in the immunohistochemical localization studies. In the meantime, the perception of the homogeneity of glutamate metabolism in organs such as the liver has been replaced by more recent, broadening concepts of its heterogeneity.

The early studies with isotopically labeled precursors administered intravenously to animals also suggested a compartmentation of glutamate/glutamine/ammonia metabolism in other organs such as the liver.[13] This was not pursued at the time. It is now clear that ammonia metabolism in the liver is heterogeneous. Glutamine synthetase appears to be localized in a small layer of perivenous cells[21] which results in a heterogeneity in glutamine and ammonia metabolism as studied by steady-state anterograde and retrograde perfusion experiments.[22] Thus, there is a periportal location of urea synthesis and a perivenous location for glutamine synthesis in the liver. Each of these processes is subject to regulation and the resulting studies have been most fruitful in better understanding ammonia metabolism in the liver and its response to various physiological effectors.[23] Häussinger[22] has proposed an intercellular "glutamine cycle" operating in the liver during ureogenesis which is to some extent reminiscent of the "glutamine cycle" of the brain. The disparate distribution of glutamine synthetase and the resulting heterogeneity of ammonia metabolism also impacts on the *in situ* activity of other enzymes which may be more homogeneously distributed, such as glutamate dehydrogenase [EC 1.4.1.3], an oxidoreductase which catalyses the NAD(P)-dependent deamination of glutamate to 2-oxoglutarate as well as the reverse reaction, the amination of 2-oxoglutarate to glutamate. The direction of the reaction can be different in different organs and under different conditions within the same organ. In the brain, the contribution of this enzyme to amino acid metabolism is not well understood but is under active investigation.[24] Studies in the brain might well profit from what has been found in experiments with other organs such as the liver. As pointed out by Sies and Häussinger,[23] ammonia production from catabolism of endogenous sources implies an increased oxidative deamination of glutamate by glutamate dehydrogenase in the periportal lobule of the liver. Conversely, perivenous glutamine synthesis from ammonia released from periportal hepatocytes requires increased glutamate formation by glutamate dehydrogenase to maintain glutamate levels. Here again there is an interesting analogy to studies in the nervous system. Berl et al.[13,25] in their pioneering studies on ^{15}N-NH$_3$ metabolism in the brain found an increased synthesis of glutamate which occurred via glutamate dehydrogenase when glutamine synthesis was stimulated by increased ammonia levels. Concomitantly, to maintain 2-oxoglutarate levels, fixation of carbon dioxide via pyruvate carboxylase was also stimulated. The astrocyte is fixed as the site where these effects occur by the fact that ^{14}C-HCO$_3$ behaves like acetate as a glutamine precursor in vivo[25] and in vitro,[26] and pyruvate carboxylase appears to be a glial enzyme.[27]

The above discussion illustrates the complexities of the regulation of glutamate metabolism in different organs. It also serves to illustrate the differences and similarities in approach which can be taken in such studies. Hopefully, the present volume will allow even more "borrowing" between investigators in this field. This interdisciplinary sharing will become even more important as research begins on the molecular biology of glutamate function and metabolism and the novel revelations expected from those studies.

REFERENCES

1. **Meister, A.,** Biochemistry of glutamate, glutamine and glutathione, in *Advances in Biochemical Physiology,* Garattini, S., Filer, L. J., Kare, H., Reynolds, W. A., and Wurtman, R. J., Eds., Raven Press, New York, 1979, 69.
2. **Krebs, H.,** Glutamine metabolism in the animal body, in *Glutamine Metabolism, Enzymology, and Regulation,* Mora, J. and Palacios, R., Eds., Academic Press, New York, 1980, 319.

3. **Balazs, R. and Cremer, J. E., Eds.,** *Metabolic Compartmentation in the Brain,* Macmillan, London, 1973.
4. **Bradford, H. F.,** *Neurotransmitter Interaction and Compartmentation,* Plenum Press, New York, 1982.
5. **Hertz, L., Kvamme, E., McGeer, E., and Schousboe, A., Eds.,** *Glutamine, Glutamate and GABA in the Central Nervous System,* Alan R. Liss, New York, 1983.
6. **Roberts, P. J., Storm-Mathesen, J., and Johnston, G. A. R., Eds.,** *Glutamate: Transmitter in the Central Nervous System,* John Wiley & Sons, New York, 1981.
7. **Meldrum, B.,** Possible therapeutic applications of antagonists of excitatory amino acid neurotransmitters, *Clin. Sci.,* 68, 113, 1985.
8. **Olney, J. W.,** Excitotoxins: an overview, in *Excitotoxins,* Vol. 39, Wenner-Gren Int. Symp. Ser., Fuxe, K., Roberts, P., and Schwarcz, R., Eds., Macmillan, London, 1983, 82.
9. **Nicklas, W. J.,** Relative contributions of neurons and glia to metabolism of glutamate and GABA, in *Glutamine, Glutamate and GABA in the Central Nervous System,* Hertz, L., Kvamme, E., McGeer, E., and Schousboe, A., Eds., Alan R. Liss, New York, 1983, 219.
10. **Benjamin, A. M.,** Control of glutaminase activity in rat brain cortex *in vitro:* influence of glutamate, phosphate, ammonium, calcium and hydrogen ions, *Brain Res.,* 208, 363, 1981.
11. **Kvamme, E.,** Enzymes of cerebral glutamine metabolism, in *Glutamine Metabolism in Mammalian Tissues,* Häussinger, D. and Sies, H., Eds., Springer-Verlag, Berlin, 1984, 32.
12. **Meister, A.,** Glutamine synthetase of mammals, *Enzymes,* 10, 699, 1974.
13. **Berl, S., Takagaki, G., Clarke, D. D., and Waelsch, H.,** Metabolic compartments *in vivo:* ammonia and glutamic acid metabolism in brain and liver, *J. Biol. Chem.,* 237, 2562, 1962.
14. **Balazs, R., Patel, A. J., and Richter, D.,** Metabolic compartments in the brain: their properties and relation to morphological structures, in *Metabolic Compartmentation in the Brain,* Balazs, R. and Cremer, J. E., Eds., Macmillan, London, 1973, 167.
15. **Norenberg, M. and Martinez-Hernandez, A.,** Fine structural localization of glutamine synthetase in astrocytes in brain, *Brain Res.,* 161, 303, 1979.
16. **Van den Berg, C. J. and Garfinkel, D.,** A simulation study of brain compartments. Metabolism of glutamate and related substances in mouse brain, *Biochem. J.,* 123, 211, 1971.
17. **Minchin, M. C. W.,** The release of amino acids synthesized from various compartmental precursors in rat spinal cord slices, *Exp. Brain Res.,* 29, 515, 1977.
18. **Krespan, B., Berl, S., and Nicklas, W. J.,** Alteration in neuronal-glial metabolism of glutamate by the neurotoxin kainic acid, *J. Neurochem.,* 38, 509, 1982.
19. **Rothstein, J. D. and Tabakoff, B.,** Alteration of striatal glutamate release after glutamine synthetase inhibition, *J. Neurochem.,* 43, 1438, 1984.
20. **Rothstein, J. D. and Tabakoff, B.,** Effects of the convulsant methionine sulfoximine on striatal dopamine metabolism, *J. Neurochem.,* 39, 452, 1982.
21. **Gebhardt, R. and Mecke, D.,** Heterogeneous distribution of glutamine synthetase among rat liver parenchymal cells *in situ* and in primary culture, *EMBO J.,* 2, 567, 1983.
22. **Häussinger, D.,** Hepatocyte heterogeneity in glutamine and ammonia metabolism and the role of an intercellular glutamine cycle during ureogenesis in perfused rat liver, *Eur. J. Biochem.,* 133, 269, 1983.
23. **Sies, H. and Häussinger, D.,** Hepatic glutamine and ammonia metabolism, in *Glutamine Metabolism in Mammalian Tissues,* Häussinger, D. and Sies, H., Eds., Springer-Verlag, Berlin, 1984, 78.
24. **Nicklas, W. J.,** Amino acid metabolism in the central nervous system: role of glutamate dehydrogenase, in *The Olivopontocerebellar Atrophies,* Duvoisin, R. C. and Plaitakis, A., Eds., Raven Press, New York, 1984, 245.
25. **Berl, S., Takagaki, G., Clarke, D. D., and Waelsch, H.,** Carbon dioxide fixation in the brain, *J. Biol. Chem.,* 237, 2570, 1962.
26. **Berl, S., Nicklas, W. J., and Clarke, D. D.,** Compartmentation of citric acid cycle metabolism in brain: labeling of glutamate, glutamine, aspartate and GABA by several radioactive tracer metabolites, *J. Neurochem.,* 17, 1009, 1970.
27. **Yu, A. C. H., Drejer, J., Hertz, L., and Schousboe, A.,** Pyruvate carboxylase activity in primary cultures of astrocytes and neurons, *J. Neurochem.,* 41, 1481, 1983.

Enzymes in Glutamine and Glutamate Metabolism

Chapter 2

GLUTAMINE SYNTHETASE

Arthur J. L. Cooper

TABLE OF CONTENTS

I. METABOLIC IMPORTANCE: OVERVIEW

Glutamine participates in a number of amide and amine transfer reactions; in addition, glutamine is a constituent of most proteins (Figure 1). The amide nitrogen of glutamine is used for the synthesis of nitrogen 3 and 9 of the purine ring, the amide of NAD^+, asparagine amide, nitrogen 1 of the imidazole ring of histidine, the pyrrole nitrogen of tryptophan, the amino groups of glucosamine-6-phosphate, guanine, cytidine and *p*-aminobenzoate, and carbamyl phosphate. Carbamyl phosphate is in turn used for the synthesis of urea, arginine, and nitrogen I of the pyrimidine ring.[3-5] In these reactions glutamine seems to play a role that could conceivably have been fulfilled by ammonia. However, ammonia is toxic to many animal tissues, particularly the central nervous system (CNS). It may be that for thermodynamic reasons ammonia cannot bind easily to most enzymes that catalyze nitrogen incorporation reactions. On the other hand, glutamine provides a "handle" that allows easy binding to glutamine amidotransferases. Glutamine thus serves as a nontoxic store of easily transferred nitrogen and of glutamate. In man (and probably in the higher apes) glutamine participates in a unique detoxification reaction: phenylacetic acid (derived from phenylalanine) is coupled with glutamine to form phenylacetylglutamine, which is excreted in the urine in large amounts.[6] Certain microorganisms and plants contain glutamate synthase, an enzyme that reductively transfers the amide nitrogen of glutamine to α-ketoglutarate (2-oxoglutarate) to yield glutamate (Figure 1).[7,8] Apparently, the combined action of glutamine synthetase and glutamate synthase is more efficient at fixing low levels of ammonia into glutamate than is glutamate dehydrogenase. Glutamate synthase has not been detected in mammalian tissues but O'Donovan and Lotspeich[9] have suggested (based on studies with L-[*amide*-15N]glutamine) that kidney cortex preparations can catalyze the transfer of the amide nitrogen of glutamine to pyruvate, oxaloacetate, and α-ketoglutarate without prior formation of free ammonia. The exact mechanism remains to be elucidated. Glutamine is a major fuel of the small intestine,[10] bone,[11] human diploid fibroblasts,[12] HeLa cells,[13] and possibly of the brain[14] (see Chapter 10). In addition glutamine is a major source of urinary ammonia (see below) while oxidation of the carbon skeleton provides an important source of energy.[15]

Despite the large number of enzymatic reactions that can potentially deplete glutamine, this amino acid is present in high concentrations in most body fluids. In man, glutamine is the amino acid of highest concentration in the blood and cerebrospinal fluid (CSF) accounting for ~20 and 67% of the plasma and CSF amino acid content, respectively.[16,17] In rats, glutamine occurs in millimolar concentrations in the brain, heart, liver, small intestine, and skeletal muscle.[18] The widespread activity of glutamine synthetase probably accounts at least in part for the high glutamine content of most tissues. In an ambitious survey, Wu[19] found that glutamine synthetase was present in several organs in all the higher vertebrates studied. Among the lower vertebrates, snakes were found to have exceedingly high activities in the brain and liver with smaller amounts in the lung and pancreas. In the newt, bullfrog, bluegill, and crappie, glutamine synthetase activity was found only in the brain, wherein it was of very high activity. In the rat, Wu[19] found high activity of glutamine synthetase in the brain, liver, kidney, and testes. He was unable to find activity in other rat organs but this may have been due to the insensitivity of the assay employed. It is now known that glutamine synthetase is present in the mammalian heart, lungs, spleen, and skeletal muscle (see below). Mammalian glutamine synthetase was first obtained in a highly purified form from preparations of the sheep brain.[20] Subsequently, the enzyme was purified from several mammalian tissues. Consult Meister[3-5] and Tate and Meister[2] for original references and for a comparison of enzymes purified from rat liver, ovine brain, rat brain, human brain, pea, *Escherichia coli*, and *Bacillus subtilis*.

E. coli glutamine synthetase is highly regulated by a complex control mechanism including

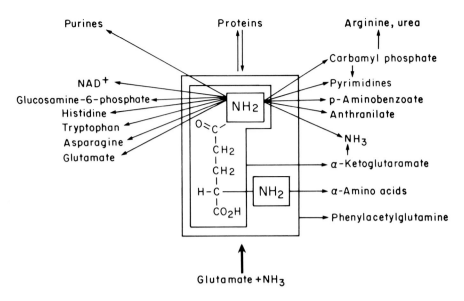

FIGURE 1. Central role of glutamine in nitrogen metabolism. The bold arrow emphasizes the fact that only one route for glutamine formation is known (the glutamine synthetase reaction) whereas glutamine breakdown is catalyzed by many enzymes. Note that some of the reactions shown only occur in microorganisms and plants. (Modified from Tate, S. S. and Meister, A., Glutamine synthetase of mammalian liver and brain, in *The Enzymes of Glutamine Metabolism,* Prusiner, S. and Stadtman, E. E., Eds., Academic Press, New York, 1973, 77.)

repression/derepression of enzyme synthesis, cumulative feedback inhibition by metabolic effectors, and by chemical interconversion (i.e., adenylation/deadenylation) of the enzyme.[21] Presumably this complex regulation is necessary to cope with a continuously changing environment. (See the discussion by Gebhardt and Mecke.[21]) There is no evidence that mammalian glutamine synthetase activity is controlled by chemical modification. On the other hand, levels of glutamine synthetase activity in normal and cancerous cultured mammalian cells from a variety of sources are greatly influenced by hormones. (See the discussions by Tate and Meister[2] and Gebhardt and Mecke.[21]) The relevance of these findings to the in vivo situation is not clear. The enzymes purified from a variety of mammalian organs are remarkably similar.[3-5] Moreover, the enzyme levels do not appear to be greatly altered in the tissues of adult rats subjected to a variety of metabolic insults. For example, we were unable to detect a change in the levels of glutamine synthetase in the brains of chronically hyperammonemic (12 to 14 week portacaval-shunted) rats.[22] However, a variety of metabolic insults have been shown to moderately alter glutamine synthetase activity in the muscle and adipose tissue (see below). Despite the above-mentioned negative findings, it is highly probable that glutamine synthetase *is* regulated in vivo. Thus, a number of important metabolites have been shown to affect the activity of purified liver and brain glutamine synthetases. This topic has been extensively reviewed by Tate and Meister[2] and is briefly summarized here. The enzymes are markedly inhibited by carbamyl phosphate, particularly in the presence of Mn^{2+}. This inhibition may play an important role in the control of the utilization of glutamine for pyrimidine synthesis. Both the liver and brain enzymes are inhibited by phosphate. This inhibition may impose a reciprocal control on the activities of glutamine synthetase and glutaminase (activated by phosphate), thus preventing a futile, energy-wasting cycle. (A futile cycle is also minimized by the different cellular/subcellular locations of these two enzymes in brain and liver.) The liver (but not the brain) enzyme is strongly activated by α-ketoglutarate providing a "feed-forward" activation whereby excess α-ketoglutarate produced by the citric acid cycle or by transamination can stimulate glutamine metabolism. The rat liver enzyme is markedly inhibited by glycine, alanine, and serine, particularly in the presence of Mn^{2+}. (The sheep brain enzyme is not affected by these compounds, whereas the rat brain enzyme is inhibited only slightly.) The α-keto analogues of glycine, alanine, and serine are substrates of the glutamine aminotransferases so that these amino acids may help to regulate the interaction between glutamine aminotransferases and glutamine synthetase. Both the rat liver and sheep brain enzyme are activated by chloride and bicarbonate at nonsaturating levels of glutamate. Apparently bicarbonate lowers the K_m value for glutamate but not for ATP.[2] Tate and Meister[2] suggested that the bicarbonate (and chloride) activation may possibly be related to the regulation of intracellular hydrogen ion concentration. This is a reasonable assumption. In the brain, bicarbonate metabolism is intimately related to H^+ homeostasis and at the same time both glutamine synthetase and carbonic anhydrase are enriched in the same cell type (see below).

II. ASSAY METHODS FOR GLUTAMINE SYNTHETASE

There have been several conflicting reports on the activity of glutamine synthetase in mammalian organs. Much of this confusion appears to have resulted from inadequate assay procedures so that it is worth commenting on the procedures employed. The most commonly employed method utilizes hydroxylamine in place of ammonia (Equation 2). The resultant L-γ-glutamylhydroxamate forms a brown color with acidic ferric chloride that absorbs in the region of 550 nm.[20,23] In studies with the sheep brain enzyme, it was found that hydroxylamine[2,23] behaves almost identically to ammonia as a substrate. However, the disadvantages are that the assay is not very sensitive and appropriate controls (e.g., those lacking ATP) must be carried out. Ehrenfeld et al.[24] have shown that some glutaminases can catalyze the conversion of glutamate to γ-glutamylhydroxamate in the absence of ATP. It is possible to measure the rate of formation of inorganic phosphate,[25] but appropriate controls for adenosine triphosphatase (ATPase) are necessary. Some workers have utilized ^{14}C-labeled glutamate followed by ion exchange chromatographic (IEC)[26] or thin layer chromatographic (TLC)[27] separation of ^{14}C-glutamine but these assays are often not very sensitive, difficult to reproduce, and are not suitable for assays of large numbers of samples. Recently, Martin et al.[28] have devised a rapid high performance liquid chromatography (HPLC) analysis; glutamine and glutamate are rapidly separated (within minutes) isochratically as the O-phthalaldehyde-2-mercaptoethanol derivatives.

It is well known that glutamine synthetase under optimal conditions catalyzes the L-glutamine-γ-glutamyltransferase reaction (Equation 3) manyfold faster than the glutamine synthetase reaction.[23] In order to increase sensitivity, many workers have employed the transferase reaction in place of the synthetase reaction and assumed that the transferase activity is solely catalyzed by glutamine synthetase. However, as cautioned by Meister et al.,[24] this conclusion is not necessarily true. For example, Lemieux et al.[29] have shown that following acidosis the synthetase activity of rat kidney was unaltered whereas the transferase activity decreased by 40%. A problem often encountered when assaying glutamine synthetase in crude preparations is the loss of ATP catalyzed by endogenous ATPases. This loss of ATP will curtail the synthetase reaction giving artificially low synthetase values. In order to circumvent this problem, several authors have advocated the use of ATP-regenerating systems. Herzfeld and Estes[30,31] have utilized phosphoenolpyruvate and pyruvate kinase as an ATP-regenerating system in the γ-glutamylhydroxamate synthetase assay mixture. However, these authors were unaware that pyruvate generated from the pyruvate kinase reaction reacts with hydroxylamine to yield an oxime that produces a brown color with acidic ferric chloride. Thus, tissues with high ATPase activity yield artificially high values of glutamine synthetase activity if the appropriate blank (i.e., minus glutamate) is not included (see Vorhaben et al.[32]). Because of the possibility of endogenous glutamate in the blank, it is preferable not to use the pyruvate kinase-regenerating system; Lemieux et al.[29] have suggested the use of creatine phosphate/creatine kinase to regenerate ATP and in our experience, this regenerating system has provided reliable activity values.

III. STRUCTURE AND CATALYTIC FUNCTION OF GLUTAMINE SYNTHETASE

Of the various preparations of glutamine synthetase isolated from mammalian tissues, most work has been carried out on the sheep brain enzyme. This enzyme has been thoroughly characterized by Meister's group and its properties have been extensively reviewed by Meister.[3-5] What follows is a brief summary of the important points.

Glutamine synthetase catalyzes the reversible formation of glutamine from glutamate, ammonia, and ATP (see Equation 1).[33] A divalent cation (Mg^{2+}, Mn^{2+}, or Co^{2+}) is required for activity. When the enzyme is incubated with L-glutamate, ammonium ions and MgATP (at a concentration of 10 mM at 37°C; pH 7.0) equilibrium is attained when about 90% of the glutamate is converted to glutamine.[33] When hydroxylamine is substituted for ammonia (Equation 2) the reaction proceeds to greater than 99% completion.

$$\text{L-Glutamate} + \text{NH}_3 + \text{ATP} \rightleftarrows \text{L-glutamine} + \text{ADP} + \text{P}_i \qquad (1)$$

$$\text{L-Glutamate} + \text{hydroxylamine} + \text{ATP} \rightleftarrows \gamma\text{-glutamylhydroxamate} + \text{ADP} + \text{P}_i \quad (2)$$

The sheep brain enzyme has a molecular weight of 392,000 and is composed of eight apparently identical subunits. The octomer possesses D_4 symmetry and is formed by isologous association of two heterologously bonded tetramers.[34] The specificity toward nucleotides is narrow. In addition to ATP only dATP is appreciably active; low activity occurs with adenosine tetraphosphate, ITP, GTP, and UTP.[35] In contrast, ammonia can be replaced by a number of nucleophiles including hydroxylamine, hydrazine, monomethyl hydrazine, methylamine, ethylamine, and glycine ethyl ester, to yield the corresponding γ-glutamyl compound.[3-5] The specificity of glutamine synthetase toward amino dicarboxylic acid substrates is unusual. The enzyme is active toward both D- and L-glutamates but is active only toward the L isomer of α-methylglutamate. Of the four β-methylglutamates, only the *threo*-β-methyl-D-glutamate is a substrate; of the γ-methylglutamates, only the *threo*-γ-methyl-L-glutamate is a substrate. L-Aspartate is neither a substrate nor an effective inhibitor, whereas both D- and L-α-aminoadipates are substrates. Furthermore, the rigid glutamate analogue, *cis*-L-1-amino-1,3-dicarboxycyclohexane (*cis*-L-cycloglutamate) is a good substrate. These, and other considerations, suggest that glutamate binds to glutamine synthetase in a fully (or almost fully) extended configuration.

The overall mechanism of the glutamine synthetase reaction is complex. An enzyme-bound acyl phosphate is thought to be an important intermediate; nucleophilic displacement of P_i by NH_3 leads to glutamine formation. In support of this hypothesis is the finding that L-methionine-SR-sulfoximine (MSO), an analogue of the tetrahedral transition state intermediate, is phosphorylated to MSO-phosphate which binds so tightly to the active site that the enzyme is rendered inactive.[36] Glutamate provides some protection against MSO inactivation but ammonia does not; glutamate (0.05 M) plus ammonia (0.05 M) provides complete protection.[36] Further evidence for formation of enzyme-bound acyl phosphate was obtained from ^{18}O studies in which scrambling of ^{18}O in the β,γ bridge to the β-nonbridge oxygens of ATP was observed; the rate of scrambling was approximately the rate of the overall enzyme-catalyzed reaction.[37] Furthermore, turnover of the *E. coli* enzyme in the presence of sodium borohydride resulted in formation of α-amino-δ-hydroxyvaleric acid.[38] Finally, glutamine synthetase catalyzes the direct phosphorylation of cycloglutamate in the absence of ammonia to yield an enzyme[cycloglutamyl phosphate][ADP] complex.[39] A list of the partial reactions catalyzed by glutamine synthetase is given below[3-5] (Equations 3 to 11).

$$\text{L-Glutamine} + \text{NH}_2\text{OH} \xrightarrow[\text{P}_i(\text{As}_i)]{\text{ADP(ATP), M}^{2+}} \text{L-}\gamma\text{-glutamylhydroxamate} + \text{NH}_3 \qquad (3)$$

$$\text{L-Glutamine} + \text{H}_2\text{O} \xrightarrow[\text{As}_i]{\text{ADP, M}^{2+}} \text{L-glutamate} + \text{NH}_3 \qquad (4)$$

$$\text{L-(or D-)Glutamate} + \text{ATP} \xrightarrow{\text{M}^{2+}} \begin{array}{l}\text{2-L-(or D-)pyrrolidone-} \\ \text{5-carboxylate} + \text{ADP} + \text{P}_i\end{array} \qquad (5)$$

$$\beta\text{-Glutamyl phosphate} + \text{ADP} \xrightarrow{\text{M}^{2+}} \beta\text{-glutamate} + \text{ATP} \qquad (6)$$

$$\text{Acetyl phosphate} + \text{ADP} \xrightarrow{\text{M}^{2+}} \text{acetate} + \text{ATP} \qquad (7)$$

$$\text{Carbamyl phosphate} + \text{ADP} \xrightarrow{\text{M}^{2+}} \text{CO}_2 + \text{NH}_3 + \text{ATP} \qquad (8)$$

$$\text{Enzyme} + \text{cycloglutamate} + \text{ATP} \xrightarrow{\text{M}^{2+}} \begin{array}{l}\text{Enzyme[cycloglutamylphosphate][ADP]} \\ + \text{P}_i\end{array} \qquad (9)$$

$$\text{Enzyme} + \text{L-MSO} + \text{ATP} \xrightarrow{\text{M}^{2+}} \text{Enzyme[L-MSOP]} + \text{ADP} \qquad (10)$$

It is known that a plant glutamine synthetase[40] and two bacterial glutamine synthetases[24,41] can catalyze exchange of the amide group of glutamine with [^{15}N]ammonia (Equation 11).

$$\text{L-Glutamine} + {}^*\text{NH}_3 \xrightarrow[\text{(where }{}^*\text{N} = {}^{13}\text{N or }{}^{15}\text{N)}]{} \text{L-[}amide\text{-}{}^*\text{N]glutamine} + \text{NH}_3 \quad (11)$$

To my knowledge, this reaction has not previously been demonstrated with the mammalian enzyme. We have now demonstrated this reaction directly with purified sheep brain glutamine synthetase (*N = ^{13}N). The rate of enzyme-catalyzed amide exchange (50 mM L-glutamine, 50 mM potassium phosphate [pH 7.2], 50 mM MgCl$_2$, 10 mM ammonia plus tracer quantities of [^{13}N]ammonia) was found to be similar to the rate of γ-glutamylhydroxamate formation (Equation 3) when labeled ammonia was replaced by hydroxylamine. We found for the rat brain enzyme that the K$_m$ value for glutamine (transferase reaction, Equation 3; 50 mM MgCl$_2$, 50 mM 2-mercaptoethanol, 50 mM potassium phosphate [pH 7.2], 100 mM NH$_2$OH, 100 μM ADP; 37°C) is ~80 mM. The K$_m$ value for glutamate (synthetase reaction, Equation 2; 50 mM imidazole-HCl [pH 7.2], 2.0 mM ATP, 50 mM MgCl$_2$, 50 mM 2-mercaptoethanol, 100 mM NH$_2$OH; 37°C) is 1.8 mM. The V$_{max}$ value for the transferase reaction was found to be 5.3 times greater than that for the synthetase reaction. However, assuming that (1) NH$_3$ behaves similarly to hydroxyalamine, (2) the relative concentrations of glutamate to glutamine in the small compartment of brain is 2:1, and (3) the γ-glutamyltransferase activity of the brain is catalyzed solely by glutamine synthetase (a reasonable assumption because the ratio of transferase to synthetase activity appears to be constant in all parts of the brain and throughout development of the brain[42]) then one can calculate[43] that 5% of the ammonia reacting at the active site of rat brain glutamine synthetase will participate in a nonproductive amide exchange reaction. However, at the physiological concentration of phosphate (2 to 3 mM) the γ-glutamyltransferase reaction is only 50% of maximal. Assuming the same is true for the amide exchange reaction, then it is probable that ≤3% of ammonia reacting at the active site of glutamine synthetase undergoes a nonproductive amide exchange reaction in the rat brain in vivo.[44] This is important since previous conclusions concerning glutamine compartmentation and rates of synthesis in the brain with [^{15}N or ^{13}N]ammonia did not take into account ammonia-glutamine amide exchange (see below).

A detailed kinetic analysis of the glutamine synthetase reaction and the partial reactions (Equations 3 to 10) together with (a) the use of space filling and Dreiding models and (b) computer analysis of substrate conformations[45] has led to a very detailed understanding of the reaction mechanism and topology of the active site.[45] A summary is as follows:

1. The enzyme possesses separate binding sites for glutamate, ATP, and ammonia, but the substrates do not bind covalently to these sites; glutamate binds in an extended conformation.
2. Ammonia binding requires prior binding of glutamate.
3. L-S-MSO binds to both the glutamate and ammonia binding sites; MSO mimics the tetrahedral intermediate with the methyl group occupying the ammonia binding site and the imine nitrogen occupying the site that normally binds the oxygen of the carboxyl group that is to be phosphorylated.
4. Formation of an enzyme-stabilized acyl phosphate intermediate is very likely; in the absence of ammonia the acyl phosphate intermediate slowly cyclizes to 2-pyrrolidone-5-carboxylate (= 5-oxoproline) + P_i.

IV. METABOLIC IMPORTANCE OF GLUTAMINE SYNTHETASE

A considerable amount of ammonia is generated in the gut of normal, healthy individuals from protein digestion, deamination reactions, and by deamidation of glutamine.[46,47] (It has long been thought that the hydrolysis of urea in the gut is also an important source of blood ammonia,[48-50] but recent studies of human volunteers administered [^{15}N]urea suggest that very little fecal ammonia is derived from endogenous urea.[51]) It is estimated that in healthy, well-nourished adults several grams of ammonia enter the portal circulation daily.[50,52] However, peripheral arterial levels of ammonia are quite low (50 to 200 μM) attesting to the efficiency with which the liver urea cycle and, to a lesser extent, glutamine synthetase remove most of the portal ammonia.[52] In addition to gut-derived ammonia, some ammonia is generated in extrasplanchnic tissues by the action of glutamate dehydrogenase, glutaminase, and AMP deaminase and to a lesser extent by other enzymes, and at least some of this ammonia is liberated to the circulation. Some ammonia is released to the urine following deamidation of glutamine by the kidneys,[53] but, as was first suggested by Nash and Benedict in 1921,[54] it is now known that the kidney is also capable of liberating ammonia to the blood. Output from the kidney may be responsible for the hyperammonemia observed in some individuals on valproate therapy.[55] With the recent interest in sports medicine it has become evident that ammonia is a major metabolic product found in the blood following vigorous exercise.[56-58] (Actually, it has been known since the 1920s that muscle extracts catalyze the rapid breakdown of AMP to IMP and ammonia.[59]) Ammonia generated in the extrasplanchnic tissues and released to the nonportal blood has a different fate than that of the gut-derived ammonia in the portal blood. Duda and Handler[60] showed that, in the brain and other organs, the major fate of ^{15}N in the rat whether administered intravenously as [^{15}N]ammonia or derived from endogenously produced [^{15}N]ammonia (as in the breakdown of D-[^{15}N]leucine), was incorporation into the amide group of glutamine. More recently, Stein et al.[61] found that, following i.v. infusion of [^{15}N]ammonia into adult volunteers, ~90% of the label in the blood was in the amide group of glutamine.

In studies from our laboratory, we have found that following an i.v. bolus injection of [^{13}N]ammonia into anesthetized rats label disappears from the blood extremely rapidly.[62] By 20 to 25 sec, about 10% of the dose remains in the blood and this remaining dose is cleared much more slowly ($t_{1/2} > 15$ min). Within seconds of administration of [^{13}N]ammonia, L-[*amide*-^{13}N]glutamine appears in the blood followed more slowly by the appearance of [^{13}N]urea; by 2 min, only 19% of the dose in the blood was found to be associated with ammonia whereas 52, 28, and 4% were found in glutamine, urea, and other components, respectively.[62] These data suggest a very rapid clearance of [^{13}N]ammonia in the first pass of the circulation. Indeed, Freed and Gelbard[63] have shown that the fractional extraction of [^{13}N]ammonia in most rat organs, with the notable exception of the brain and lung, is 0.7 to 1.0. Following the rapid uptake of labeled ammonia, there is a second phase in which labeled metabolites appear in the blood. The early appearance of labeled glutamine attests to the widespread distribution of glutamine synthetase in rat organs. The slower appearance of label in urea is a reflection of the limited distribution of the complete urea cycle (almost totally confined to the liver). A picture emerges in which the major fate of ammonia in the portal vein is incorporation into urea within the liver with smaller amounts in glutamine. Conversely, the major fate of systemic blood ammonia is initial rapid incorporation into glutamine in extrahepatic tissues. Because urea synthesis is irreversible, whereas glutamine synthesis is not, the nitrogen present in systemic blood ammonia will eventually appear in urea. Factors that govern the partitioning of ammonia nitrogen between glutamine (amide) and urea have been extensively studied by Phromphetcharat et al.[64] with particular emphasis on interorgan participation and on the change in partitioning that accompanies acidosis.

Shröck and Goldstein[65] estimate that in the normal rat glutamine is released from muscle to the bloodstream at the rate of 0.28 μmol/min/100 g body weight. In the acidotic rat the rate was found to be 0.57 μmol/min/100 g body weight. (In the acidotic rat, a significant portion of the glutamine release was from the liver.) From continuous infusion experiments with L-[1-^{14}C]glutamine, Squires and Brosnan[66] estimate a turnover of ~130 μmol/hr/100 g for whole-body glutamine in normal and acidotic rats. By combining the two sets of data, Squires and Brosnan estimate as much as one quarter of the turnover of the glutamine pool in the rat can be accounted for by release into the blood stream.[66] Thus, glutamine plays important roles as a nontoxic carrier of easily transferable nitrogen and in the maintenance of interorgan nutritional balance. Efficient interorgan transport systems have evolved to make the most effective use of circulatory "materials". One organ may donate to the circulation a compound that is a nonessential product of a metabolic process but that is a nutritional requirement of another organ. For example, the gut and kidney utilize glutamine as a major energy source, whereas smooth muscle exports glutamine as a product of branched-chain amino acid metabolism. (For reviews of general interorgan amino acid nutrition, see Christensen,[67] and of the role of branched-chain amino acid in interorgan nutrition, see Harper et al.[68])

The effects of hormonal (and other) manipulations on the activity of glutamine synthetase in normal and cancerous cell lines in culture have been the subject of much research. However, space limitations do not permit an adequate treatment of this topic. Therefore, in the remainder of the section I will discuss the role of glutamine synthetase in individual organs in vivo and some recent findings on the compartmentation of glutamine synthetase in the liver. I will also discuss some ot the findings of studies in which [^{13}N]ammonia has been used as a tracer.

The use of ^{13}N as a tracer is not generally familiar to most biochemists. ^{13}N is a positron-emitting isotope with a half-life of 9.96 min — suitable for short-term metabolic studies.

The isotope is potentially available with an extremely high specific activity so that true (i.e., undisturbed steady state) tracer studies are relatively easy to carry out. Moreover, the resulting γ-radiation (from positron-electron annihilation) can be used for external detection and in vivo quantitation. (For a detailed review of ^{13}N as a tracer, see Reference 69.)

A. Brain

In early work, Waelsch and co-workers[70,71] investigated the metabolic fate of L-[U-^{14}C]glutamate and concluded, from the specific activities of isolated glutamate and glutamine, that glutamate metabolism is compartmented in the brain. In later experiments [^{15}N]ammonia was infused into the right common carotid artery of cats and the incorporation of label into the α-amino group of glutamate and both nitrogens of glutamine was determined for the brain and liver.[72] The resulting relative ^{15}N-enrichment in the brain was found to be as follows: glutamine (amide) > glutamine (amine) > glutamate. Since the only known route to glutamine is the glutamine synthetase reaction, with glutamate as a precursor, and since at least some glutamate must have been generated by reductive amination of α-ketoglutarate, one might have expected that the enrichment of glutamine (amine) should be less than that in glutamate. In order to explain the ^{15}N-enrichment data, the authors proposed that blood-borne ammonia is converted to glutamine in the brain in a small, rapidly turning over compartment of glutamate which is distinct from a more slowly turning over large glutamate compartment.[72] In contrast to the brain, the liver was shown to contain a single kinetically-defined compartment of glutamate metabolism. However, it is now known that the liver does indeed contain separate metabolic (i.e., cellular) compartments; see the following section. In order to obtain significant increases above the natural background of ^{15}N (~0.4%) in metabolites, Berl et al.[72] used large, nonphysiological quantities of [^{15}N]ammonia. In more recent experiments, Cooper et al.[73] used tracer levels of [^{13}N]ammonia in awake rats. The authors confirmed that ammonia metabolism is indeed compartmented in the brain. In addition, they showed that on entering the brain 98% or more of ammonia is incorporated into glutamine (amide), and that the rate of this reaction in the small compartment is extremely rapid ($t_{1/2} \leq 3$ sec). It was also found that (1) ammonia entering the brain from the CSF is converted to glutamine in the small compartment and (2) inhibition of brain glutamine synthetase by prior administration of methionine sulfoximine results in a labeling pattern more reminiscent of a single compartment, i.e., following carotid artery infusion of [^{13}N]ammonia, the specific activity of L-[^{13}N]glutamate was greater than that of L-[*amine*-^{13}N]glutamine. The absolute amount of label retained by the brain compared to normal controls was also greatly diminished, suggesting that the less efficient trapping of [^{13}N]ammonia following MSO treatment results in an increase in back-diffusion of label from the brain to the blood.

By the early 1960s it was also apparent that the brain contained at least two distinct tricarboxylic acid cycles (see References 74 and 75). Initially the anatomical basis for the kinetically defined compartment was uncertain. However, much circumstantial evidence began to accumulate that suggested glial and neuronal elements contributed to the small and large compartments, respectively. (For a review see Reference 76.) The most compelling evidence that the glia represent the small compartment was provided by the elegant work of Norenberg and associates.[77,78] These authors, by using an immunohistochemical method, showed that glutamine synthetase is concentrated in the astrocytes in the brain and in the equivalent cell type in the retina.[79] There is also some evidence that glutamine synthetase occurs in neurons,[80] especially the nerve endings.[81] The glutamine synthetase of the nerve endings may contribute to the small glutamate/ammonia pool.[75] Nevertheless, there is no doubt that the astrocytes represent the major source of brain glutamine synthetase. Bradbury[82] has emphasized the special anatomical relationship between astrocytes and neurons. Proximally, astrocytic end-feet ensheath the capillaries whereas distally they abut onto neurons;

the astrocytes also underlie the ependymal layer. Thus, astrocytes are in a position to act as a physiological buffer between neurons and the blood compartment on the one hand and neurons and the CSF on the other. (The unique biochemical and physiological roles of the astrocytes have been reviewed.[83])

Cooper et al.[73] determined the brain uptake index (BUI) of [^{13}N]ammonia relative to a freely diffusible marker (^{14}C-labeled butanol) following a bolus injection into the carotid artery of rats. The BUI was independent of the ammonia concentration in the bolus over a 1000-fold range. In other experiments, it was found that the BUI was independent of ammonia concentration but dependent on the pH of the bolus.[84,85] These data suggest that there is no saturable carrier for ammonia across the blood-brain barrier and that ammonia diffuses from the blood to the brain largely as the free base (NH_3). Raichle and Larson[86] calculate that some ammonia (~25%) diffuses as ammonium (NH_4^+).

The unique characteristic of the blood-brain barrier (i.e., tight junctions) allows for the exclusion of large and/or polar molecules and for the selective uptake of blood-borne metabolites by carrier-mediated processes. However, in the case of freely diffusible molecules, such as ammonia, there is no exclusion at the epithelium of the capillary walls. Since ammonia is potentially toxic to the CNS, it makes sense for the glutamine synthetase to be located in astrocytes just beneath the capillary epithelium. From its location in the brain, glutamine synthetase may be regarded as an "enzymatic barrier" between blood and neurons. This is obviously a very effective barrier as judged by the rapidity with which blood-borne [^{13}N]ammonia is incorporated into glutamine (within seconds) in the rat brain and the very little back-diffusion (<3%) of labeled ammonia from the brain to the blood in both the rat and the monkey.[85-87] Under hyperammonemic conditions (portacaval shunting or urease treatment) the turnover of the total ammonia pool to glutamine in the astrocytes is considerably slowed.[22] Nevertheless, even under these conditions of hyperammonemia the glutamine synthetase is still the only important route for the cerebral detoxification of blood-borne ammonia.[22]

In addition to its role as an agent of detoxification, glutamine synthetase also plays an important role in the maintenance of carbon and nitrogen homeostasis in the brain (Figure 2). There appears to be a net output of glutamine from brain astrocytes to the blood (although not everyone is in agreement on this) and to CSF and from astrocytes to neurons, which may counterbalance the net uptake of ammonia and other amino acids. (For a discussion, see Cooper and Plum.[76]) Moreover, it seems probable that glial glutamine synthetase plays a central role in the recirculation of carbon derived from amino acid neurotransmitters (Figure 2). These neurotransmitter cycles are discussed more fully in Chapter 15, Volume II.

It is possible that ammonia (and hence glutamine synthetase) plays a role in H^+ homeostasis. Hindfelt and Siesjö[94] have shown that the brain is able to buffer against lactic acidosis associated with ammonium acetate infusion and suggest that this is due to a passive influx of ammonia from blood. On the other hand, Kelley and Kazemi[95] suggest that ammonia production by the CNS is an important buffer mechanism for controlling brain and CSF pH. Although there are many reactions in the brain that can give rise to ammonia, there are probably only three major routes: glutaminase, glutamate dehydrogenase, and the purine nucleotide cycle, the last being the most important according to Schultz and Lowenstein.[96] It is difficult to envisage how these enzymes can respond to an increase in H^+ concentration to yield more ammonia. Perhaps a clue is in the recent findings that the glia represent the major site of ion homeostasis in the brain.[97,98] Bicarbonate is thought to be a major buffer in the brain and indeed the glial cells are rich in carbonic anhydrase.[99] As lactate accumulates during ischemia, there is a depletion of HCO_3^- [98] and as already mentioned, bicarbonate is a very effective activator of glutamine synthetase. Thus, bicarbonate depletion in the astrocytes may decrease the activity of glutamine synthetase, thereby increasing the level of ammonia in these cells. In fact, ammonia levels in the brain rise during ischemia/hypoxia.

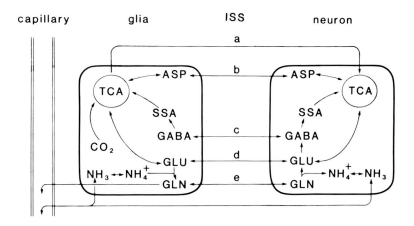

FIGURE 2. The important role of glutamine synthetase in the detoxification of ammonia and amino acid neurotransmitter metabolism; $\overrightarrow{d} \rightarrow \overrightarrow{e}$, the "Glutamine Cycle" proposed by Benjamin and Quastel;[88,89] $\overrightarrow{e} \rightarrow \overleftarrow{c}$, the "Glutamine, Glutamate, GABA Cycle" proposed by Van Den Berg;[74] $\overrightarrow{d} \rightarrow \overrightarrow{a}$, release of glutamate from neurons to glia followed by return of carbon to neurons as α-ketoglutarate and malate.[90] Note that the glia contain a high affinity uptake system for aspartate[91] and that, via the TCA cycle there are at least two routes for return of carbon to the neurons, i.e., $\overrightarrow{a}$ and $\overrightarrow{d}$. Note also that the glia are rich in the anaplerotic enzyme, pyruvate carboxylase,[92] so that CO_2 fixation provides a means of replenishing carbon lost from the small TCA cycle (as α-ketoglutarate, oxaloacetate, or malate). This enzyme, apparently accounts in part for the increase in (glutamate plus glutamine) in the brains of hyperammonemic rats compared to controls.[93] The various pathways are discussed more fully by Shank and Aprison in Volume II. SSA, succinic semialdehyde; ISS, interstitial fluid.

(See the discussion by Cooper and Plum.[76]) However, the hypothesis of a decrease in glutamine synthetase activity due to bicarbonate depletion leads to the question "Why would the brain utilize a potential toxin as buffer?" Perhaps the production of ammonia by inhibition of glutamine synthetase is a "last-ditch" defense against a drastic accumulation of H^+ ions during ischemia.

Van Gelder[100] has proposed that the glial glutamine synthetase and carbonic anhydrase enzymes play an important role in osmoregulation in the CNS. He suggested that carbonic anhydrase activity increases glial volume which in turn is offset by glutamine synthesis; glutamine release is accompanied by osmoequivalent quantities of water. Van Gelder has also proposed that carbonic anhydrase and glutamine synthetase activities are metabolically linked in the choroid plexus; carbonic anhydrase-mediated influx of water into the choroid plexus is offset by synthesis of glutamine which upon release is accompanied by water transfer to the CSF. Thus, the glutamine synthetase of the CNS plays an important role not only for the detoxification of ammonia and for the maintenance of neurotransmitter cycles but also possibly for the regulation of pH and water balance. Clearly, much work still needs to be carried out to further define the metabolic roles of this important enzyme in the CNS.

B. Liver

Glutamine synthetase activity is relatively high in the liver[2,19] and it has long been recognized that glutamine synthetase and the urea cycle play an important role in the detoxification of ammonia. Early tracer studies gave no hint of any compartmentation of these systems. However, within the last few years it has become apparent that the liver contains cells with markedly different enzyme profiles and that this segregation plays an important role in nitrogen homeostasis and pH regulation. It is now known that the urea cycle enzymes

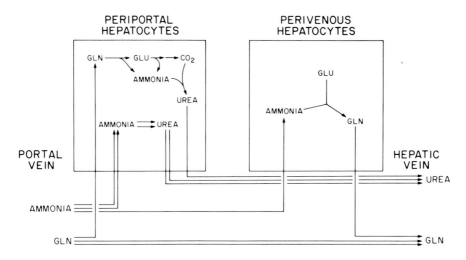

FIGURE 3.   Ureogenesis in the liver according to Häussinger and Gerok.[101,102] Glutamine synthetase is located in the perivenous hepatocytes whereas glutaminase and the urea cycle enzymes are predominantly located in the periportal hepatocytes. The glutamine cycle results in an effective utilization of ammonia. Urea synthesis is improved by additional substrate supply for urea synthesis by periportal glutamine degradation whereas glutamine is resynthesized in the perivenous hepatocytes from ammonia that escapes urea synthesis in the periportal hepatocytes. According to Häussinger and Gerok, under normal conditions approximately two thirds of portal ammonia is converted to urea and one third to glutamine. Recent work from our laboratory suggests that the ratio may be closer to 10:1.[102a] Glutamate loss by conversion to glutamine in the perivenous hepatocytes is partially offset by uptake from the blood.

and glutaminase are predominantly located in the periportal cells whereas glutamine synthetase is exclusively located in a small population of perivenous cells[101] (Figure 3). (See References 21 and 102 for reviews.) Glutamate appears to be selectively taken up from the blood by the perivenous cells,[103] glutamate-alanine aminotransferase activity is enriched in the periportal cells,[104,105] and glutamate dehydrogenase activity is higher in the perivenous cells.[105] As pointed out by Häussinger and Gerok,[102] carbamyl phosphate synthetase (the rate-limiting step of the urea cycle) has a relatively high K_m for ammonia (1 to 2 mM)[106] whereas the K_m exhibited by rat liver glutamine synthetase is lower (0.3 mM).[107] The urea cycle is thus a relatively low affinity/high capacity system for ammonia removal whereas glutamine synthetase is a higher affinity/lower capacity system for ammonia removal.[102] The two systems ensure effective removal of ammonia during passage through the liver (Figure 3). Häussinger and Gerok have also stressed the importance of the hepatic glutamine cycle for the regulation of pH. It is thought that the major pathway for HCO_3^- removal is hepatic urea synthesis.[108,109] In acidosis urea production by the liver is decreased whereas glutamine production is increased.[64] This leads to a decreased removal of bicarbonate. Conversely, in alkalosis urea synthesis is increased and glutamine synthesis is diminished. This has the effect of increasing the rate of bicarbonate removal.[102] This response of liver glutamine synthetase to acidosis is thought to be intimately linked to the secretion of NH_4^+ by the kidney (see the following section).

In liver disease, brain function is compromised. There have been many suggestions as to the toxin(s) responsible. However, there seems to be little doubt that ammonia is a major toxin.[76] Part of the increased ammonia generally (but not always) found in the blood of patients with liver disease may be due to extrahepatic shunting of blood from the gut to the systemic circulation. It is also probable that ammonia-detoxifying enzymes are also reduced in activity in the damaged liver. Häussinger and Gerok[110] have shown that, in CCl_4-damaged rat liver, perivenous glutamine synthetase activity is greatly diminished, whereas the periportal urea cycle enzymes are unaffected. However, others[111] have shown a diminished output of urea from CCl_4-damaged rat liver, and carbamyl phosphate synthetase and arginase activities have been shown to be significantly decreased in biopsy material from patients with alcoholic hepatitis.[112] Häussinger and Gerok[102,113] have suggested that alkalosis associated with liver disease may be due to diminished bicarbonate removal as urea. Thus a rational treatment designed to counteract both the hyperammonemia and alkalosis of patients with liver disease might involve a regimen designed to stimulate what is left of the urea cycle and glutamine synthetase in the liver and to stimulate extrahepatic glutamine synthetase.

C. Kidney

It has been known for over 50 years that rat, guinea pig, and rabbit kidneys contain glutamine synthetase.[114] Glutamine synthetase activity is also present in sheep,[19] mice,[115] and hamster[115] kidneys, but is of low (or undetectable) activity in dog[29] and human kidneys.[19,29] Krebs et al.[116] estimated that, in the rat, the kidney is a major source of circulating glutamine. Burch et al.[115] have pointed out that the wide species variability of kidney glutamine synthetase may be related to urine acidity. In man and dogs the urine is usually acidic, requiring large excretion of ammonium ions. In rodents and lagomorphs, on the other hand, the urine is usually neutral or alkaline. Thus, this group may use glutamine synthetase to retrieve ammonium not needed in the urine. Quantitative biochemical analyses of different regions of the rat kidney following either a glutamine or glutamate load suggest that the synthesis and degradative pathways of glutamine metabolism are segregated in the kidney.[117] Indeed, analysis of glutamine synthetase in different parts of rat nephron dissected from freeze-dried microtome slices, showed that the enzyme was confined essentially to the proximal straight segment.[115] Moreover, although the activity of glutamine synthetase in the whole kidney is only moderate, it is of extremely high activity in this segment. In the rabbit, highest glutamine synthetase activity was found in both proximal convoluted and straight tubules with some activity in glomeruli and distal straight tubules. Curiously, in the rat the proximal and distal tubules produce ammonia from glutamine; in acidosis there is a very marked production of ammonia from the proximal tubules.[118] These results are consistent with an important role for glutamine synthetase in the control of the release of ammonium ion excretion from the proximal tubule in the rat kidney. (For a recent review on ammonia transport in the kidneys see Reference 119.)

As discussed above, it has long been known that glutamine (amide) is an important source of urinary ammonia. More recently, glutamate has also been recognized as an important secondary source of urinary ammonia, particularly in the acidotic rat. Ammonia from glutamate could arise from the glutamate dehydrogenase reaction[120] and/or purine nucleotide cycle (via aspartate)[121]. However, in the dog kidney, it has been shown that the increased ammonia excretion associated with metabolic acidosis is derived almost entirely from glutamine.[122] Clearly there are species differences in the way the kidney excretes ammonium ion and in the activities of enzymes that utilize or dispose of ammonia. It seems clear that in the rat, at least, metabolic acidosis is associated with increased ammonia excretion and decreased glutamine synthesis, whereas in alkalosis ammonia excretion is diminished, glutamine synthesis is enhanced, and glutamine is added to renal venous blood.[123]

Within the last few years it has become evident that glutamine levels are regulated to serve the varying needs of different organs under differing metabolic conditions. In mammals glutamine synthetase plays an important role in the maintenance of nitrogen and H^+ ion homeostasis. Welbourne, Phromphetcharat, and co-workers[64,124] have elaborated on this idea; a summary is as follows: metabolic acidosis results in a diminished plasma glutamine ($\sim 60\%$ of normal) and elevated ammonia. Despite the reduced glutamine, the kidney and gut are still able to effectively utilize glutamine. However, instead of releasing alanine (which it does under normal conditions) the gut releases ammonia. Since glutamine plus alanine is a good source of urea, the decreased concentration of these amino acids in the portal vein of acidotic animals ensures a switch from ureogenesis to glutamine formation and decreased glucose formation in the liver. Conversely, acidosis promotes renal glutamine conversion to ammonia (in the rat, at least in part, by decreasing glutamine synthesis) and an increase in bicarbonate and glucose formation. In the recovery phase, glutamine synthesis (particularly in the muscle, see below) is enhanced and plasma glutamine levels rise; the gut reverts to releasing alanine. The higher levels of portal vein alanine and circulating glutamine (and decreased portal ammonia) promote liver ureogenesis and gluconeogenesis. In the kidney gluconeogenesis and ammonia production are decreased. Thus, there appears to be a reciprocal response of the liver and kidney to glutamine/ammonia metabolism. This reciprocity (at least in rodents and lagomorphs) may be due, in part, to the different responses to acidosis of glutamine synthetase activity in the kidney and liver.

D. Skeletal Muscle

The specific activity of glutamine synthetase in the muscle is relatively low[125] However, due to the large mass of muscle compared to other tissues in the body, the formation of glutamine by the muscle is appreciable. In fact, it is probable that the muscle is the major site of glutamine synthesis.[65] Lockwood et al.[126] obtained two-dimensional body scans of patients with liver disease and normal volunteers following an injection of [^{13}N]ammonia. From an estimate of uptake of label in various organs, the authors concluded that as much as 50% of circulating ammonia is removed by the skeletal musculature. This reliance on the muscle for glutamine synthesis has clinical implications for diseases in which muscle wasting is a problem. For example, it has recently been shown that patients with liver cirrhosis develop the catabolic state of starvation in response to food withdrawal more rapidly than do normal volunteers.[127] The attempt to maintain energy balance by mobilization of amino acids may contribute to the muscle wasting and hyperammonemia commonly seen in these patients. The hyperammonemia may thus be at least in part a consequence of increased amino acid metabolism and decreased glutamine synthetase activity.

The muscle is an important source of amino acids released to the circulation and a large proportion (25 to 30%) is glutamine formed *de novo*.[128] As Durschlag and Smith[129] point out, glutamine carbon is derived from many potential precursors, including circulating amino acids and amino acids released by the breakdown of muscle proteins and glucose — many amino acids as well as free ammonia can provide the nitrogen. Durschlag and Smith[129] also make several other important points. Glutamine released from skeletal muscle may serve as (1) a vehicle for removing excess ammonia, (2) a gluconeogenic precursor, (3) a source of renal ammonia for buffering urinary acid, and (4) a metabolic fuel for the small intestine. Perhaps because of this multiplicity of reactions glutamine release from the skeletal muscle occurs during both the absorptive and postabsorptive states. Finally, there seems to be a direct relationship between glutamine output from the muscle and glutamine uptake by the kidney. (Consult Durschlag and Smith[129] for original references; see also the previous section.)

It is not known at present what mechanisms control the acidosis and other metabolic conditions that increase the output of glutamine from the muscle. Several groups are tackling this problem by using muscle cells in culture.[129,130] King et al.[131] have shown that administration of chloride salts or induction of diabetic ketoacidosis increased the maximum activity of glutamine synthetase in the rat skeletal muscle in vivo. Starvation and administration of adrenal steroids also increased the activity of the enzyme in the muscle. The basis for the increase in activity is not known, but may be due to an increased synthesis of protein, a chemical modification of the enzyme, or both. Clearly much remains to be accomplished in determining what factors regulate the increased activity of glutamine synthetase in one organ and down-regulation in another in response to changing metabolic needs.

Recently Golden et al.[132] have used ^{15}N tracer kinetics to investigate ammonia metabolism in the healthy adult human male. They calculate that the muscle is indeed the major organ of glutamine synthesis; rate of synthesis in the muscle was estimated at 52 mmol/hr with a $t_{1/2}$ for turnover of $\sim$5 hr. This synthesis was counterbalanced by an equivalent loss to the extracellular fluid (ECF). The ECF was calculated to contain 6.5 mmol of glutamine with a very rapid turnover ($t_{1/2}$ $\sim$5 min). About 98% of the glutamine (51 mmol/hr) was estimated to be utilized by the intestine and other organs with only about 2% utilized by the kidney (1.1 mmol/hr). Nevertheless, glutamine provided a major source of urinary ammonia (63%). The utilization of glutamine by the adult human kidney seems rather small in light of the above discussion of the proposed interrelationship between liver and kidney glutamine metabolism. However, in chronically acidotic human subjects, the utilization of glutamine by the kidney reached 6.1 mmol/hr[133] or about 12% of the glutamine production rate calculated by Golden et al.[132] Thus, in the human, as noted for other species, there is a marked increase in glutamine utilization by the kidney in response to acidosis.

[15]N has two inherent disadvantages as a tracer for studying nitrogen metabolism, i.e., a natural background of 0.4% and a relatively tedious analysis procedure. In addition, experiments on humans can only be limited to the sampling of easily accessible body fluids. Since ^{13}N is radioactive with no natural background and a short half-life, it should be almost ideal for tracing short-term nitrogen metabolism in humans *in situ* with an external detector. However, experiments relating to human muscle nitrogen metabolism have been somewhat limited. In addition to the above-mentioned study by Lockwood et al.,[126] there is one other study of [^{13}N]ammonia disposition in the human muscle. Thus, in a study by Schelstraete et al.[134] of a patient with right-sided static tremor up to 8.5 times the uptake of label was noted in some of the right-sided muscles compared to the contralateral normal limb. It is probable that the high uptake of label was related to the increased blood flow produced by the continuous rhythmic exercise of the tremulous muscle. The high uptake of label suggests effective metabolic trapping even in the hyperactive state. Presumably, the trapping is due to metabolic conversion to glutamine.

Finally, glutamine synthetase from the rat skeletal muscle has been highly purified and its kinetic properties have been compared to enzymes isolated from the liver, brain, and spleen.[135] The skeletal muscle enzyme appears to have a lower K_m value for ATP than previously characterized (i.e., brain and liver) preparations and to be more susceptible to inhibition by ADP. Rowe[135] suggested that this difference in sensitivity to regulation by adenine nucleotides may be a reflection of the different role this enzyme plays in different tissues. Since glutamine synthetase in the brain is concerned with the detoxification of ammonia, neutralization of neurotransmitter glutamate, and possibly regulation of water and pH, it is important that high activity of the brain enzyme be maintained under a variety of metabolic conditions. On the other hand, it seems reasonable to assume that muscle glutamine synthetase is under tighter metabolic control by ATP and ADP; nucleotide interactions could provide a mechanism for the decreased utilization of high energy phosphate bonds for the formation of glutamine when energy demands are high for muscle contraction. Clearly, an understanding of the regulatory mechanisms governing muscle glutamine synthetase activity in vivo are of great importance in understanding whole-body nitrogen homeostasis.[135]

E. Heart

Glutamine production by the mammalian heart was first reported in 1959 by Doell and Felts[136] in studies with perfused rabbit hearts, and more recently, by Davidson and Sonnenblick[137] with perfused rat hearts. Nevertheless, there has been some controversy as to whether or not heart tissue contains glutamine synthetase. Wu[19] was unable to detect glutamine synthetase activity in hearts from several species of mammal (limit of detection 10 μmol/hr/g wet weight; 37°C). Lund[138] was unable to detect activity in the rat heart (limit of detection 30 μmol/hr/g wet weight). Iqbal and Ottaway[125] were unable to demonstrate activity in the rat heart that met the criteria of linearity with respect to incubation time and homogenate concentration. (Herzfeld and Estes[31] report a value > 200 μg/hr/g but this value is too large). On the other hand, Trush[139] reported glutamine synthetase activities for rat, rabbit, and cat hearts of 3.4, 4.4, and 4.1 μmol/hr/g, respectively; 40°C) and Rowe[135] has reported a value of 6.4 μmol/hr/g for the rat heart and comparable values for mouse, rabbit, sheep, pig, and beef hearts. Rowe has purified the enzyme from the pig heart and has studied its kinetic properties. With the actual purification, the controversy as to whether or not the heart contains glutamine synthetase can be put to rest — it does! Moreover, recent ^{13}N studies suggest that the heart converts ammonia to glutamine very effectively.

In 1971 Hunter and Monahan[140] reported ''striking scans of the myocardium'' following i.v. injection of [^{13}N]ammonia into dogs and humans. Monahan et al.[141] subsequently reported that administration of [^{13}N]ammonia to dogs by inhalation or by s.c. injection also yielded heart images. Harper et al. reported a high first-pass extraction of [^{13}N]ammonia in the human heart[142] and 90% extraction in the dog heart.[143] Other workers have also found appreciable uptake of label in the heart following administration of [^{13}N]ammonia to mice,[144,145] rabbits,[144] dogs,[146] rhesus monkeys,[147] and humans[148,149] (see also below). Freed and Gelbard[63] calculate that the first-pass extraction of [^{13}N]ammonia through the heart in anesthetized rats is ~70%.

Schelbert et al.[150,151] studied ^{13}N-extraction and label retention in the hearts of pentobarbitol-sedated, passively ventilated dogs, using an open-chest preparation. Bergmann et al.[152] studied the extraction of [^{13}N]ammonia in rabbit hearts perfused retrogradely through the aorta with a modified Krebs-Henseleit buffer, either with or without added sheep erythrocytes in a noncirculating system. Krivokapich et al.[153,154] studied [^{13}N]ammonia extraction in perfused intraventricular septa of rabbit hearts, maintained at either 28 or 37°C and paced by electrical stimulation at 42 or 72 beats per min, respectively; perfusion was by the septal artery. (These studies[150-154] have been discussed in detail by Cooper et al.[69]) A complex and nonlinear relationship between blood flow and retention of label was found. Generally, the fraction of label retained (or more accurately, the slow clearance phase extrapolated to zero time) on passage of the bolus through the heart was in the range of 0.5 to 0.8. The slow release of label from the heart presumably reflected metabolism of [^{13}N]ammonia to a relatively nondiffusible product (see below) as was previously demonstrated for the rat brain.[73] In several of the above-mentioned studies, the investigators noted that prior treatment with MSO caused a diminution of retention of label by the heart following administration of [^{13}N]ammonia.[143,151,154] These results strongly suggest that ammonia on entry into the heart from the blood is rapidly converted to the only slowly ''releasable'' glutamine; but on poisoning with MSO there is much less efficient trapping of [^{13}N]ammonia and a large portion of the label once taken up is free to return from the heart to the blood. (These findings are similar to our observations that label derived from [^{13}N]ammonia is less effectively retained in the rat brain poisoned with MSO than in the normal rat brain.[73]) Conversion of [^{13}N]ammonia to L-[*amide*-^{13}N]glutamine in the heart has now been directly demonstrated. Krivokapich et al.[154] used a combination of acid extraction, HPLC analysis, and glutaminase treatment of rabbit heart tissue, isolated and deproteinized 6 min following administration of [^{13}N]ammonia. In two separate experiments ~67 and 78% of the label were found in glutamine amide, and 27 and 15%, respectively, in unmetabolized ammonia. In the 5 to 6 min effluent fractions, 11 and 15% of the label were found in glutamine (amide), respectively, whereas 88 and 84% were in ammonia, respectively. When the perfusate contained 1 m*M* MSO the greatly reduced label content of the septa at 6 min was composed mostly of ammonia, only 27% of the label in the septa was in glutamine and 98% of the label in the effluent was in ammonia. Taken together, the experiments of Krivokapich et al.[154] clearly demonstrate the *de novo* synthesis of glutamine in the rabbit heart and its preferential retention compared to extracted ammonia. Moreover, these authors provided indirect evidence for compartmentation of ammonia/glutamine metabolism in the heart. A comparison of the retention and uptake of label derived from L-[*amide*-¹³N]glutamine and [¹³N]ammonia (which as noted is converted to L-[*amide*-¹³N]glutamine) showed that the fate of L-glutamine *entering* the tissue is considerably different from that generated *within* the tissue. Moreover, [¹³N]ammonia arising from the deamidation of extracted L-[*amide*-¹³N]glutamine in the perfused septum was preferentially released, with respect to glutamine, into the perfusion medium.[154] The anatomical basis for the compartmentation of ammonia/glutamine metabolism in the heart remains to be established.

In two recent reports, [¹³N]ammonia, together with an external imaging device, was used to study heart function in normal adults and in adults with heart disease.[155,156] Marshall et al.[155] assume that retention of label by the heart is related to blood flow. This assumption may be valid under normal conditions; but since retention of label is contingent on conversion of ammonia to glutamine, and glutamine synthetase requires ATP, a decrease of ATP in severely damaged tissues may result in a decreased retention of label in the heart for a given blood flow than in normal tissue. (See the discussion by Cooper et al.[69]) Rauch et al.[157] also caution against [¹³N]ammonia uptake as an indicator of myocardial blood flow. These authors suggest that in addition to blood flow, factors such as membrane integrity, pH gradients, and possibly the bicarbonate exchange system will affect uptake of label. Nevertheless, the use of [¹³N]ammonia to qualitatively and noninvasively assess heart function in humans seems promising.

In conclusion, ammonia is readily extracted from the circulation (50 to 90% depending on species and blood flow) in a single pass through the heart and is rapidly converted to metabolites (principally glutamine), possibly in a distinct metabolic compartment. This rapid metabolism of ammonia by glutamine synthetase has provided a clinical basis for the evaluation of heart function using [¹³N]ammonia as a tracer.

F. Lung

Recent studies with [¹³N]ammonia suggest that the lung may also be an important organ for the metabolism of circulating ammonia. Freed and Gelbard[63] found that 12 sec following i.v. [¹³N]ammonia administration, approximately 20% of the injected dose in pentobarbital-anesthetized rats was in the lungs. More than 80% of this dose was released within the next 10 min. HPLC analysis showed that at 6 sec ~24% of the dose in the lung was in glutamine and at 2 min ~75% was in glutamine (less than 1% was in glutamate plus aspartate).[62] Since more than 70% of the dose present at 2 min was released by 10 min after injection, it was clear that most of the labeled glutamine in the lung at 2 min was recirculated to the rest of the body. At 2 min the percentage of label in the blood as glutamine was ~50% but the relative concentration of label in the lungs as glutamine was *30* times that in the blood. It seems highly unlikely that the lung could concentrate glutamine from the blood to such an extent in so short a time. It seemed reasonable to us that the lung can actually synthesize glutamine *de novo*[62] and, indeed, we showed that the isolated lung can make ¹³N-labeled glutamine from [¹³N]ammonia. It is interesting to note that 25 years ago Berl and colleagues[158] concluded that lung glutamine rapidly equilibrates with plasma glutamine. This finding is certainly in agreement with the rapid loss of label from the rat lung 2 to 10 min after administration of [¹³N]ammonia noted by Freed and Gelbard.[63] Berl et al.[158] discussed the idea that the lung may be a major source of plasma glutamine but then rejected the idea. As discussed above, our data do show that the lung almost certainly donates glutamine to the blood, but the exact amount contributed to the plasma by this route remains to be determined.

Having established that glutamine synthetase must be present in the rat lung, we conducted a literature search and found contradictory reports on the enzyme activity in lung. Wu[19] was unable to detect activity in the lungs of four species of mammals, three species of birds, and a turtle. He did, however, find moderate activity in the snake lung. Lund[138] was unable to detect activity in the rat lung, but Knox et al.[159] found a value of 5.4 ± 1.2 μmol/hr/g (25°C) in the rat lung. El-Asmar and Greenburg[160] found an activity of 6.8 μmol/hr/mg protein (37°C) in the mouse lung. This value is of the same order as the mouse brain (11.6 μmol/hr/mg protein) and the mouse liver (2.0 μmol/hr/mg protein).[160] Herzfeld and Estes[31] reported a value of 98 ± 66 μmol/hr/g for the rat lung, but they used the inappropriate phosphoenolpyruvate-regenerating system in their assay. Using this technique we also obtained relatively high values; but using the more appropriate phosphocreatine regenerating system, we obtained a value of ~12 μmol/hr/g,[62] a value similar to that previously reported by Knox et al.[159] for the rat lung. It seems reasonable that the value for rat lung glutamine synthetase is in the range of 4 to 12 μmol/hr/g, which is similar to the specific activity in the heart and skeletal muscle.[135.]

A few studies have been reported on the uptake of [13N] label by human lungs following i.v. injection of [13N]ammonia as assessed by an external imaging device.[142,143,148,156] It appears that uptake of label by the lung is increased and the washout prolonged in heavy smokers compared to nonsmokers[143,148] and in patients with obstructive lung disease.[156] In view of our findings on the metabolic fate of [13N]ammonia in rat lungs, it seems reasonable to believe that this tracer may be of clinical value in assessing pulmonary metabolic function.

The lung alveoli are known to contain small amounts of gaseous ammonia[161] presumably arising from nonionic diffusion from arterial blood.[162] However, in an experiment in which [13N]ammonia was collected in a metabolic chamber, following i.v. injection of [13N]ammonia into a rat, the recovered label was only ~1 ppm of the original dose,[62] suggesting that only a minute fraction of blood ammonia is lost through respiration. Interestingly, the reverse route, i.e., from the surrounding atmosphere to the rat blood, has been demonstrated. At 100 ppm environmental ammonia, only a small increase in blood ammonia was noted; but at a higher concentration blood ammonia levels rose significantly.[163] On prolonged exposure blood ammonia levels declined, suggesting an adaptive response in the rat. It is known that at very high concentrations of ammonia in the environmental atmosphere, significant lung damage occurs in rats and mice.[163] The role of glutamine synthetase in protecting the lung at modest environmental levels of ammonia should be evaluated. Some species of cave bats can withstand for prolonged periods environmental concentrations of ammonia that are ten times the lethal concentration in humans.[164,165] Mucus in the respiratory tract may afford protection,[165] but it would be of interest to measure the levels of glutamine synthetase in the lungs and other organs of bats.

In summary, the lung contains glutamine synthetase and this enzyme may be responsible for converting up to 30% of blood ammonia to glutamine. Its role in this capacity was heretofore unrecognized.

G. Adipose Tissue

In 1975 Miller[166] briefly reported that adipose tissues contain high glutamine synthetase activity. The specific activity in this tissue was found to be tenfold greater than that in the muscle and of the same order of magnitude as that in the brain and the liver. Once again, there is evidence of compartmentation. The specific activity is twofold greater in isolated adipocytes than in the adipose tissue itself suggesting the activity is localized in the fat cell. Miller[166] suggests that >25% of the rapidly metabolized glutamine pool may be derived from the adipocytes. Miller also makes the point that "glutamine synthetase…is a potentially strategic target for hormonal regulation of nitrogen metabolism since it links numerous catabolic processes to a multitude of biosynthetic pathways." In streptozotocin-diabetic rats the enzyme activity rose twofold in the muscle and adipocytes (but not in the brain, liver, and kidney) compared to controls. Since 1975 Miller and associates have studied the response of glutamine synthetase in adipocytes to a variety of external manipulations including exposure to different hormones. For a recent paper see Miller et al.[167] (This paper also contains a summary of the response of glutamine synthetase in other cell lines to environmental hormonal manipulations.)

V. CONCLUDING REMARKS

Glutamine synthetase is a crucial enzyme for the maintenance of nitrogen homeostasis. Its activity appears to be finely regulated in vivo in response to continuously fluctuating amino acid levels in the various body constituents. An increase in its activity in one organ due to a given metabolic demand may be matched by a decrease in activity in another organ. On the face of it, the activity of glutamine synthetase in a given organ is often not that impressive when measured under optimal conditions in vitro compared to other metabolically important enzymes of glutamate metabolism (e.g., glutamate dehydrogenase, glutamate aspartate-aminotransferase, and glutamate-alanine aminotransferase) when also assayed under optimal conditions. However, it appears that glutamine synthetase activity is often compartmented within distinct cells so that the specific activity in these specialized cells becomes quite high. This certainly is true in the brain, liver, kidney, adipose tissue, and is probably true in the heart. Moreover, this strategic localization of the enzyme provides an efficient local utilization of ammonia, a separation from glutaminase (a juxtaposition to this enzyme could result in a wasteful futile cycle), and a physical basis for various glutamine cycles (e.g., in the brain and liver).

ACKNOWLEDGMENTS

I thank Drs. William H. Horner and James C. K. Lai for their helpful suggestions, Dr. Richard Kraig for his help with Figure 2, Dr. H. Ronald Zielke for suggesting the ^{13}N-amide exchange experiments, Timothy Hearn for comments on the manuscript, and Carol Hopkins for preparing the manuscript. Work cited from the author's laboratory was supported in part by NIH grant DK 16739.

REFERENCES

1. **Cooper, A. J. L., Vergara, F., and Duffy, T. E.,** Cerebral glutamine synthetase, in *Glutamine, Glutamate, and Gaba in the Central Nervous System,* Hertz, L., Kvamme, E., McGeer, E. G., and Schousboe, A., Eds., Alan R. Liss, New York, 1983, 77.
2. **Tate, S. S. and Meister, A.,** Glutamine synthetases of mammalian liver and brain, in *The Enzymes of Glutamine Metabolism,* Prusiner, S. and Stadtman, E. E., Eds., Academic Press, New York, 1973, 77.
3. **Meister, A.,** Glutamine synthetase of mammals, in *The Enzymes,* Vol. 10, 3rd ed., Boyer, P. D., Ed., Academic Press, New York, 1974, 699.
4. **Meister, A.,** Catalytic mechanism of glutamine synthetase; overview of glutamine metabolism, in *Glutamine, Metabolism, Enzymology, and Regulation,* Meister, A., Ed., Academic Press, New York, 1980, 1.
5. **Meister, A.,** Enzymology of glutamine, in *Glutamine Metabolism in Mammalian Tissues,* Haüssinger, D. and Sies, H., Eds., Springer-Verlag, Berlin, 1984, 3.
6. **Moldave, K. and Meister, A.,** Synthesis of phenylacetylglutamine by human tissues, *J. Biol. Chem.,* 229, 463, 1957.
7. **Tempest, D. W., Meers, J. L., and Brown, C. M.,** Synthesis of glutamate in *Aerobacter aerogenes* by a hitherto unknown route, *Biochem. J.,* 117, 405, 1970.
8. **Miflin, B. J. and Lea, P. J.,** Amino acid metabolism, *Annu. Rev. Plant Physiol.,* 28, 299, 1977.
9. **O'Donovan, D. J. and Lotspeich, W. D.,** The role of the amide group of glutamine in renal biosynthesis of amino acids, *Enzymologia,* 36, 301, 1969.
10. **Windmueller, H. G. and Spaeth, A. E.,** Respiratory fuels and nitrogen metabolism *in vivo* in small intestine of fed rats, *J. Biol. Chem.,* 255, 107, 1980.

11. **Biltz, R. M., Letteri, J. M., Pellegrino, E. D., and Pinkus, L.,** Glutamine: a new metabolic substrate, in *Regulation of Phosphate and Mineral Metabolism,* Vol. 151, Massry, S. G., Letteri, J. M., and Ritz, E., Eds., (Advances in Experimental Medicine and Biology), Plenum Press, New York, 1982, 423.

12. **Zielke, H. R., Ozand, P. T., Tildon, J. T., Sevdalian, D. A., and Cornblath, M.,** Reciprocal regulation of glucose and glutamine utilization by cultured human diploid fibroblasts, *J. Cell. Physiol.,* 95, 41, 1980.

13. **Reitzer, L. J., Wice, B. M., and Kennell, D.,** Evidence that glutamine, not sugar, is the major energy source for cultured HeLa cells, *J. Biol. Chem.,* 254, 2669, 1979.

14. **Tildon, J. T. and Roeder, L. M.,** Glutamine oxidation by dissociated cells and homogenates of rat brain; kinetics and inhibitor studies, *J. Neurochem.,* 42, 1069, 1984.

15. **Pitts, R. F.,** Production of CO_2 by the intact functioning kidney of the dog, in *Medical Clinics of North America, Vol. 59, Symp. Renal Metabolism,* Baruch, S., Ed., W. B. Saunders, Philadelphia, 1973, 507.

16. **Record, C. O., Buxton, B., Chase, R. A., Curzon, G., Murray-Lyon, I. M., and Williams, R.,** Plasma and brain amino acids in fulminant hepatic failure and their relationship to hepatic encephalopathy, *Eur. J. Clin. Invest.,* 6, 387, 1976.

17. **Ferraro, T. N. and Hare, T. A.,** Triple-column ion-exchange physiological amino acid analysis with fluorescent detection: baseline characterization of human cerebrospinal fluid, *Anal. Biochem.,* 143, 82, 1984.

18. **Herbert, J. D., Coulson, R. A., and Hernandez, T.,** Free amino acids in the caiman and rat, *Comp. Biochem. Physiol.,* 17, 583, 1966.

19. **Wu, C.,** Glutamine synthetase. I. A comparative study of its distribution in animals and its inhibition by DL-allo-δ-hydroxylysine, *Comp. Biochem. Physiol.,* 8, 335, 1963.

20. **Pamiljans, V., Krishnaswamy, P. R., Dumville, G., and Meister, A.,** Studies on the mechanism of glutamine synthesis; isolation and properties of the enzyme from sheep brain, *Biochemistry,* 1, 153, 1962.

21. **Gebhardt, R. and Mecke, D.,** Cellular distribution and regulation of glutamine synthetase in liver, in *Glutamine Metabolism in Mammalian Tissues,* Haüssinger, D. and Sies, H., Eds., Springer-Verlag, Berlin, 1984, 98.

22. **Cooper, A. J. L., Mora, S. N., Cruz, N. F., and Gelbard, A. S.,** Cerebral ammonia metabolism in hyperammonemic rats, *J. Neurochem.,* 44, 1716, 1985.

23. **Rowe, W. B., Ronzio, R. A., Wellner, V. P., and Meister, A.,** Glutamine synthetase (sheep brain), *Methods Enzymol.,* 17A, 900, 1970.

24. **Ehrenfeld, E., Marble, S. J., and Meister, A.,** Enzymatic synthesis of γ-glutamylhydroxamic acid from glutamic acid and hydroxylamine, *J. Biol. Chem.,* 238, 3711, 1963.

25. **Fiske, C. H. and Subbarow, Y.,** The colorimetric determination of phosphorus, *J. Biol. Chem.,* 66, 375, 1925.

26. **Prusiner, S. and Milner, L.,** A rapid radioactive assay for glutamine synthetase, glutaminase, asparagine synthetase, and asparaginase, *Anal. Biochem.,* 37, 429, 1970.

27. **Pahuja, S. L. and Reid, T. W.,** Radioisotope assay for glutamine synthetase using thin-layer chromatography, *J. Chromatogr.,* 235, 249, 1982.

28. **Martin, F., Suzuki, A., and Hirel, B.,** A new high-performance liquid chromatography assay for glutamine synthetase and glutamate synthase in plant tissues, *Anal. Biochem.,* 125, 24, 1982.

29. **Lemieux, G., Baverel, G., Vinay, P., and Wadoux, P.,** Glutamine synthetase and glutamyltransferase in the kidney of man, dog, and rat, *Am. J. Physiol.,* 231, 1068, 1976.

30. **Herzfeld, A.,** The distinction between γ-glutamylhydroxamate synthetase and L-glutamine-hydroxylamine glutamyltransferase activities in rat tissues. Studies *in vitro, Biochem. J.,* 133, 49, 1973.

31. **Herzfeld, A. and Estes, N. A., III,** The distinction between γ-glutamylhydroxamate synthetase and L-glutaminehydroxylamine glutamyltransferase activities in rat tissues. Studies *in vivo, Biochem. J.,* 133, 59, 1973.

32. **Vorhaben, J. E., Wong, L., and Campbell, J. W.,** Assay for glutamine synthetase activity, *Biochem. J.,* 135, 893, 1973.

33. **Levintow, L. and Meister, A.,** Reversibility of the enzymatic synthesis of glutamine, *J. Biol. Chem.,* 209, 265, 1954.

34. **Haschemeyer, R. H.,** Electron microscopy of enzymes, *Adv. Enzymol.,* 33, 71, 1970.

35. **Wellner, V. P. and Meister, A.,** Binding of adenosine triphosphate and adenosine diphosphate by glutamine synthetase, *Biochemistry,* 5, 872, 1966.

36. **Ronzio, R. A., Rowe, W. B., and Meister, A.,** Studies on the mechanism of inhibition of glutamine synthetase by methionine sulfoximine, *Biochemistry,* 8, 1066, 1969.

37. **Midelfort, C. F. and Rose, I. A.,** A stereochemical method for detection of ATP terminal phosphate transfer in enzymatic reactions, *J. Biol. Chem.,* 251, 5881, 1976.

38. **Todhunter, J. A. and Purich, D. L.,** Use of the sodium borohydride reduction technique to identify a γ-glutamyl phosphate intermediary in the *Escherichia coli* glutamine synthetase reaction, *J. Biol. Chem.,* 250, 3505, 1975.

39. **Tsuda, Y., Stephani, R. A., and Meister, A.,** Direct evidence for the formation of an acyl phosphate by glutamine synthetase, *Biochemistry,* 10, 3186, 1971.

40. **Stumpf, P. K., Loomis, W. D., and Michelson, C.,** Amide metabolism in higher plants. I. Preparation and properties of a glutamyl transphorase from pumpkin seedlings, *Arch. Biochem.,* 30, 126, 1951.

41. **Waelsch, H., Owades, P., Bordek, E., Grossowicz, N., and Schou, M.,** The enzyme-catalyzed exchange of ammonia with the amide group of glutamine and asparagine, *Arch. Biochem.,* 27, 237, 1950.

42. **Berl, S.,** Glutamine synthetase. Determination of its distribution in brain during development, *Biochemistry,* 5, 916, 1966.

43. **Segel, H.,** *Enzyme Kinetics,* John Wiley & Sons, New York, 1975, 103.

44. **Cooper, A. J. L.,** unpublished results.

45. **Gass, J. D. and Meister, A.,** Computer analysis of the active site of glutamine synthetase, *Biochemistry,* 9, 1380, 1970.

46. **Windmueller, H. G. and Spaeth, A. E.,** Uptake and metabolism of plasma glutamine by the small intestine, *J. Biol. Chem.,* 249, 5070, 1974.

47. **Weber, F. L., Jr. and Veach, G. L.,** The importance of the small intestine in gut ammonium production in the fasting dog, *Gastroentrology,* 77, 235, 1979.

48. **Walser, M. and Bodenlos, L. J.,** Urea metabolism in man, *J. Clin. Invest.,* 38, 1617, 1959.

49. **Walser, M.,** Use of isotopic urea to study the distribution and degradation of urea in man, in *Proc. Int. Colloquium on the Urea and Kidney,* Schmidt-Nielson, B., Ed., Excerpta Medica, Amsterdam, 1968, 421.

50. **Summerskill, W. H. J. and Wolpert, E.,** Ammonia metabolism in the gut, *Am. J. Clin. Nutr.,* 23, 633, 1970.

51. **Wrong, O. M., Vince, A. J., and Waterlow, J. C.,** The contribution of endogenous urea to fecal ammonia in man, determined by ^{15}N labelling of plasma urea, *Clin. Sci.,* 68, 193, 1985.

52. **Lund, P., Brosnan, J. T., and Eggleston, L. V.,** Regulation of ammonia in mammalian tissues, in *Essays in Cell Metabolism,* Bartley, W., Kornberg, H. L., and Quayle, J. R., Eds., Wiley-Interscience, London, 1970, 167.

53. **Tannen, R. L.,** Ammonia metabolism, *Am. J. Physiol.,* 235, F265, 1978.

54. **Nash, T. P., Jr. and Benedict, S. R.,** The ammonia content of the blood and its bearing on the mechanism of the acid neutralization in the animal organism, *J. Biol. Chem.,* 48, 463, 1921.

55. **Warter, J. M., Brandt, Ch., Marescaux, Ch., Rumbach, L., Michelletti, G., Chabrier, G., Krieger, J., and Imler, M.,** The renal origin of sodium valproate-induced hyperammonemia in fasting humans, *Neurology,* 33, 1136, 1983.

56. **Babit, P., Mathews, S. M., Wolman, S. E., Halliday, D., Millward, D. J., Mathews, D. E., and Rennie, M. J.,** Blood and ammonia accumulation and leucine oxidation during exercise, *Int. Ser. Sports Sci.,* 13, 345, 1983.

57. **Babij, P., Mathews, S. M., and Rennie, M. J.,** Changes in blood ammonia, lactate, and amino acids in relation to workload during bicycle ergometer exercise in man, *Eur. J. Appl. Physiol. Occup. Physiol.,* 50, 405, 1983.

58. **Banister, E. W., Allen, M. E., Mekjavic, I. B., Singh, A. K., Legge, B., and Mutch, B. J. C.,** The time course of ammonia and lactate accumulation in blood during bicycle exercise, *Eur. J. Appl. Physiol. Occup. Physiol.,* 51, 195, 1983.

59. **Schmidt, G.,** Über fementative Desaminierung im Muskel, *Z. Physiol. Chem.,* 179, 243, 1928.

60. **Duda, G. D. and Handler, P.,** Kinetics of ammonia metabolism *in vivo, J. Biol. Chem.,* 232, 303, 1958.

61. **Stein, T. P., Leskiw, M. J., and Wallace, H. W.,** Metabolism of parenterally administered ammonia, *J. Surg. Res.,* 21, 17, 1976.

62. **Freed, B. R. and Cooper, A. J. L.,** in preparation.

63. **Freed, B. R. and Gelbard, A. S.,** Distribution of ^{13}N following intravenous injection of [^{13}N]ammonia in the rat, *Can. J. Physiol. Pharmacol.,* 60, 60, 1982.

64. **Phromphetcharat, V., Jackson, A., Dass, P. D., and Welbourne, T. C.,** Ammonia partitioning between glutamine and urea: interorgan participation in metabolic acidosis, *Kidney Int.,* 20, 598, 1981.

65. **Shröck, H. and Goldstein, L.,** Interorgan relationships for glutamine metabolism in normal and acidotic rats, *Am. J. Physiol.,* 240, E519, 1981.

66. **Squires, E. J. and Brosnan, J. T.,** Measurements of the turnover rate of glutamine in normal and acidotic rats, *Biochem. J.,* 210, 277, 1983.

67. **Christensen, H. N.,** Interorgan amino acid nutrition, *Physiol. Rev.,* 62, 1193, 1982.

68. **Harper, A. E., Miller, R. H., and Block, K. P.,** Branched-chain amino acid metabolism, *Annu. Rev. Nutr.,* 4, 409, 1984.

69. **Cooper, A. J. L., Gelbard, A. S., and Freed, B. R.,** ^{13}N as a biological tracer, *Adv. Enzymol.,* 57, 251, 1985.

70. **Lajtha, A., Berl, S., and Waelsch, H.,** Amino acid and protein metabolism of the brain. IV. The metabolism of glutamic acid, *J. Neurochem.,* 3, 322, 1959.

71. **Berl, S., Lajtha, A., and Waelsch, H.,** Amino acid and protein metabolism. VI. Cerebral compartments of glutamic acid metabolism, *J. Neurochem.,* 7, 186, 1961.

72. **Berl, S., Takagaki, G., Clarke, D. D., and Waelsch, H.,** Metabolic compartments *in vivo*. Ammonia and glutamic acid metabolism in brain and liver, *J. Biol. Chem.,* 237, 2562, 1962.

73. **Cooper, A. J. L., McDonald, J. M., Gelbard, A. S., Gledhill, R. F., and Duffy, T. E.,** The metabolic fate of ^{13}N-labeled ammonia in rat brain, *J. Biol. Chem.,* 254, 4982, 1979.

74. **Van Den Berg, C. J.,** A model of compartmentation in the brain based on glucose and acetate metabolism, in *Metabolic Compartmentation in the Brain,* Balázs, R. and Cremer, J. E., Eds., Macmillan, London, 1973, 137.

75. **Lai, J. C. K., Walsh, J. M., Dennis, S. C., and Clark, J. B.,** Compartmentation of citric acid cycle and related enzymes in distinct populations of rat brain mitochondria, in *Metabolic Compartmentation and Neurotransmitters,* Berl, S., Clarke, D. D., and Schneider, D., Eds., Plenum Press, New York, 1975, 487.

76. **Cooper, A. J. L. and Plum, F.,** Biochemistry and physiology of cerebral ammonia, *Physiol. Rev.,* 67, 440, 1987.

77. **Martinez-Hernandez, A., Bell, K. P., and Norenberg, M. D.,** Glutamine synthetase: glial localization in brain, *Science,* 195, 1356, 1977.

78. **Norenberg, M. D. and Martinez-Hernandez, A.,** Fine structural localization of glutamine synthetase in astrocytes of rat brain, *Brain Res.,* 161, 303, 1979.

79. **Riepe, R. E. and Norenberg, M. D.,** Müller cell localization of glutamine synthetase in rat retina, *Nature,* 268, 654, 1977.

80. **Weiler, C. T., Nyström, B., and Hamberger, A.,** Glutaminase and glutamine synthetase activity in synaptosomes, bulk isolated glia and neurons, *Brain Res.,* 160, 539, 1979.

81. **Dennis, S. C., Lai, J. C. K., and Clark, J. B.,** The distribution of glutamine synthetase in subcellular fractions of rat brain, *Brain Res.,* 197, 469, 1980.

82. **Bradbury, M.,** *The Concept of a Blood-Brain Barrier,* John Wiley & Sons, Chichester, 1979.

83. **Hertz, L.,** Astrocytes, in *Handbook of Neurochemistry,* Vol. 1., 2nd ed., Lajtha, A., Ed., Plenum Press, New York, 1982, 319.

84. **Lockwood, A. H., Finn, R. D., Campbell, J. A., and Richman, T. B.,** Factors that affect the uptake of ammonia by the brain: the blood-brain pH gradient, *Brain Res.,* 181, 259, 1980.

85. **Cooper, A. J. L., Duffy, T. E., McDonald, J. M., and Gelbard, A. S.,** ^{13}N as a tracer for studying ammonia uptake and metabolism in the brain, in *Short Lived Radionuclides in Chemistry and Biology,* Vol. 197, Root, J. W. and Krohn, K. A., Eds., Advances in Chemistry Series, American Chemical Society, Washington, D. C., 1981, 369.

86. **Raichle, M. E. and Larson, K. B.,** The significance of the NH_3-NH_4^+ equilibrium on the passage of ^{13}N-ammonia from blood to brain. A new regional residue detection model, *Clin. Res.,* 48, 913, 1981.

87. **Phelps, M. E., Hoffman, E. J., and Raybaud, C.,** Factors which affect cerebral uptake and retention of $^{13}NH_3$, *Stroke,* 8, 694, 1977.

88. **Benjamin, A. M. and Quastel, J. H.,** Locations of amino acids in brain slices from the rat. Tetrodotoxin-sensitive release of amino acids, *Biochem. J.,* 128, 631, 1972.

89. **Benjamin, A. M. and Quastel, J. H.,** Metabolism of amino acids and ammonia in rat brain cortex slices *in vitro:* a possible role of ammonia in brain function, *J. Neurochem.,* 25, 197, 1975.

90. **Shank, R. P. and Campbell, G. LeM.,** α-Ketoglutarate and malate uptake and metabolism by synaptosomes. Further evidence for an astrocyte-to-neuron metabolic shuttle, *J. Neurochem.,* 42, 1153, 1984.

91. **Hertz, L.,** Functional interactions between neurons and astrocytes. I. Turnover and metabolism of putative amino acid transmitters, *Progr. Neurobiol.,* 13, 277, 1979.

92. **Yu, A. C. H., Drejer, J., Hertz, L., and Schousboe, A.,** Pyruvate carboxylase activity in primary cultures of astrocytes and neurons, *J. Neurochem.,* 41, 1484, 1983.

93. **Berl, S., Takagaki, G., Clarke, D. D., and Waelsch, H.,** Carbon dioxide fixation in the brain, *J. Biol. Chem.,* 237, 2570, 1962.

94. **Hindfelt, B. and Siesjö, B. K.,** Cerebral effects of acute ammonia intoxication. I. The influence on intracellular and extracellular acid-base parameters, *Scand. J. Clin. Lab. Invest.,* 28, 353, 1971.

95. **Kelley, M.A. and Kazemi, H.,** Role of ammonia as a buffer in the central nervous system, *Resp. Physiol.,* 22, 345, 1974.

96. **Schultz, V. and Lowenstein, J. M.,** The purine nucleotide cycle. Studies of ammonia production and interconversion of adenine and hypoxanthine nucleotides and nucleosides by rat brain *in situ, J. Biol. Chem.,* 253, 1938, 1978.

97. **Kraig, R. P., Pulsinelli, W. A., and Plum, F.,** Hydrogen ion buffering during complete brain ischemia, *Brain Res.,* 342, 281, 1985.

98. **Kraig, R. P., Pulsinelli, W. A., and Plum, F.,** Carbonic acid buffer changes during complete brain ischemia, *Am. J. Physiol.,* 250, R348, 1986.

99. **Giacobini, E.,** A cytochemical study of carbonic anhydrase in the nervous system, *J. Neurochem.,* 9, 169, 1962.

100. **Van Gelder, N. M.,** Metabolic interactions between neurons and astroglia: glutamine synthetase, carbonic anhydrase, and water balance, in *Basic Mechanisms of Neuronal Hyperexcitability,* Jasper, H. H. and Van Gelder, N. M., Eds., Alan R. Liss, New York, 1983, 5.

101. **Häussinger, D.,** Hepatocyte heterogeneity in glutamine and ammonia metabolism and the role of an intercellular glutamine cycle during ureogenesis in perfused rat liver, *Eur. J. Biochem.,* 133, 269, 1983.

102. **Häussinger, D. and Gerok, W.,** New concepts in hepatic ammonia metabolism and pH regulation, in *Advances in Hepatic Encephalopathy and Urea Cycle Diseases,* Kleinberger, G., Ferenci, P., Reiderer, P., and Thaler, H. S., Eds., S. Karger, Basel, 1984, 113.

102a. **Cooper, A. J. L., Nieves, E., Coleman, E. A., Filc-DeRicco, S., and Gelbard, A. S.,** Short-term metabolic fate of [^{13}N]ammonia in rat liver *in vivo, J. Biol. Chem.,* 262, 1073, 1987.

103. **Häussinger, D. and Gerok, W.,** Hepatocyte heterogeneity in glutamate uptake by isolated perfused rat liver, *Eur. J. Biochem.,* 136, 421, 1983.

104. **Quistorff, B.,** Gluconeogenesis in periportal and perivenous hepatocytes of rat liver, isolated by a new high-yield digitoxin/collagenase perfusion technique, *Biochem. J.,* 229, 221, 1985.

105. **Väänänen, H., Salaspuro, M., and Lindros, K.,** The effect of chronic ethanol ingestion on ethanol metabolizing enzymes in isolated periportal and perivenous hepatocytes, *Hepatology,* 4, 862, 1984.

106. **Lusty, C. J.,** Carbamoylphosphate synthetase I of rat-liver mitochondria, *Eur. J. Biochem.,* 85, 373, 1978.

107. **Deuel, T. F., Louie, M., and Lerner, A.,** Glutamine synthetase from rat liver. Purification, properties and preparation of specific antisera, *J. Biol. Chem.,* 253, 6111, 1978.

108. **Atkinson, D. E. and Camien, M. N.,** The role of urea synthesis in the removal of metabolic bicarbonate and the regulation of blood pH, *Curr. Top. Cell. Regul.,* 21, 261, 1982.

109. **Oliver, J., Koelz, A. M., Costello, J., and Bourke, E.,** Acid-base induced alterations in glutamine metabolism and ureogenesis in perfused muscle and liver of the rat, *Eur. J. Clin. Invest.,* 7, 445, 1977.

110. **Häussinger, D. and Gerok, W.,** Hepatocyte heterogeneity in ammonia metabolism: impairment of glutamine synthesis in CCl_4 induced liver cell necrosis with no effect on urea synthesis, *Chem.-Biol. Interact.,* 48, 191, 1984.

111. **Perez, G., Rietberg, B., and Schiff, E.,** Amino acid release by isolated perfused cirrhotic livers, *Life Sci.,* 23,2533, 1978.

112. **Maier, K.-P., Volk, B., Hoppe-Seyler, G., and Gerok, W.,** Urea-cycle enzymes in normal liver and in patients with alcoholic hepatitis, *Eur. J. Clin. Invest.,* 4, 193, 1974.

113. **Gerok, W. and Häussinger, D.,** Ammonia detoxication and glutamine metabolism in severe liver disease and its role in the pathogenesis of hepatic coma, in *Glutamine Metabolism in Mammalian Tissues,* Häussinger, D. and Sies, M., Eds., Springer-Verlag, Berlin, 1984, 257.

114. **Krebs, H. A.,** Metabolism of amino acids. IV. The synthesis of glutamine from glutamic acid and ammonia, and the enzymic hydrolysis of glutamine in animal tissues, *Biochem. J.,* 29, 1951, 1935.

115. **Burch, H. B., Choi, S., McCarthy, W. Z., Wong, P. Y., and Lowry, O. H.,** The location of glutamine synthetase within the rat and rabbit nephron, *Biochem. Biophys. Res. Commun.,* 82, 498, 1978.

116. **Nishiitsutsuji-Uwo, J. M., Ross, B. D., and Krebs, H. A.,** Metabolic activities of the isolated perfused rat kidney, *Biochem. J.,* 103, 852, 1967.

117. **Burch, H. B., Chan, A. W. K., Alvey, T. R., and Lowry, O. H.,** Localization of glutamine accumulation and tubular reabsorption in rat nephron, *Kidney Int.,* 14, 406, 1978.

118. **Good, D. W. and Burg, M. B.,** Ammonia production by individual segments of the rat nephron, *J. Clin. Invest.,* 73, 602, 1984.

119. **Good, D. W. and Knepper, M. A.,** Ammonia transport in the mammalian kidney, *Am. J. Physiol.,* 248, F459, 1985.

120. **Schoolwerth, A. C., Nazar, B. L., and LaNue, K. F.,** Glutamate dehydrogenase activation and ammonia formation by rat kidney mitochondria, *J. Biol. Chem.,* 253, 6177, 1978.

121. **Bogusky, R. T. and Aoki, T. T.,** Early events in the initiation of ammonia formation in kidney, *J. Biol. Chem.,* 258, 2795, 1983.

122. **Halperin, M. L., Vinay, P., Gougoux, A., Pichette, C., and Jungas, R. L.,** Regulation of the maximum rate of renal ammoniagenesis in the acidotic dog, *Am. J. Physiol.,* 248, F607, 1985.

123. **Damian, A. C. and Pitts, R. F.,** Rates of glutaminase 1 and glutamine synthetase reactions in rat kidney *in vivo, Am. J. Physiol.,* 218, 1249, 1970.

124. **Welbourne, T. C. and Phromphetcharat, V.,** Renal glutamine metabolism and hydrogen ion homeostasis, in *Glutamine Metabolism in Mammalian Tissues,* Haüssinger, D. and Sies, H., Eds., Springer-Verlag, Berlin, 1984, 161.

125. **Iqbal, K. and Ottaway, J. H.,** Glutamine synthetase in muscle and kidney, *Biochem. J.,* 119, 145, 1970.

126. **Lockwood, A. H., McDonald, J. M., Reiman, R. E., Gelbard, A. S., Laughlin, J. S., Duffy, T. E., and Plum, F.,** The dynamics of ammonia metabolism in man. Effects of liver disease and hyperammonemia, *J. Clin. Invest.,* 63, 449, 1979.

127. **Owen, O. E., Trapp, V. E., Reichard, G. A., Jr., Mozzoli, M. A., Moctezuma, J., Paul, P., Skutches, C. L., and Boden, G.,** Nature and quantity of fuels consumed in patients with alcoholic cirrhosis, *J. Clin. Invest.,* 72, 1821, 1983.

128. **Marliss, E. B., Aoki, T. T., Pozefsky, T., Most, A. S., and Cahill, G. F., Jr.,** Muscle and splanchnic glutamine and glutamate metabolism in postabsorptive and starved man, *J. Clin. Invest.,* 50, 814, 1971.

129. **Durschlag, R. P. and Smith, R. J.,** Regulation of glutamine production by skeletal muscle cells in culture, *Am. J. Physiol.,* 248, C442, 1985.

130. **Pardridge, W. M. and Casanello-Ertl, D.,** Effects·of glutamine deprivation on glucose and amino acid metabolism in tissue culture, *Am. J. Physiol.,* 236, E234, 1979.

131. **King, P. A., Goldstein, L., and Newsholme, E. A.,** Glutamine synthetase activity of muscle in acidosis, *Biochem. J.,* 216, 523, 1983.

132. **Golden, M. H. N., Jahoor, P., and Jackson, A. A.,** Glutamine production rate and its contribution to urinary ammonia in normal man, *Clin. Sci.,* 62, 299, 1982.

133. **Owen, E. E. and Robinson, R. R.,** Amino acid extraction and ammonia metabolism by the human kidney during prolonged administration of ammonium chloride, *J. Clin. Invest.,* 42, 263, 1963.

134. **Schelstraete, K., Simons, M., Deman, J., Vermuelen, F. L., Goethals, P., and Bratzlavsky, M.,** Visualization of muscles involved in unilateral tremor using ^{13}N-ammonia and positron emission tomography, *Eur. J. Nucl. Med.,* 7, 422, 1982.

135. **Rowe, W. B.,** Glutamine synthetase (muscle), *Methods Enzymol.,* 113, 199, 1985.

136. **Doell, R. G. and Felts, J. M.,** Metabolism of glutamic acid in the perfused rabbit heart, *Am. J. Physiol.,* 197, 138, 1959.

137. **Davidson, S. and Sonnenblick, E. H.,** Glutamine production by the isolated perfused rat heart during ammonium chloride perfusion, *Cardiovasc. Res.,* 9, 295, 1975.

138. **Lund, P.,** A radiochemical assay, for glutamine synthetase, *Biochem. J.,* 118, 35, 1970.

139. **Trush, G. P.,** Enzymes of glutamine metabolism in myocardium, *Ukr. Biokhim. Zh.,* 35, 713, 1963; as translated in *Fed. Proc. (Trans. Suppl.),* 23, 1305, 1964.

140. **Hunter, W. W., Jr. and Monahan, W. G.,** ^{13}N-Ammonia: a new physiologic radiotracer for nuclear medicine, *J. Nucl. Med.,* 12, 368, 1972.

141. **Monahan, W. G., Tilbury, R. S., and Laughlin, J. S.,** Uptake of ^{13}N-labeled ammonia, *J. Nucl. Med.,* 13, 274, 1972.

142. **Harper, P. V., Lathrop, K. A., Krizek, H., Lembares, N., Stark, V., and Hoffer, P. B.,** Clinical feasibility of myocardial imaging with [13]NH$_3$, *J. Nucl. Med.,* 13, 278, 1972.

143. **Harper, P. V., Schwartz, J., Beck, R. N., Lathrop, K. A., Lembares, N., Krizek, H., Gloria, I., Dinwoodie, R., McLaughlin, A., Stark, V. J., Bekerman, C., Hoffer, P. B., Gottschalk, A., Resnekov, L., Al-Sadir, J., Mayorga, A., and Brooks, H. L.,** Clinical myocardial imaging with nitrogen-13 ammonia, *Radiology,* 108, 613, 1973.

144. **Cohen, M. B., Spolter, L., MacDonald, N. S., Masuoka, D. T., Laws, S., Neely, H. H., and Takahashi, T.,** Production of nitrogen-13-labeled amino acids by enzymic synthesis, in *Radiopharmaceuticals and Labelled Compounds, Vol. 1,* International Atomic Energy Agency, Vienna, 1973, 483.

145. **Lathrop, K. A., Harper, P. V., Rich, B. H., Dinwoodie, R., Krizek, H., Lembares, N., and Gloria, I.,** Rapid incorporation of short-lived cyclotron-produced radionuclides into radiopharmaceuticals, in *Radiopharmaceuticals and Labeled Compounds, Vol. 1,* International Atomic Energy Agency, Vienna, 1973, 471.

146. **Gelbard, A. S., Clarke, L. P., McDonald, J. M., Monahan, W. G., Tilbury, R. S., Kuo, T. Y. T., and Laughlin, J. S.,** Enzymatic synthesis and organ distribution studies with ^{13}N-labeled glutamine and L-glutamic acid, *Radiology,* 116, 127, 1975.

147. **Gelbard, A. S., McDonald, J. M., Reiman, R. E., and Laughlin, J. S.,** Species differences in myocardial localization of ^{13}N-labeled amino acids, *J. Nucl. Med.,* 16, 529, 1975.

148. **Walsh, W. F., Harper, P. V., Resnekov, L., and Fill, H.,** Noninvasive evaluation of regional myocardial perfusion in 112 patients using a mobile scintillation camera and intravenous nitrogen-13 labeled ammonia, *Circulation,* 54, 266, 1976.

149. **Gelbard, A. S., Benua, R. S., Reiman, R. E., McDonald, J. M., Vomero, J. J., and Laughlin, J. S.,** Imaging of the human heart after administration of L-[^{13}N] glutamate, *J. Nucl. Med.,* 21, 988, 1980.

150. **Schelbert, H. R., Phelps, M. E., Hoffman, E. J., Huang, S.-C., Selin, C. E., and Kuhl, D. E.,** Regional myocardial perfusion assessed with N-13 labeled ammonia and positron emission computerized axial tomography, *Am. J. Cardiol.,* 43, 209, 1979.

151. **Schelbert, H. R., Phelps, M. E., Huang, S.-C., MacDonald, N. S., Hansen, H., Selin, C., and Kuhl, D. E.,** N-13 ammonia as an indicator of myocardial blood flow, *Circulation,* 63, 1259, 1981.

152. **Bergmann, S. R., Hack, S., Tewson, T., Welch, M. J., and Sobel, B. E.,** The dependence of accumulation of [13]NH$_3$ by myocardium on metabolic factors and its implications for quantitative assessment of perfusion, *Circulation,* 61, 34, 1980.

153. **Krivokapich, J., Huang, S.-C., Phelps, M. E., MacDonald, N. S., and Shine, K. I.,** Dependence of $^{13}NH_3$ myocardial extraction and clearance on flow and metabolism, *Am. J. Physiol.,* 242, H536, 1982.

154. **Krivokapich, J., Barrio, J. R., Phelps, M. E., Watanabe, C. R., Keen, R. E., Padgett, H. C., Douglas, A., and Shine, K. I.,** Kinetic characterization of $^{13}NH_3$ and [^{13}N]glutamine metabolism in rabbit heart, *Am. J. Physiol.,* 246, H267, 1984.

155. **Marshall, R. C., Tillisch, J. H., Phelps, M. E., Huang, S.-C., Carson, R., Henze, E., and Schelbert, H. R.,** Identification and differentiation of resting myocardial ischemia and infarction in man with positron computed tomography, ^{18}F-labeled fluorodeoxyglucose, and N-13 ammonia, *Circulation,* 67, 766, 1983.

156. **Tamaki, N., Senda, M., Yonekura, Y., Saji, H., Kodama, S., Konishi, Y., Ban, T., Kambara, H., Kawai, C., and Torizuka, K.,** Dynamic positron computed tomography of the heart with a high sensitivity positron camera and nitrogen-13 ammonia, *J. Nucl. Med.,* 26, 567, 1985.

157. **Rauch, B., Helus, F., Grunze, M., Braunwell, E., Mall, G., Hasselbach, W., and Kübler, W.,** Kinetics of ^{13}N-ammonia uptake in myocardial single cells indicating potential limitations in its applicability as a marker of myocardial blood flow, *Circulation,* 71, 387, 1985.

158. **Berl, S., Lajtha, A., and Waelsch, H.,** Studies of glutamic acid metabolism in the central nervous system, in *Chemical Pathology of the Nervous System,* Folch-Pi, J., Ed., Pergamon Press, Elmsford, N.Y., 1961, 361.

159. **Knox, W. E., Kupchik, H. Z., and Liu, L. P.,** Glutamine and glutamine synthetase in fetal, adult, and neoplastic rat tissues, *Enzyme,* 12, 88, 1971.

160. **El-Asmar, F. A. and Greenberg, D. M.,** Studies on the mechanism of inhibition of tumor growth by the enzyme glutaminase, *Cancer Res.,* 26, 116, 1966.

161. **Jacquez, J. A., Poppell, J. W., and Jeltsch, R.,** Partial pressure of ammonia in alveolar air, *Science,* 129, 269, 1959.

162. **Robin, E. D., Travis, D. M., Bromberg, P. A., Forkner, C. E., Jr., and Tyler, J. M.,** Ammonia excretion by mammalian lung, *Science,* 129, 270, 1959.

163. **Schaerdel, A. D., White, W. J., Lang, C. M., Dvorchik, B. H., and Bohner, K.,** Localized and systemic effects of environmental ammonia in rats, *Lab. Anim. Sci.,* 33, 40, 1983.

164. **Riedesel, M. L.,** Blood physiology, in *Biology of Bats,* Vol. 3, Wimsatt, W. A., Ed., Academic Press, New York, 1977, 500.

165. **Studier, E. H.,** Studies on the mechanisms of ammonia tolerance in the guano bat, *J. Exp. Zool.,* 163, 79, 1966.

166. **Miller, R. E.,** Adipose tissue and skeletal muscle glutamine synthetase in normal and diabetic rats, *Diabetes,* 24, 416, 1975.

167. **Miller, R. E., Pope, S. R., DeWille, J. W., and Burns, D. M.,** Insulin decreases and hydrocortisone increases the synthesis of glutamine synthetase in cultured 3T3-L1 adipocytes, *J. Biol. Chem.,* 258, 5405, 1983.

Chapter 3

GLUTAMINE AMINOTRANSFERASES AND ω-AMIDASES

Arthur J. L. Cooper

TABLE OF CONTENTS

I. INTRODUCTION

Several reviews on the glutamine aminotransferases (transaminases) have been published previously. The interested reader should consult Cooper and Meister[1-4] for accounts of the discovery, characterization, and possible physiological roles of the glutamine aminotransferases. In this review I will concentrate on the more recent work on the occurrence and physiological roles of the glutamine aminotransferases.

The glutamine aminotransferases catalyze the transfer of the α-amino group of L-glutamine to a suitable α-keto acid acceptor, yielding α-ketoglutaramate and an L-amino acid. Although the reaction is reversible, L-glutamine utilization is favored because either α-ketoglutaramate spontaneously cyclizes or it is converted to α-ketoglutarate (2-oxoglutarate) by ω-amidase (Figure 1). Glutamine aminotransferase and ω-amidase activities are widely distributed in rat organs (see below). These activities have also been detected in a wide variety of organisms. (For reviews see Cooper and Meister[1,2,4].) The widespread occurrence of the glutamine aminotransferase-ω-amidase pathway attests to the metabolic importance of this pathway.

II. GLUTAMINE AMINOTRANSFERASES IN RAT TISSUES

In the original characterization, in which pyruvate was used as the amine acceptor, it was concluded that glutamine aminotransferase activity was largely confined to the rat liver.[5,6] Later Kupchik and Knox[7] claimed that, on the contrary, the specific activity of glutamine aminotransferase was much higher in the rat kidney than in the rat liver. However, these authors used low levels of phenylpyruvate as the α-keto acid substrate. The apparent contradiction was resolved when Cooper and Meister[8] showed that the kidney and the liver contain distinct glutamine aminotransferase enzymes which were named glutamine aminotransferases K and L, respectively. Both enzymes exhibit broad specificity toward L-amino acids and α-keto acids, but from a consideration of the most active substrates the L type may be regarded as a fully reversible glutamine-methionine aminotransferase whereas the K type may be regarded as a fully reversible glutamine (aromatic amino acid) methionine aminotransferase.[1-4,8,9] In addition, glyoxylate, despite its high degree of hydration, is a moderately good substrate of both enzymes. Despite certain similarities in substrate specificities, there are a number of assays that can distinguish between the L- and K-glutamine aminotransferases. Glutamine aminotransferase L can effectively utilize L-albizziin (see Figure 2) in place of glutamine whereas L-albizziin is a very poor substrate of glutamine aminotransferase K.[2,10,11] The α-keto acid analogue of albizziin cyclizes and dehydrates in a base to generate the strongly UV-absorbing compound, 2-imidazolinone-4-carboxylate (Figure 2). This strong absorbance provides the basis for a convenient assay for glutamine aminotransferase L. Although both K and L enzymes can utilize phenylpyruvate as substrate, the K enzyme has a much higher affinity for phenylpyruvate. The K activity can be distinguished from the L-type activity by measuring the rate of disappearance of phenylpyruvate in reaction mixtures containing glutamine and low concentrations of phenylpyruvate (0.4 mM).[8] Alternatively, glutamine aminotransferase K may be assayed using the substrate pair, phenylalanine and α-keto-γ-methiolbutyrate.[12] At the end of the reaction KOH is added to a final concentration of 3 M. Phenylpyruvate has a very high extinction coefficient at 320 nm in 3 M KOH (ϵ = 24,000) whereas that due to α-keto-γ-methiolbutyrate is negligible. Details of the various assay procedures for glutamine aminotransferases K and L and ω-amidase may be found in Volume 113 of *Methods in Enzymology*.[13-15] All three activities are widespread in rat tissues (Table 1) and, where the subcellular distribution has been determined, are present in both mitochondrial and cytosolic fractions (Table 2).

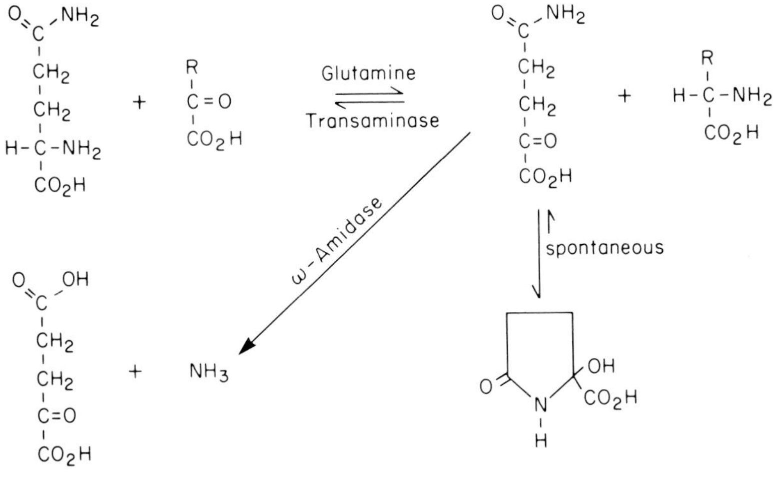

FIGURE 1.   Reactions catalyzed by glutamine aminotransferases (transaminases) and ω-amidase. (From Cooper, A. J. L. and Meister, A., *Chemical and Biological Aspects of Vitamin B₆ Catalysis*, Evangelopoulos, A. E., Ed., Alan R. Liss, New York, 1984, 3. With permission.)

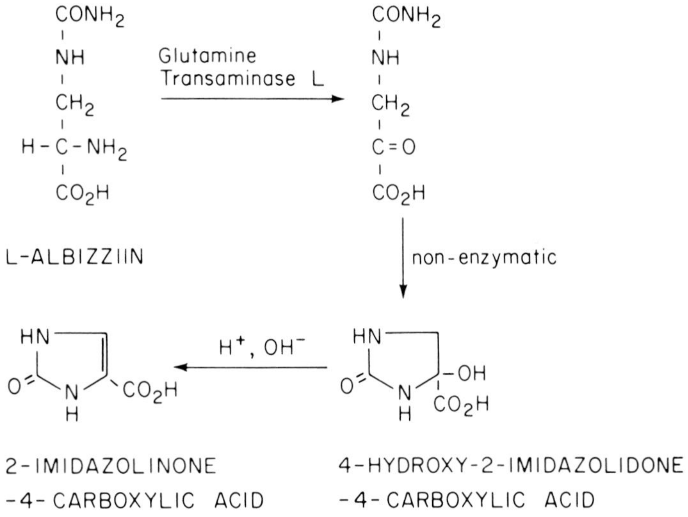

FIGURE 2.   Transamination of L-albizziin with a suitable α-keto acid acceptor catalyzed by glutamine aminotransferase L (glutamine transaminase L). (From Cooper, A. J. L. and Meister, A., *Chemical and Biological Aspects of Vitamin B₆ Catalysis*, Evangelopoulos, A. E., Ed., Alan R. Liss, New York, 1984, 3. With permission.)

III. ω-AMIDASE: DISTRIBUTION STRUCTURE AND CATALYTIC PROPERTIES

Early studies by Meister and colleagues[18-20] showed that ω-amidase activity is widespread in rat tissues (see also Tables 1 and 2), Novikoff hepatoma, yeast, *Escherichia coli, Streptococcus faecalis,* spinach leaves, and lettuce leaves. The enzyme was purified 40-fold from the rat liver and its catalytic activity was extensively studied[18-20] (see below). Subsequently, ω-amidases from *Bacillus subtilus* and *Thermus aquaticus* YT-1 were characterized by

Table 1

**ACTIVITIES OF GLUTAMINE AMINOTRANSFERASE AND
ω-AMIDASE IN RAT TISSUES (μmol/hr/g; 37°C)**

| Tissue | Glutamine aminotransferase L | | Glutamine aminotransferase K | | ω-Amidase |
	L-ALB-glyox assay	L-ALB-αKMB assay	GLN-PP assay	PHE-αKMB assay	
Liver	90	110	35	42	1200
Kidney	3	3	135	145	750
Brain	2	2	9	12	60
Heart	6	5	15	14	189
Skeletal muscle	2	2	9	8	113
Spleen	1	2	19	19	160
Pancreas	3	3	22	16	450
Testes	2	2	13	10	58
Small intestine	3	2	6	7	111
Lung	2	2	9	8	171
Red blood cells	<0.5	<0.5	1	1	2

Note: Adult male Wistar rats (~350 g) were decapitated; the organs were quickly removed, weighed, and disrupted in 5 vol of ice-cold 10 mM potassium phosphate buffer, pH 7.2. The homogenates were freeze-thawed twice and the precipitate was removed by centrifugation at 20,000 g for 15 min. The activities (average of three determinations) are due to both cytosolic and mitochondrial components. The activities in this series are similar to those published previously except that glutamine aminotransferase K activity is higher in hearts, lungs, spleen, skeletal muscle, and testes than reported in Reference 2. ALB, albizziin; αKMB, α-keto-γ-methiolbutyrate; PP, phenylpyruvate; glyox, glyoxylate.

Ramaley et al.[21,22] and a bacterial ω-amidase (actually named 5-hydroxy-N-methylpyroglutamate synthetase) was isolated and studied by Hersh.[23-25] Later Hersh purified an ω-amidase from the soluble fraction of the rat liver to apparent homogeneity,[26,27] although Cooper et al.[15] later obtained a preparation of even higher specific activity. The enzyme has an apparent molecular weight of 58,000 and can be dissociated into two identical subunits.[26]

The catalytic properties of cytosolic rat liver ω-amidase may be summarized as follows:[18-20,26,27] the enzyme catalyzes hydrolysis of 4- and 5-carbon dicarboxylic monoamides (such as α-ketoglutaramate, α-ketosuccinamate, glutaramate, and succinamate), and a variety of glutarate esters. It will also hydrolyze succinylhydroxamate but is inactive toward glutamine and asparagine. The enzyme catalyzes hydroxamate formation from the reaction of hydroxylamine with glutarate, succinamate, or glutarate esters (hydroxaminolysis). The enzyme can also catalyze a weak methanolysis of glutaramate and an aminolysis (with CH_3NH_2) of glutaramate and glutaramate esters. Hersh[27] suggests that the catalytic properties of ω-amidase may be explained in part by the ability of the enzyme to form an acyl-enzyme intermediate. Hersh was unable to detect ω-amidase-catalyzed hydrolysis of N-methyl-α-ketoglutaramic acid[26,27] whereas Meister[18] observed a slow rate of hydrolysis. Most likely the extreme tendency of N-methyl-α-ketoglutaramate to cyclize promotes the unusual reversal of amide hydrolysis. Meister[18] observed that with α-ketosuccinamic acid (open-chain form) as a substrate the pH optimum is broad (pH 5 to 9) whereas with α-ketoglutaramate as a substrate, the pH optimum is much narrower (pH 8.5 to 9.0). Hersh[26,27] explained this observation by showing that below pH 8.0 the ring opening of the cyclic form of α-ketoglutaramate becomes rate limiting.

Although ω-amidase purified from the cytosolic fraction of the rat liver has a wide substrate

Table 2
SUBCELLULAR DISTRIBUTION OF GLUTAMINE
AMINOTRANSFERASE AND ω-AMIDASE IN RAT TISSUE[a]

Tissue	Glutamine aminotransferases		ω-Amidase[e]
	K Type: GLN-phenylpyru-vate[b] or PHE-α-KMB[c] aminotransferase activity	L Type: ALB-glyoxylate aminotransferase activity[d]	
Forebrain			
Cytosol	1.1[b] 1.3[c]	3.1	20
Particulate[f]	9.9[b] 12.1[c]	1.1	4
Liver			
Cytosol	26[b]	75	1070
Mitochondria	13[b]	25	350
Kidney			
Cytosol	133[b]	3	750
Mitochondria	16[b]	<2	100
Pancreas			
Cytosol	~5[g]	N.D.	N.D.
Mitochondria	~5[g]	N.D.	N.D.

[a]   The glutamine aminotransferase activities of the liver and kidney are from Cooper and Meister,[2] and the ω-amidase activities of liver are from Cooper et al.[15] The ω-amidase activities of the kidney and forebrain are previously unpublished data. The pancreas values are estimated from the data of Lenzen et al.;[16] all activities are expressed as μmol/hr/g wet weight at 37°C. ALB: L-albizziin, α-KMB: α-keto-γ-methiolbutyrate, N.D.: not determined.

[b]   20 mM L-Glutamine, 0.4 mM sodium phenylpyruvate, 200 mM ammediol-HCl buffer, pH 9.0 (except where noted).

[c]   20 mM L-Phenylalanine, 5 mM α-keto-γ-methiolbutyrate, 10 mM 2-mercaptoethanol, 200 mM ammediol-HC1 buffer, pH 9.0

[d]   20 mM L-Albizziin, 20 mM sodium glyoxylate, 200 mM glycylglycine buffer, pH 8.5

[e]   20 mM Barium α-ketoglutaramate, 10 mM 2-mercaptoethanol, 100 mM Tris-HCl buffer, pH 8.5.

[f]   The forebrain was fractionated according to the method of Lai and Clark.[17] Most of the particulated glutamine aminotransferase K activity (assay[c]) was in the nonsynaptosomal mitochondrial fraction with approximately 39% in the synaptosomal fraction. Of the activity in the synaptosomal fraction, approximately 65% was in the mitochondria and 35% was in the soluble fraction. The data indicate that overall the soluble enzyme represents ~20% of the total glutamine aminotransferase K activity in rat forebrain. Traces of L-type glutamine aminotransferase and ω-amidase were also detected in nonsyntosomal mitochondria and synatosomes. The mitochondrial fractions were freeze-thawed three times to insure the release of the bound enzyme.

[g]   2 mM L-Glutamine, 5 mM sodium phenylpyruvate.

specificity, it would seem that α-ketoglutaramate is the predominant natural substrate. Thus, α-ketoglutaramate has been detected in the rat liver, kidney, and brain.[28] Moreover, both glutamine aminotransferase activity and ω-amidase activity are widespread in rat tissues and there is a rough parallel between glutamine aminotransferase activity and ω-amidase activity (Table 1). This finding suggests that ω-amidase is present to ensure hydrolysis of α-ketoglutaramate. (Although α-ketosuccinamate does occur in vivo, it is probably less important than α-ketoglutaramate as a substrate. Asparagine aminotransferase is mostly in the liver with smaller amounts in kidney and is of lower inherent activity than either of the glutamine aminotransferases.) It should be pointed out that the apparent K_m of ~3 mM exhibited by rat liver ω-amidase for α-ketoglutaramate[26] is not particularly impressive at first sight, but Hersh has shown that at physiological pH the concentration of open-chain α-ketoglutaramate is only 0.3%. Thus, the true K_m may be of the order of 10 μM ("total" α-ketoglutaramate is present in rat tissues in the micromolar range). Although at physiological pH values the

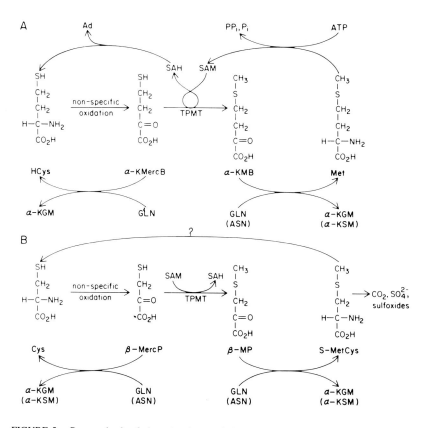

FIGURE 5.   Proposed role of glutamine (asparagine) aminotransferases in (A) the salvage of α-keto-γ-mercaptobutyrate and (B) in the salvage/partial salvage of β-mercaptopyruvate. Note that, although *S*-methylcysteine is an important constituent of some plants, it is generally not considered to be a metabolically important amino acid in mammals (although it may be an important product of xenobiotic transformations).[63] In large amounts, *S*-methylcysteine is toxic.[64] Nevertheless, there are a few studies which show that following administration to experimental animals the methyl group of *S*-methylcysteine is readily converted to CO_2[63,65,66] and that sulfate and various sulfoxides accumulate in the urine.[67] At present it is not known how much *S*-methylcysteine is converted to cysteine but *S*-methylcysteine cannot replace cysteine in vivo.[66] Met: L-methionine, Cys: L-cysteine, HCys: homocysteine, SAH: *S*-adenosylhomocysteine, SAM: *S*-adenosylmethionine, Ad: adenine, α-KGM: α-ketoglutaramate, α-KSM: α-ketosuccinamate, α-KMB: α-keto-γ-methiolbutyrate, α-KMercB: α-keto-γ-mercaptobutyrate, β-MercP: β-mercaptopyruvate, β-MP: β-methiolpruvate, TPMT: thiopurine-*S*-methyltransferase.

$$\text{D,L-α-Hydroxy-γ-methiolbutyrate} \xrightarrow[\substack{\text{D- or L-α-hydroxy}\\\text{acid dehydrogenases}}]{} \text{α-keto-γ-methiolbutyrate}$$

$$\xrightarrow[\text{Gln (Asn)aminotransferases}]{} \text{L-methionine} \tag{8}$$

These reactions are of economic importance. Soybean protein is now processed for livestock and human consumption in large quantities. However, soy protein is low in methionine. Direct addition of L-methionine is expensive and leads to unappetizing flavors due to degradation in the gut and release of volatile sulfides. After considerable testing of various sulfur compounds as less objectionable precursors of L-methionine, calcium D,L-α-hydroxy-γ-methiolbutyrate ("Hydroxy methionine analogue", HMA) has been found to be a safe additive to feedstocks in lieu of methionine. (For a discussion see Cooper and Meister[4] and Cooper.[47]) The conversion of HMA to α-keto-γ-methiolbutyrate has been well characterized

E. Other Metabolic Functions

It is conceivable that mitochondrial and soluble forms of the glutamine aminotransferases play a role in the transport of amino acids. In such a transport system, α-keto acids might be formed on one side of the membrane (or within it) to be reaminated on the other. By utilizing an α-ketoglutarate-linked aminotransferase on one side of the membrane and a glutamine-linked aminotransferase on the other, a directionality will be imparted because of the virtually irreversible nature of the latter reaction. To my knowledge, this possibility has not yet been investigated.

Lenzen et al.[16] have provided evidence that phenylpyruvate is a powerful initiator of insulin secretion. These authors suggest that although phenylpyruvate is not a fuel, transamination of phenylpyruvate with glutamate or glutamine in the pancreatic B cells will yield the Krebs cycle intermediate, α-ketoglutarate. As B-cell preparations transaminate glutamine at very low levels of phenylpyruvate, it is likely that glutamine aminotransferase K is responsible for this activity. It would be interesting to measure the in vivo levels of circulating and pancreatic phenylpyruvate in order to ascertain whether or not glutamine aminotransferase K plays a role in regulation of insulin secretion in vivo.

F. Function(s) in Microorganisms and Plants

Although the glutamine aminotransferase-ω-amidase pathway is present in microorganisms and plants[3] little is known about its physiological role. However, Mora et al.[87,88] have suggested that the combined action of glutamate dehydrogenase, glutamine synthetase, glutamine aminotransferase, and ω-amidase in *Neurospora crassa* provides a glutamine cycle for the incorporation of ammonium nitrogen into amino acids:

$$\alpha\text{-Keto acid} + \text{L-glutamine} \rightleftarrows \text{L-amino acid} + \alpha\text{-ketoglutaramate} \tag{4}$$

$$\alpha\text{-Ketoglutaramate} \rightarrow \alpha\text{-ketoglutarate} + NH_3 \tag{5}$$

$$\alpha\text{-Ketoglutarate} + NH_3 + NAD(P)H + H^+ \rightleftarrows \text{L-glutamate} + NAD(P)^+ \tag{12}$$

$$\text{L-Glutamate} + NH_3 + ATP \rightleftarrows \text{L-glutamine} + ADP + P_i \tag{6}$$

$$\text{Sum: } \alpha\text{-Keto acid} + NH_3 + NAD(P)H + ATP + H^+ \rightarrow$$

$$\text{L-amino acid} + NAD(P)^+ + ADP + P_i \tag{13}$$

G. Use of α-Keto Acids to "Spare" Nitrogen

It was independently suggested by Schloerb[89] and by Richards et al.[90] that α-keto acid mixtures administered in the diet of patients with uremia might spare nitrogen. Since 1966, there have been many studies on the use of α-keto acid (or their equivalent) mixtures in patients with a variety of disorders including uremia, urea cycle disorders, obesity, and liver disease. (See the general discussion by Cooper and Meister,[1] the recent book edited by Walser and Williamson,[91] and the discussion of principles by Walser.[92]) Presumably, such therapy reduces accumulation of urea by directing nitrogen from the urea pathway to amino acid synthesis by pathways involving transamination.

Although glutamate-linked aminotransferases probably play a role in this nitrogen "sparing" effect of α-keto acid mixtures, there is strong evidence that the glutamine aminotransferases are also important. When isolated rat liver preparations were perfused with solutions containing the α-keto acid analogues of valine, isoleucine, leucine, methionine, and phenylalanine, substantial increases in the corresponding L-amino acids were found in the effluent.[93] Analysis of freeze-clamped tissue after such treatment suggested a marked decrease in glutamine levels sufficient to account for the increase in amino acid nitrogen in the effluent. Although perfused muscle was effective in converting α-keto acids to the corresponding amino acids, the level of glutamine remained unchanged, whereas levels of glutamate and alanine decreased.[93] In the case of skeletal muscle, there is little glutamine aminotransferase activity (Table 1). We will mention just two clinical studies which also suggest involvement of the glutamine aminotransferases in the nitrogen-sparing effect of α-keto acid mixtures. After administration of α-keto acid mixtures to patients with portal systemic encephalopathy, blood glutamine levels fell; glutamate levels were unaffected.[94] Plasma levels of glutamine decreased markedly in a patient with argininosuccinic aciduria following administration of a mixture of α-keto and α-hydroxy acids.[95]

There are several pathways whereby glutamine could act to spare nitrogen. Equation 7 yields an essentially irreversible net transfer of glutamate amine nitrogen to α-keto acids thus depleting the urea cycle of a source of nitrogen. Glutamate may be regenerated by α-ketoglutarate-linked aminotransferases or possibly by the glutamate dehydrogenase reaction. Inclusion of a reductive amination of α-ketoglutarate would yield a glutamine cycle similar to that described above for microorganisms, in which there is a net reductive amination of α-keto acids (Equation 13). It is not clear to what extent such a glutamine cycle operates in mammals. Glutamate dehydrogenase has a high K_m for ammonia (10 to 40 mM),[96,97] and ammonia levels are generally low (100 to 300 μM). In addition, it is by no means clear whether the equilibrium position in vivo is in favor of net ammonia utilization. However, under conditions of extreme hyperammonemia or decreased nitrogen intake, it is possible that the glutamate dehydrogenase reaction may be driven toward glutamate formation. Whatever the mechanism, it seems certain that the glutamine aminotransferases play an important role in the nitrogen-sparing mechanism of α-keto (or α-hydroxy) acid mixtures.

VI. CONCLUDING REMARKS

The importance of glutamine (amide) as a source of nitrogen in a large number of biosynthetic reactions is widely recognized; however, the importance of glutamine (amine) for the maintenance of amino acid homeostasis has often been overlooked. This review has stressed the importance of the glutamine aminotransferase-ω-amidase pathway for the salvage of essential amino acid carbon and sulfur and as a possible source of ammonia in the liver and kidney.

Since completion of the original manuscript three relevant papers on glutamine aminotransferase have been published. Dowton and Kennedy[98] have shown that glutaminase is absent from the flight muscle and head of the fleshfly but that glutamine-phenylpyruvate aminotransferase and ω-amidase activity is high in these tissues.

Ricci et al.[99] have purified an enzyme from the bovine liver, which, from its subunit structure (2 identical subunits each of ~47,000 mol wt) and substrate specificity, is almost certainly glutamine aminotransferase K. These authors showed that the enzyme is capable of effectively transaminating L-cystathionine, L-cystine, L-lanthionine, and S-aminethyl-L-cysteine. The corresponding α-keto acids are converted nonenzymatically to 6- or 7-membered unsaturated heterocylic compounds.

Not only is glutamine aminotransferase interesting in its broad substrate specificity toward glutamine, phenylalanine (and tyrosine), and sulfur-containing amino acids, but to complicate matters still further it now seems that cytosolic rat kidney glutamine aminotransferase K is identical to rat kidney cytosolic cysteine conjugate β-lyase (previously considered to be a distinct enzyme).[100] Thus, Stevens et al.[100] have shown that the lyase has a molecular weight of 100,000, is composed of 2 identical subunits and copurifies with glutamine aminotransferase K. Glutamine aminotransferase K transaminates S-1,2-dichlorovinyl-L-cysteine (DCVC) (by now it should be apparent that *S*-substituted cysteines are good substrates for glutamine aminotransferase K) in the presence of a suitable α-keto acid such as α-keto-γ-methiolbutyrate, to *S*-(1,2-dichlorovinyl)-3-mercapto-2-oxopropionic acid. However, β elimination also competes with the usual transamination step eventually yielding pyruvate, ammonia, and 1,2-dichlorovinyl mercaptan. (In the absence of an α-keto acid acceptor the β-elimination reaction is slowed because a transamination reaction results in the pyridoxamine 5′-phosphate form of the enzyme that cannot react further with amino acid substrate.) DCVC, and related compounds are kidney toxins. It seems that, while under normal circumstances glutamine aminotransferase K may act to salvage potentially toxic α-keto acids, when confronted with certain cysteine conjugates glutamine aminotransferase K becomes a liability by converting such amino acids in part to highly toxic fragments.

ACKNOWLEDGMENT

Work cited from the author's laboratory was supported in part by NIH grant DK 16739.

REFERENCES

1. **Cooper, A. J. L. and Meister, A.,** The glutamine transaminase-ω-amidase pathway, *Crit. Rev. Biochem.,* 4, 281, 1977.
2. **Cooper, A. J. L. and Meister, A.,** Comparative studies of glutamine transaminases from rat tissues, *Comp. Biochem. Physiol. B,* 69, 137, 1981.
3. **Cooper, A. J. L. and Meister, A.,** Glutamine transaminases, in *Chemical and Biological Aspects of Vitamin B₆ Catalysis,* Evangelopoulos, A. E., Ed., Alan R. Liss, New York, 1984, 3.
4. **Cooper, A. J. L. and Meister, A.,** Glutamine and asparagine transaminases, in *Transaminases,* Christen, P. and Metzler, D. E., Eds., John Wiley & Sons, New York, 1985, 396.
5. **Meister, A. and Tice, S. V.,** Transamination from glutamine to α-keto acids, *J. Biol. Chem.,* 187, 173, 1950.
6. **Meister, A., Sober, H. A., Tice, S. V., and Fraser, P. E.,** Transamination and associated deamidation of asparagine and glutamine, *J. Biol. Chem.,* 197, 319, 1952.
7. **Kupchik, H. Z. and Knox, W. Z.,** Assays of glutamine and its aminotransferase with the enol-borate of phenylpyruvate, *Arch. Biochem. Biophys.,* 136, 178, 1970.
8. **Cooper, A. J. L. and Meister, A.,** Isolation and properties of a new glutamine transaminase from rat kidney, *J. Biol. Chem.,* 249, 2554, 1973.
9. **Cooper, A. J. L. and Meister, A.,** Isolation and properties of highly purified glutamine transaminase, *Biochemistry,* 11, 661, 1972.
10. **Cooper, A. J. L. and Meister, A.,** Activity of glutamine transaminase toward L-γ-glutamylhydrazones of α-keto acids, *J. Biol. Chem.,* 248, 8489, 1973.
11. **Cooper, A. J. L. and Meister, A.,** Action of liver glutamine transaminase and L-amino acid oxidase on several glutamine analogs, *J. Biol. Chem.,* 248, 8499, 1973.
12. **Cooper, A. J. L.,** Purification of soluble and mitochondrial glutamine transaminase K from rat kidney: use of a sensitive assay involving transamination between L-phenylalanine and α-keto-γ-methiolbutyrate, *Anal. Biochem.,* 89, 451, 1978.
13. **Cooper, A. J. L. and Meister, A.,** Glutamine transaminase L from rat liver, *Methods Enzymol.,* 113, 338, 1985.
14. **Cooper, A. J. L. and Meister, A.,** Glutamine transaminase K from rat kidney, *Methods Enzymol.,* 113, 344, 1985.
15. **Cooper, A. J. L., Duffy, T. E., and Meister, A.,** α-Keto acid ω-amidase from rat liver, *Methods Enzymol.,* 113, 350, 1985.
16. **Lenzen, S., Rustenbeck, I., and Panten, U.,** Transamination of 3-phenylpyruvate in pancreatic B-cell mitochondria, *J. Biol. Chem.,* 259, 2043, 1984.
17. **Lai, J. C. K. and Clark, J. B.,** Preparation of synaptic and nonsynaptic mitochondria from mammalian brain, *Methods Enzymol.,* 55F, 51, 1979.
18. **Meister, A.,** Preparation and enzymatic reactions of the keto analogues of asparagine and glutamine, *J. Biol. Chem.,* 200, 571, 1953.

19. **Meister, A., Levintow, L., Greenfield, R. E., and Abendshein, P. A.,** Hydrolysis and transfer reactions catalyzed by ω-amidase preparations, *J. Biol. Chem.,* 215, 441, 1955.
20. **Meister, A.,** Glutaminase, asparaginase and α-keto acid ω-amidase, *Methods Enzymol.,* 2, 380, 1955.
21. **Ramaley, R. F., Fernald, N., and DeVries, T.,** Dicarboxylate ω-amidase of *Bacillus subtilis*-168: evidence for a membrane-associated form, *Arch. Biochem. Biophys.,* 153, 88, 1972.
22. **Fernald, N. J. and Ramaley, R. F.,** Purification and properties of dicarboxylate ω-amidase from *Bacillus subtilis* 168 and *Thermus aquaticus* YT-1, *Arch. Biochem. Biophys.,* 153, 95, 1972.
23. **Hersh, L. B.,** 5-Hydroxy-*N*-methylpyroglutamate synthetase. Purification and mechanism of action, *J. Biol. Chem.,* 245, 3526, 1970.
24. **Hersh, L. B.,** 5-Hydroxy-*N*-methylpyroglutamate synthetase. Evidence for an α-ketoglutaryl enzyme intermediate from partitioning studies, *J. Biol. Chem.,* 246, 6803, 1971.
25. **Hersh, L. B.,** The effect of aliphatic alcohols and organic solvents on reactions catalyzed by 5-hydroxy-*N*-methylpyroglutamate synthetase, *J. Biol. Chem.,* 246, 7804, 1971.
26. **Hersh, L. B.,** Rat liver ω-amidase purification and properties, *Biochemistry,* 10, 2884, 1971.
27. **Hersh, L. B.,** Rat liver ω-amidase. Kinetic evidence for an acyl-enzyme intermediate, *Biochemistry,* 11, 2251, 1972.
28. **Duffy, T. E., Cooper, A. J. L., and Meister, A.,** Identification of α-ketoglutaramate in rat liver, kidney, and brain: relationship to glutamine transaminase and ω-amidase activities, *J. Biol. Chem.,* 249, 7603, 1974.
29. **Yoshida, T.,** Purification and some properties of soluble and mitochondrial glutamine-keto acid aminotransferase isozymes, *Vitamins,* 35, 227, 1967.
30. **MacPhee, K. G. and Schuster, S. M.,** Properties of cytosolic and mitochondrial hepatic ω-amidase, *Fed. Proc., Fed. Am. Soc. Exp. Biol.,* 42 (Abstr.) 1967, 1983.
31. **Rowsell, E. V., Carnie, J. A., Snell, K., and Taktak, B.,** Assays for glyoxylate aminotransferase activities, *Int. J. Biochem.,* 3, 247, 1972.
32. **Guha, S. R., Chakravati, M. S., and Ghosh, J. J.,** Glutamine-α-keto acid transaminase-deamidase activity in mammalian brain, *Ann. Biochem. Exp. Med.,* 18, 103, 1959.
33. **Benuck, M., Stern, F., and Lajtha, A.,** Transamination of amino acids in homogenates of rat brain, *J. Neurochem.,* 18, 1555, 1971.
34. **Benuck, M., Stern, F., and Lajtha, A.,** Regional and subcellular distribution of aminotransferases in rat brain, *J. Neurochem.,* 19, 949, 1972.
35. **Van Leuven, F.,** Highly purified glutamine transaminase from brain. Physical and kinetic properties, *Eur. J. Biochem.,* 58, 153, 1975.
36. **Van Leuven, F.,** Glutamine transaminase from brain tissue: further studies on kinetic properties and specificity of the enzyme, *Eur. J. Biochem.,* 65, 271, 1976.
37. **Cooper, A. J. L. and Gross, M.,** The glutamine transaminase-ω-amidase system in rat and human brain, *J. Neurochem.,* 28, 771, 1977.
38. **Kurokawa, M., Sakamoto, T., and Kato, M.,** A rapid isolation of nerve-ending particles from brain, *Biochim. Biophys. Acta,* 94, 307, 1965.
39. **Bowsher, R. R. and Henry, D. P.,** Purification of soluble tyrosine transaminase from rat brain, *Fed. Proc., Fed. Am. Soc. Exp. Biol.,* 44 (Abstr.) 1632, 1985.
40. **Duffy, T. E., Vergara, F., and Plum, F.,** α-Ketoglutaramate in hepatic encephalopathy, *Res. Publ. Assoc. Res. Nerv. Ment. Dis.,* 53, 39, 1974.
41. **Vergara, F., Plum, F., and Duffy, T. E.,** α-Ketoglutaramate. Increased concentrations in the cerebrospinal fluid in patients in hepatic coma, *Science,* 183, 81, 1974.
42. **Cooper, A. J. L., Dhar, A. K., Kutt, H., and Duffy, T. E.,** Determination of 2-pyrrolidone-5-carboxylic and α-ketoglutaramic acids in human cerebrospinal fluid by gas chromatography, *Anal. Biochem.,* 103, 118, 1980.
43. **Mattson, W. J., Jr., Iob, V., Sloan, M., Coon, W. W., Turcotte, J. G., and Child, C. G., III,** Alterations of individual free amino acids in brain during acute hepatic coma, *Surg. Gynecol. Obstet.,* 130, 263, 1970.
44. **Van Sande, M., Mardens, Y., Adriaenssens, K., and Lowenthal, A.,** The free amino acids in human cerebrospinal fluid, *J. Neurochem.,* 17, 125, 1970.
45. **Record, C. O., Buxton, B., Chase, R. A., Curzon, G., Murray-Lyon, I. M., and Williams, R.,** Plasma and brain amino acids in fulminant hepatic failure and their relationship to hepatic encephalopathy, *Eur. J. Clin. Invest.,* 6, 387, 1976.
46. **Steele, R. D. and Benevenga, N. J.,** Identification of 3-methylthiopropionic acid as an intermediate in mammalian methionine metabolism *in vitro, J. Biol. Chem.,* 253, 7844, 1978.
47. **Cooper, A. J. L.,** Biochemistry of the sulfur-containing amino acids, *Annu. Rev. Biochem.,* 52, 187, 1983.
48. **Livesey, G.,** Methionine degradation: "anabolic and catabolic", *TIBS,* 9, 27, 1984.

49. **Livesey, G. and Lund, P.**, Methionine metabolism via the transamination pathway in liver, *Biochem. Soc. Trans.*, 8, 540, 1980.

50. **Herbert, J. D., Coulson, R. A., and Hernandez, T.**, Free amino acids in the caiman and rat, *Comp. Biochem. Physiol.*, 17, 583, 1966.

51. **Cooper, A. J. L., Haber, M. T., and Meister, A.**, On the chemistry and biochemistry of 3-mercaptopyruvic acid, the α-keto acid analog of cysteine, *J. Biol. Chem.*, 257, 816, 1982.

52. **Cooper, A. J. L. and Meister, A.**, Enzymatic oxidation of L-homocysteine, *Arch. Biochem. Biophys.*, 239, 556, 1985.

53. **Cammarata, P. S. and Cohen, P. P.**, The scope of the transamination reaction in tissues, *J. Biol. Chem.*, 187, 439, 1950.

54. **Ikeda, T., Konishi, Y., and Ichihara, A.**, Transaminase of branched-chain amino acids. XI. Leucine (methionine) transaminase of rat liver mitochondria, *Biochim. Biophys. Acta*, 445, 622, 1976.

55. **Backlund, P. S., Jr., Chang, C. P., and Smith, R. A.**, Identification of 2-keto-4-methylthiobutyrate as an intermediate compound in methionine biosynthesis from 5'-methylthioadenosine, *J. Biol. Chem.*, 257, 4196, 1982.

56. **Cahill, W. M. and Rudolph, G. G.**, The replacement of *dl*-methionine in the diet of the rat with its α-keto acid analogue, *J. Biol. Chem.*, 145, 201, 1942.

57. **Miller, J. E. and Litwack, G.**, Purification, properties, and identity of liver mitochondrial tyrosine aminotransferase, *J. Biol. Chem.*, 246, 3234, 1971.

58. **Ubuka, T., Yuasa, S., Ishimoto, Y., and Shimomura, M.**, Desulfuration of L-cysteine through transamination and transsulfuration in rat liver, *Physiol. Chem. Phys.*, 9, 241, 1977.

59. **Meister, A., Fraser, P. E., and Tyce, S. V.**, Enzymatic desulfuration of β-mercaptopyruvate to pyruvate, *J. Biol. Chem.*, 206, 561, 1954.

60. **Sörbo, B.**, Enzymic transfer of sulfur from mercaptopyruvate to sulfite or sulfinates, *Biochim. Biophys. Acta*, 24, 324, 1957.

61. **Donahue, J. G. and Henry, D. P.**, Endogenous substrates for thiopurine S-methyltransferase: formation of S-methylcysteine and methionine *in vitro*, *Fed. Proc., Fed. Am. Soc. Exp. Biol.*, 43 (Abstr.) 464, 1984.

62. **Cooper, A. J. L.**, Asparagine transaminase from rat liver, *J. Biol. Chem.*, 252, 2032, 1977.

63. **Landry, T. D., Gushow, T. S., Langvardt, P. W., Wall, J. M., and McKenna, M. J.**, Pharmokinetics and metabolism of inhaled methyl chloride in the rat, *Toxicol. Appl. Pharmacol.*, 68, 473, 1983.

64. **Benevenga, N. J., Yeh, M.-H., and Lalich, J. J.**, Growth depression and tissue reaction to the conversion of excess dietary methionine and S-methylcysteine, *J. Nutr.*, 106, 1714, 1976.

65. **Horner, W. H. and Kuchinskas, E. J.**, Metabolism of methyl-labeled S-methylcysteine in the rat, *J. Biol. Chem.*, 234, 2935, 1959.

66. **Case, G. L. and Benevenga, N. J.**, Evidence for S-adenosylmethionine independent catabolism of methionine in the rat, *J. Nutr.*, 106, 1721, 1976.

67. **Sklan, N. M. and Barnsley, E. A.**, The metabolism of S-methyl-L-cysteine in the rat, *Biochem. J.*, 107, 217, 1968.

68. **Langer, B. W., Jr.**, The biochemical conversion of 2-hydroxy-4-methylthiol-butyric acid into methionine by the rat *in vitro*, *Biochem. J.*, 95, 683, 1965.

69. **Dibner, J. J. and Knight, C. D.**, Conversion of 2-hydroxy 4-(methylthio)butanoic acid to L-methionine in the chick; a stereospecific pathway, *J. Nutr.*, 114, 1716, 1984.

70. **Shrawder, E. and Martinez-Carrion, M.**, Evidence of phenylalanine transaminase activity in the isoenzymes of aspartate aminotransferase, *J. Biol. Chem.*, 247, 2486, 1972.

71. **King, S. and Phillips, A. T.**, Aromatic aminotransferase activity of rat brain cytoplasmic and mitochondrial aspartate aminotransferase, *J. Neurochem.*, 30, 1399, 1978.

72. **Jacoby, G. A. and La Du, B. N.**, Studies on the specificity of tyrosine-α-ketoglutarate transaminase, *J. Biol. Chem.*, 239, 419, 1964.

73. **Meister, A., Undenfriend, S., and Bessman, S. P.**, Diminished phenylketonuria in phenylpyruvic oligophrenia after administration of L-glutamine, L-glutamate or L-asparagine, *J. Clin. Invest.*, 35, 619. 1956.

74. **Collier, V. U., Butler, D. O., and Mitch, W. E.**, Metabolic effects of L-phenyllactate in perfused kidney, liver, and muscle, *Am. J. Physiol.*, 238, E450, 1980.

75. **Hargrove, J. L. and Granner, D. K.**, Biosynthesis and intracellular processing of tyrosine aminotransferase, in *Transaminases,* Christen, P. and Metzler, D., Eds., John Wiley & Sons, New York, 1985, 511.

76. **Fellman, J. H., Vanbellinghen, P. J., Jones, R. T., and Koler, R. D.**, Soluble and mitochondrial forms of tyrosine aminotransferase. Relationship to human tyrosinemia, *Biochemistry*, 8, 615, 1961.

77. **Lund, P. and Watford, M.**, Glutamine as a precursor of urea, in *The Urea Cycle,* Grisolia, S., Báguena, R., and Mayor, F., Eds., John Wiley & Sons, New York, 1976, 479.

78. **Häussinger, D., Stehle, T., and Gerok, W.**, Glutamine metabolism in isolated perfused rat liver. The transamination pathway, *Biol. Chem. Hoppe-Seyler*, 366, 527, 1985.

79. **Schoolwerth, A. C., Nazar, B. L., and LaNue, K. F.**, Glutamate dehydrogenase activation and ammonia formation by rat kidney mitochondria, *J. Biol. Chem.*, 253, 6177, 1978.

80. **Kunin, A. S. and Tannen, R. L.,** Regulation of glutamate metabolism by renal cortical mitochondria, *Am. J. Physiol.,* 237, F55, 1979.

81. **Pitts, R. F., DeHaas, J., and Klein, J.,** Relation of renal amino and amide nitrogen extraction to ammonia production, *Am. J. Physiol.,* 204, 187, 1963.

82. **Goldstein, L.,** Pathways of glutamine deamination and their control in rat kidney, *Am. J. Physiol.,* 213, 983, 1967.

83. **Fine, A., Scott, J., and Bourke, E.,** Studies on the glutamine aminotransferase-ω-amidase pathway in human kidney *in vitro, J. Lab. Clin. Med.,* 80, 591, 1972.

84. **Kopyt, N. and Narins, R. C.,** Stimulation by acidosis of a new renal ammoniagenic pathway, *Clin. Res.,* 23 (Abstr.) 367A, 1975.

85. **Tannen, R. L.,** Ammonia metabolism, *Am. J. Physiol.,* 235, F265, 1978.

86. **Cooper, A. J. L.,** unpublished observation.

87. **Espín, G., Palacios, R., and Mora, J.,** Glutamine metabolism in nitrogen-starved conidia of *Neurospora crassa, J. Gen. Microbiol.,* 115, 59, 1979.

88. **Calderon, J., Morett, E., and Mora, J.,** ω-Amidase pathway in the degradation of glutamine in *Neurospora crassa, J. Bacteriol.,* 161, 807, 1985.

89. **Schloerb, P. R.,** Essential L-amino acid administration in uremia, *Am. J. Med. Sci.,* 252, 650, 1966.

90. **Richards, P., Metcalfe-Gibson, A., Ward, E. E., Wrong, O., and Houghton, B. J.,** Utilisation of ammonia nitrogen for protein synthesis in man, and the effects of protein restriction and uraemia, *Lancet,* 2, 845, 1967.

91. **Walser, M. and Williamson, J. R., Eds.,** *Metabolism and Clinical Implications of Branched Chain Amino and Keto Acids,* (Developments in Biochemistry Series, Vol. 18), Elsevier/North-Holland, New York, 1981.

92. **Walser, M.,** Principles of keto acid therapy in uremia, *Am. J. Clin. Nutr.,* 31, 1756, 1978.

93. **Walser, M., Lund, P., Ruderman, N. B., and Coulter, A. W.,** Synthesis of essential amino acids from their α-keto analogues by perfused rat liver and muscle, *J. Clin. Invest.,* 52, 2856, 1973.

94. **Maddrey, W. C., Weber, F. L., Jr., Coulter, A. W., Chura, C. M., Chapanis, N. P., and Walser, M.,** Effects of keto-analogues of essential amino acids in portal-systemic encephalopathy, *Gastroenterology,* 65, 190, 1976.

95. **Böhles, H., Harms, D., Heid, H., Schmid, D., and Fekl, W.,** Treatment of argininosuccinic aciduria with keto analogues of essential amino acids, *Am. J. Clin. Nutr.,* 31, 1808, 1978.

96. **Frieden, C.,** Glutamic dehydrogenase. III. The order of substrate addition in the enzymatic reaction, *J. Biol. Chem.,* 234, 2891, 1959.

97. **Chee, P. Y., Dahl, J. L., and Fahien, L. A.,** The purification and properties of rat brain glutamate dehydrogenase, *J. Neurochem.,* 33, 53, 1979.

98. **Dowton, M. and Kennedy, I. R.,** Glutamine metabolism in fleshfly (*Parasarcophaga crassipalpis*) tissues, *Comp. Biochem. Physiol. B,* 85, 593, 1986.

99. **Ricci, G., Nardini, M., Federici, G., and Cavallini, D.,** The Transamination of L-cystathionine, L-cystine and related compounds by a bovine kidney transaminase, *Eur. J. Biochem.,* 157, 57, 1986.

100. **Stevens, J. L., Robbins, J. D., and Byrd, R. A.,** A purified cysteine conjugate β-lyase from rat kidney cytosol. Requirement for an α-keto acid or an amino acid oxidase for activity and identity with soluble glutamine transaminase K, *J. Biol. Chem.,* 261, 15529, 1986.

Chapter 4

GLUTAMINASES

Elling Kvamme, Gerd Svenneby, and Ingeborg Aasland Torgner

TABLE OF CONTENTS

I. INTRODUCTION

Glutaminase catalyzes the hydrolytic deamidation of glutamine: glutamine $+ H_2O \rightarrow$ glutamate $+ NH_3^+$.

The following enzymes are most commonly included in the glutaminase family:

1. Phosphate-activated glutaminase (PAG), phosphate-dependent glutaminase (PDG), and L-glutamine amidohydrolase (EC 3.5.1.2). Since only the kidney, brain, and liver glutaminases have been thoroughly investigated and liver glutaminase is described in Chapter 11, our review will mostly deal with kidney and brain PAG.
2. Maleate-activated glutaminase (MAG), phosphate-independent glutaminase (PIG), and γ-glutamyl transferase (EC 2.3.2.2) (see Chapter 9).
3. Glutaminase II, which is an old term that has been referred to in the literature, is no longer in use. Two enzymes, glutamine aminotransferase (EC 2.6.1.15) and ω-amidase (EC 3.3.1.3) are involved, operating in a sequence (see Chapter 3).

II. HISTORICAL BACKGROUND

Glutaminase was first discovered by Krebs[1] in 1935 and he distinguished among a "brain type" and a "hepatic type" of the enzyme. The property of being phosphate activated was discovered by Errera and Greenstein[2] in 1949. Otey et al.[3] solubilized PAG in 1954 and the enzyme was partially purified (about 300-fold) in 1958.[4,5] We purified pig kidney[6] and pig brain[7] PAG to homogeneity in 1970 making use of the property of the enzyme to solubilize and polymerize in a reversible manner. Rat kidney,[9,10] pig brain,[11] and rat brain[20] PAG was later extensively purified, and PAG from the cow[12] was partially purified using modifications of our method. Our purification methods were also improved.[8,13]

III. PURIFICATION AND ASSAY

In principle, pig kidney PAG is purified by phosphate buffer extraction of frozen homogenate followed by fractionation by Na_2SO_4 and repeated solubilizations and precipitations in Tris-HCl buffer and phosphate-borate buffer, respectively. The purification of PAG from the pig brain is essentially similar, starting with an acetone powder extract. By this method the enzyme is 14,000- to 16,000-fold purified. The final specific activity (micromole of product formed per minute per milligram of protein) of the final phosphate-borate precipitated PAG is 400 to 500 and that of the Tris-HCl solubilized enzyme 120 to 130.[13]

When purifying rat kidney PAG, isolated mitochondria are used as a starting material. The enzyme is treated with digitonin, fractionated with Na_2SO_4, followed by repeated filtrations through Sepharose® columns equilibrated with phosphate-tetraborate pyrophosphate buffer or Tris-HCl pyrophosphate buffer, respectively, [10] and finally the active fractions eluted from the latter column are precipitated with $(Na_4)_2SO_4$.

The initial rate of the PAG reaction can be assayed by measuring ammonia formed from glutamine by coupling to the glutamate dehydrogenase reaction whereby NADH oxidation is measured. This method is useful using purified enzymes. Alternatively, glutamate accumulated in a fixed time can be measured[13] by chromatography (column,[14,15] paper,[8] or high performance liquid[16]) or by using enzymatic methods. A useful enzymatic method is based on coupling to the glutamate dehydrogenase reaction and fluorometric monitoring of the NADH formed.[17]

IV. MOLECULAR PROPERTIES

Pig kidney or brain PAG has a molecular weight of 130 to 150 kdaltons when solubilized in Tris-HCl buffer and keeping the protein concentration below 0.1 mg/ml. At higher protein concentration and with phosphate present PAG will dimerize, but polymers are also found.[6,7] Borate added to phosphate will also cause the enzyme to polymerize, forming insoluble polymers of 1500 to 2000 kdaltons. The major forms of PAG are the Tris-HCl enzyme (monomeric), the phosphate enzyme (dimeric), and the phosphate-borate enzyme (polymeric), but an additional membrane-bound insoluble form of pig brain PAG has been suggested.[11] The molecular weight of rat kidney PAG is reported to be 160 kdaltons and this enzyme dimerizes and polymerizes similarly to pig kidney and brain PAG.[18]

By sodium dodecyl sulfate (SDS) polyacrylamide gel electrophroresis we found that pig kidney PAG contains two subunits of 64 and 57 kdaltons, respectively, whereas pig brain PAG has only one subunit of 64 kdaltons. Recent investigations revealed, however, that the 57 kdalton subunit is a degradation product of that of 64 kdaltons. Following SDS polyacrylamide gel electrophoresis of rat renal PAG, a series of bands which ranged in the molecular weight from 48 to 49 kdaltons were obtained, resulting from partial proteolysis.[19] Immunoblot analyses of rat brain PAG as performed by Haser et al.[20] suggest that this enzyme contains two subunits of 65 and 68 kdaltons, respectively, in a ratio of 4:1. Similarly, we found two immunoreactive bands of 64 kdaltons, or close to 64 kdaltons, and 67 kdaltons in the rat brain using antibodies raised against pig brain PAG and immunoblotting analysis of SDS-treated samples.[21] Molecular weights of 64 kdaltons only were observed using the immunoblotting technique of kidney and brain PAG from all other vertebrates investigated, i.e., man, monkey, pig, mouse, cow, rabbit, cat, fish (cod and salmon), and bird (chicken) and also from that of mouse cerebral cortex interneurons (mainly GABA-ergic) and cerebellar granule cells (glutamatergic) as well as astrocytes. However, no PAG-like immunoreactivity was found in lobster ganglion, yeast, and *Escherichia coli.*[21] PAG thus seems to be a rather conservative enzyme.

Electron micrographs appear to be similar for pig brain and kidney PAG.[7,22,23] Negative staining of the Tris-HCl enzyme reveals particles with a diameter of about 60 Å and a length of about 82 Å. If the shape is considered prolate ellipsoidal, the molecular weight is calculated to be 125.5 kdaltons. In high magnification micrographs (negative staining 2% uranyl acetate) a number of the molecules showed the presence of a stain-filled cleft, apparently dividing each molecule into two parts.[23] On addition of phosphate to the Tris-HCl enzyme an elongated dimer composed of two Tris-HCl enzyme molecules became a major component, and after addition of phosphate-borate buffer, long double-stranded helical polymers were formed.

V. CATALYTIC PROPERTIES

A. Activators

The main activators of solubilized and purified renal and brain PAG appear to be phosphate and phosphorylated compounds[3-12,25,27,39] such as riboflavin phosphate and trinucleotides.[25] Organic aniones, e.g., succinate, citrate, malonate, and maleate, also activate purified pig kidney and brain PAG, but the activation is less pronounced than that of phosphate.[27-29] Furthermore, kidney, brain, lymphoid tissue, and bone PAG in nonpurified tissue preparations, such as homogenates, mitochondria,[24,26,30-33,52] synaptosomes,[34-37] and astrocytes[38] are affected by these activators.

A different type of activator sensitizes PAG to activation by phosphate. This is exemplified by the effect of the dye Bromothymol Blue on pig kidney and brain PAG. In low concentrations the dye enhances the activation by phosphate, whereas it inhibits the enzyme activity at higher concentrations,[6,39,40] but phosphate protects against this inhibition.[40] The effects

of malate, 2-oxoglutarate, glutamine, and glutamate and increased phosphoenolpyruvate carboxykinase activity in acidosis.[97] Moreover, inhibition of gluconeogenesis by blocking phosphoenolpyruvate carboxykinase restores malate concentration and prevents the raise in ammonia production without affecting the acidification of the urine.[98] Furthermore, blocking of the citric acid cycle by adding fluorocitrate[99] or fluroacetate[100] to renal slices reduces the levels of 2-oxoglutarate whereby glutamate consumption and glutamine metabolism are stimulated.

In certain acidotic conditions ketoacids and acyl-CoA derivatives may be increased, compounds which are shown to have a profound regulatory effect on purified renal PAG (see Section V). The possibility that such compounds may be instrumental in increasing the ammonia production in such conditions has hitherto been largely overlooked.

D. Lymphocytes and Cancer Cells

Glutamine is believed to be a major energy source in a variety of cells, such as ascites tumor cells,[101] lymphocytes prepared from rat mesenteric lymphnodes[102] or rat thymus,[103] cultured HeLa cells,[104] human diploid fibroblasts,[105,106] and a variety of other vertebrate cells.[107] Glutamine appears particularly to be a major respiratory fuel for rapidly dividing cells, but the amount of glutamine utilized is decreased when glucose is added.[108,109] Glutamine is also the amino acid that exists in the highest concentration in blood plasma, extracellular fluid, and in optimal culture media.

PAG is a primary enzyme for cellular glutamine utilization and the amount of glutamate formed by PAG was increased fivefold in the proliferating thymocytes.[110] The PAG activity of several rat hepatomas was linearly correlated with growth rate and degree of malignancy.[111] Interestingly, lymphocytes possess high activities of PAG which is increased by an immunological challenge in vivo[102] and the activity increased by more than 50% after mitogenic stimulation by concanavalin A. Moreover, glutamine stimulated glycolysis in lymphocytes.[112] The major end products of glutamine metabolism in these cells are glutamate, aspartate, and ammonia[113] similarly to other cells such as Ehrlich ascites tumor cells.[114] However, the latter cells produced only glutamate under anaerobic conditions and glutamine utilization was markedly reduced by anaerobiosis. Glutamine utilized by lymphocytes in the blood stream is probably derived from the skeletal muscle and it has been hypothesized that this is one reason for increased rates of muscle protein degradation during injury, infection, burns, and surgery when the activity of both the immune system and cellular repair processes are increased.[113]

VIII. CONCLUSION

PAG from the kidney and brain has been purified to homogeneity. It has a molecular weight of 130 to 160 kdaltons, but may form polymers of 1500 to 2000 kdaltons with a threefold increase in specific activity, Furthermore, using antibodies raised against PAG and the immunoblotting technique, renal and brain PAG of all vertebrates investigated have a subunit in common of 64 kdaltons and appears to be a conservative enzyme. PAG has allosteric properties, demonstrates complex kinetic behavior, and is affected by a great variety of activators and inhibitors. Main activators are phosphate, phosphorylated compounds which promote phosphate activation, such as calcium and acyl-CoA derivatives, whereas main inhibitors are protons and the reaction products glutamate and ammonia.

In the brain two enzyme forms with distinct kinetic properties have been detected, a soluble and particulate form. PAG in intact kidney mitochondria and brain synaptosomes has also been found to be inhibited by sulfhydryl reagents which are impermeable to the inner mitochondrial membrane, and this finding could not be explained by inhibition of the phosphate or glutamine carriers. Only a small fraction of the potential activity of PAG is likely to be expressed in vivo and it is likely that the renal enzyme is normally under inhibition.

PAG, which is a general mitochondrial enzyme, has been found all over the brain, but appears to be enriched in cortical areas. PAG is also enriched in the distal portion of the nephron and PAG protein as well as enzyme activity in the rat kidney are increased during chronic acidosis. PAG is believed to play an important role in the production of transmitter glutamate in the central nervous system and of ammonia in the kidney, but its alleged involvement in certain pathological conditions, such as Huntington's disease is unclear.

REFERENCES

1. **Krebs, H. A.,** Metabolism of amino-acids. IV. The synthesis of glutamine from glutamic acid and ammonia, and the enzymic hydrolysis of glutamine in animal tissues, *Biochem. J.,* 29, 1951, 1935.
2. **Errera, M. and Greenstein, J. P.,** Phosphate-activated glutaminase in kidney and other tissues, *J. Biol. Chem.* 178, 495, 1949.
3. **Otey, M. C., Birnbaum, S. M., and Greenstein, J. P.,** Solubilized kidney glutaminase I, *Arch. Biochem. Biophys.,* 49, 245, 1954.
4. **Klingman, J. D. and Handler, P.,** Partial purification and properties of renal glutaminase, *J. Biol. Chem.,* 232, 369, 1958.
5. **Sayre, F. W. and Roberts, E.,** Preparation and some properties of a phosphate-activated glutaminase from kidneys, *J. Biol. Chem.,* 233, 1129, 1958.
6. **Kvamme, E., Tveit, B., and Svenneby, G.,** Glutaminase from pig renal cortex. I. Purification and general properties, *J. Biol. Chem.,* 245, 1871, 1970.
7. **Svenneby, G.,** Pig brain glutaminase: purification and identification of different enzyme forms, *J. Neurochem.,* 17, 1591, 1970.
8. **Kvamme, E. and Svenneby, G.,** Phosphate-activated glutaminase in brain, in *Research Methods in Neurochemistry,* Vol. 3, Marks, N. and Rodnight, R., Eds., Plenum Press, New York, 1976, 277.
9. **Huang, Y.-Z. and Knox, W. E.,** A comparative study of glutaminase isozymes in rat tissues, *Enzyme,* 21, 408, 1976.
10. **Curthoys, N. P., Kuhlenschmidt, T., and Godfrey, S. S.,** Regulation of renal ammoniagenesis. Purification and characterization of phosphate-dependent glutaminase from rat kidney, *Arch. Biochem. Biophys.,* 174, 82, 1976.
11. **Nimmo, G. A. and Tipton, K. F.,** Purification of soluble glutaminase from pig brain, *Biochem. Pharmacol.,* 29, 359, 1980.
12. **Chiu, J. F. and Boeker, E. A.,** Cow brain glutaminase: partial purification and mechanism of action, *Arch. Biochem. Biophys.,* 196, 493, 1979.
13. **Kvamme, E., Torgner, I. A. and Svenneby, G.,** Glutaminase from mammalian tissues, in *Methods in Enzymology,* Vol. 113, Colowick, S. P. and Kaplan, N. O., Eds., Academic Press, New York, 1985, 241.
14. **Prusiner, S. and Milner, L.,** A rapid radioactive assay for glutamine synthetase, glutaminase, asparagine synthetase, and asparaginase, *Anal. Biochem.,* 37, 429, 1970.
15. **Shapiro, R. A., Morehouse, R. F., and Curthoys, N. P.,** Inhibition of glutamate of phosphate-dependent glutaminase of rat kidney, *Biochem. J.,* 207, 561, 1982.
16. **Martin, F., Suzuki, A., and Hirel, B.,** A new high-performance liquid chromatography assay for glutamine synthetase and glutamate synthetase in plant tissues, *Anal. Biochem.,* 125, 24, 1982.
17. **Curthoys, N. P. and Lowry, O. H.,** The distribution of glutaminase isoenzymes in the various structures of the nephron in normal, acidotic, and alkalotic rat kidney, *J. Biol. Chem.,* 248, 162, 1973.
18. **Godfrey, S., Kuhlenschmidt, T., and Curthoys, N. P.,** Correlation between activation and dimer formation of rat renal phosphate-dependent glutaminase, *J. Biol. Chem.,* 252, 1927, 1977.
19. **Clark, V. M. and Curthoys, N. P.,** Cause of subunit heterogeneity in purified rat renal phosphate-dependent glutaminase, *J. Biol. Chem.,* 254, 4939, 1979.
20. **Haser, W. G., Shapiro, R. A., and Curthoys, N. P.,** Comparison of the phosphate-dependent glutaminase obtained from rat brain and kidney, *Biochem. J.,* 229, 399, 1985.
21. **Svenneby, G., Kvamme, E., Schousboe, A., and Torgner, I. A.,** Phosphate activated glutaminase-like immunoreactivity in the nervous system from different species and in different neuronal cell types and in astrocytes, *Neurochem. Int.,* 10, 79, 1987.

22. **Olsen, B. R., Svenneby, G., and Kvamme, E.,** Formation and ultrastructure of enzymatically active polymers of pig renal glutaminase, *J. Mol. Biol.,* 52, 239, 1970.

23. **Olsen, B. R., Torgner, I. A., Christensen, T. B., and Kvamme, E.,** Ultrastructure of pig renal glutaminase. Evidence for conformational changes during polymer formation, *J. Mol. Biol.,* 74, 239, 1973.

24. **Weil-Malherbe, H. and Beall, G. D.,** Riboflavin 5'-phosphate: a potent activator of brain glutaminase, *J. Neurochem.,* 17, 1101, 1970.

25. **Weil-Malherbe, H.,** Modulators of glutaminase activity, *J. Neurochem.,* 19, 2257, 1972.

26. **Ardawi, M. S. M. and Newsholme, E. A.,** Intracellular localization and properties of phosphate-dependent glutaminase in rat mesenteric lymphnodes, *Biochem. J.,* 217, 289, 1984.

27. **Svenneby, G., Tveit, B., and Kvamme, E.,** Glutaminase from pig renal cortex. II. Activation by inorganic and organic anions, *J. Biol. Chem.,* 245, 1878, 1970.

28. **Svenneby, G.,** Time and temperature dependent activation of pig brain glutaminase, *J. Neurochem.,* 19, 165, 1972.

29. **Svenneby, G.,** Activation of pig brain glutaminase, *J. Neurochem.,* 18, 2201, 1971.

30. **Greenstein, J. P. and Leuthardt, F. M.,** Effect of phosphate and other anions on the enzymatic desamidation of various amides, *Arch. Biochem. Biophys.,* 17, 105, 1948.

31. **O'Donovan, D. J. and Lotspeich, W. D.,** Activation of kidney mitochondrial glutaminase by inorganic phosphate and organic acids, *Nature,* 212, 930, 1966.

32. **Katunuma, N., Tomino, I., and Nishino, H.,** Glutaminase isozymes in rat kidney, *Biochem. Biophys. Res. Commun.,* 22, 321, 1966.

33. **Weil-Malherbe, H.,** Activators and inhibitors of brain glutaminase, *J. Neurochem.,* 16, 855, 1969.

34. **Bradford, H. F. and Ward, H. K.,** On glutaminase activity in mammalian synaptosomes, *Brain Res.,* 110, 115, 1976.

35. **Kvamme, E. and Olsen, B. E.,** Evidence for two species of mammalian phosphate-activated glutaminase having different regulatory properties, *FEBS Lett.,* 107, 33, 1979.

36. **Kvamme, E. and Olsen, B. E.,** Evidence for compartmentation of synaptosomal phosphate-activated glutaminase, *J. Neurochem.,* 36, 1916, 1981.

37. **Kvamme, E. and Lenda, K.,** Regulation of glutaminase by exogenous glutamate, ammonia and 2-oxo-glutarate in synaptosomal enriched preparation from rat brain, *Neurochem. Res.* 7, 667, 1982.

38. **Kvamme, E., Svenneby, G., Hertz, L., and Schousboe, A.,** Properties of phosphate activated glutaminase in astrocytes cultured from mouse brain, *Neurochem. Res.,* 7, 761, 1982.

39. **Kvamme, E., Tveit, B., and Svenneby, G.,** Glutaminase from pig kidney, an allosteric protein, *Biochem. Biophys, Res. Commun.* 20, 566, 1965.

40. **Kvamme, E. and Torgner, I. A.,** Phosphate-dependent effects of palmityl-CoA and stearyl-CoA on phosphate-activated pig brain and pig kidney glutaminase, *FEBS Lett.,* 47, 244, 1974.

41. **Kvamme, E. and Torgner, I. A.,** The effect of acetyl-coenzyme A on phosphate-activated glutaminase from pig kidney and brain, *Biochem. J.,* 137, 525, 1974.

42. **Kvamme, E. and Torgner, I. A.,** Regulatory effects of fatty acyl-coenzyme A derivatives on phosphate-activated pig brain and kidney glutaminase *in vitro, Biochem. J.,* 149, 83, 1975.

43. **Benjamin, A. M.,** Control of glutaminase activity in rat brain cortex *in vitro:* influence of glutamate, phosphate, ammonium, calcium and hydrogen ions, *Brain Res.,* 208, 363, 1981.

44. **Kvamme, E.,** Regulation of pig kidney phosphate-activated glutaminase, in *Renal Glutamine Metabolism,* Tannen, R. L., Goldstein, L., Lemieux, G., Simpson, D., and Vinay, P., Eds., (Contributions to Nephrology Series, Vol. 31, Berlyne, M., Giovannetti, S., and Thomas, S., Eds.), S. Karger, Basel, 1982, 60.

45. **Kvamme, E., Svenneby, G., and Torgner, I. A.,** Calcium stimulation of glutamine hydrolysis in synaptosomes from rat brain, *Neurochem. Res.,* 8, 25, 1983.

46. **Hovhannessian, V. S., Buniatian, H. C., Mkrdumova, G. S., and Badalian, L. L.,** The participation of thyroxine in the interaction of the isoenzymes of brain glutaminase and certain features of its action, *Vopr. Biokhim. Mozga,* 6, 5, 1970.

47. **Badalian, L. L., Buniatian, H. Ch., and Hovhannessian, V. S.,** Effect of glutamic acid in the interaction of various activators of brain glutaminase, *Vopr. Biokhim. Mozga,* 10, 40, 1975.

48. **Sahagian, J. J. and Hovhannisian, V. S.,** Effect of different modulators on the activity of rat kidney mitochondrial glutaminase and role of thyroid hormones in this process, *Biol. J. Armenii,* 35, 264, 1982.

49. **Kritschevskaya, A. A., Gerschenovitsch, Z., and Scherbatzker, S.,** Ammonia formation from amides by the brain and liver homogenates under increased oxygen pressure, *Biochimija,* 64, 459, 1959.

50. **Hovhannessian, V. S., Buniatian, H. C., Badalian, L. L., and Mkrdumova, G. S.,** On the isoenzymes of the glutaminase system of brain mitochondrial fraction, *Vopr. Biokhim. Mozga,* 5, 5, 1969.

51. **Durozard, D. and Baverel, G.,** Stimulation of glutamine metabolism by 3-aminopicolinate in isolated dog kidney-cortex tubules, *Biochem. J.,* 210, 483, 1983.

52. **Biltz, R. M., Pellegrino, E. D., Letteri, J. M., and Pinkus, L. M.,** Inorganic phosphate, pyrophosphate and the diphosphonates activate bone (calvaria) glutaminase, *Adv. Exp. Med. Biol.,* 178, 217, 1984.

53. **Tveit, B., Svenneby, G., and Kvamme, E.,** Kinetic properties of glutaminase from pig renal cortex, *Eur. J. Biochem.,* 14, 337, 1970.
54. **Shapiro, R. A., Clark, V. M., and Curthoys, N. P.,** Inactivation of rat renal phosphate-dependent glutaminase with 6-diazo-5-oxo-L-norleucine, *J. Biol. Chem.,* 254, 2835, 1979.
55. **Morehouse, R. F. and Curthoys, N. P.,** Properties of rat renal phosphate-dependent glutaminase coupled to Sepharose, *Biochem. J.,* 193, 709, 1981.
56. **Nimmo, G. A. and Tipton, K. F.,** Time-dependent activation and inactivation of pig brain glutaminase, *Biochem. Pharmacol.,* 30, 1635, 1981.
57. **Tannen, R. L. and Kunin, A. S.,** Influence of pyruvate on ammonia metabolism by renal cortical mitochondria, *Kidney Int.,* 22, 280, 1982.
58. **Mikirtumova, K. S., Hairapetiab, H. L., Hovhannessian, V. S., and Buniatian, H. C.,** The effect of diethylstylboestrol and steroid hormones on glutaminase activity on rat brain mitochondrial fractions, *Vopr, Biokhim. Mozga,* 11, 17, 1976.
59. **Clark, V. M., Shapiro, R. A., and Curthoys, N. P.,** Comparison of the hydrolysis and the covalent binding of 6-diazo-5-oxo-L-[6-^{14}C]norleucine by renal phosphate-dependent glutaminase, *Arch. Biochem. Biophys.,* 213, 232, 1982.
60. **Kvamme, E., Svenneby, G., and Tveit, B.,** Molecular aspects of glutaminase, in *The Regulation of Enzyme Activity and Allosteric Interactions,* Kvamme, E. and Pihl, A., Eds., Universitetsforlaget, Oslo, 1968, 89.
61. **Svenneby, G., Roberg, B., Hogstad, S., Torgner, I. A., and Kvamme, E.,** Phosphate activated glutaminase in the crude synaptosomal fraction (P2 fraction) from human brain cortex, *J. Neurochem.,* 47, 1351, 1986.
62. **Nimmo, G. A. and Tipton, K. F.,** Kinetic comparisons between soluble and membrane-bound glutaminase preparations from pig brain, *Eur. J. Biochem.,* 117, 57, 1981.
63. **Torgner, I. Aa., Kvamme, E., Merino, S., Svenneby, G.,** Two kinetically distinguishable forms of phosphate activated glutaminase in human brain, in *Molecular Basis of Neural Function,* Tuček, S., Štipek, S., Štastny, F., and Křivánek, J., Eds., European Society for Neurochemistry, Praque, 1986, 192.
64. **Butterworth, J., Yates, C. M., and Reynolds, G. P.,** Distribution of phosphate-activated glutaminase, succinic dehydrogenase, pyruvate dehydrogenase and τ-glutamyl transpeptidase in post-mortem brain from Huntington's disease and agonal cases, *J. Neurol. Sci.,* 67, 161, 1985.
65. **Nehling, A. and Lehr, P. R.,** Glutaminase activity in the chick central nervous system during postnatal growth, *Comp. Biochem. Physiol.,* 618, 65, 1978.
66. **Svenneby, G. and Storm-Mathisen, J.,** Immunological studies on phosphate activated glutaminase, in *Glutamine, Glutamate, and GABA in the Central Nervous System,* Hertz, L., Kvamme, E., McGeer, E. G., and Schousboe, A., Eds., Alan R. Liss, New York, 1983, 69.
67. **Storm-Mathisen, J., Leknes, A. K., Bore, A. T., Vaaland, J. L., Edminson, P., Haug, F.-M. S., and Ottersen, O. P.,** First visualization of glutamate and GABA in neurones by immunocytochemistry, *Nature,* 301, 517, 1983.
68. **Altschuler, R. A., Monaghan, D. T., Haser, W. G., Wenthold, R. J., Curthoys, N. P., and Cotman, C. W.,** Immunocytochemical localization of glutaminase-like and aspartate aminotransferase-like immunoreactivities in the rat and guinea pig hippocampus, *Brain Res.,* 330, 225, 1985.
69. **Wenthold, R. J., Skaggs, K. K., and Altschuler, R. A.,** Immunocytochemical localization of aspartate aminotransferase and glutaminase immunoreactivities in the cerebellum. *Brain Res.,* 363, 371, 1986.
70. **Monaghan, P. L., Beitz, A. J., Larson, A. A., Altschuler, R. A., Madl, J. E., and Mullett, M. A.,** Immunocytochemical localization of glutamate-, glutaminase- and aspartate aminotransferase-like immunoreactivity in the rat deep cerebellar nuclei, *Brain Res.,* 363, 364, 1986.
71. **Beitz, A. J., Larson, A. A., Monaghan, P., Altschuler, R. A., Mullett, M. M., and Madl, J. E.,** Immunocytochemical localization of glutamate, glutaminase and aspartate aminotransferase in neurons of the pontine nuclei of the rat, *J. Neurosci.,* 17, 741, 1986.
72. **Cangro, C. B., Sweetnam, P. M., Wrathall, J. R., Haser, W. B., Curthoys, N. P., and Neale, J. H.,** Localization of elevated glutaminase immunoreactivity in small DRG neurons, *Brain Res.,* 336, 158, 1985.
73. **Altschuler, R. A., Wenthold, R. J., Schwartz, A. M., Haser, W. G., Curthoys, N. P., Parakkal, M. H., and Fex, J.,** Immunocytochemical localization of glutaminase-like immunoreactivity in the auditory nerve, *Brain Res.,* 291, 173, 1984.
74. **Fex, J., Kachar, B., Rubio, J. A., Parakkal, M. H., and Altshuler, R. A.,** Glutaminase-like immunoreactivity in the organ of corti of guinea pig, *Hearing Res.,* 17, 101, 1985.
75. **Donoghue, J. P., Wenthold, R. J., and Altschuler, R. A.,** Localization of glutaminase-like and aspartate aminotransferase-like immunoreactivity in neurons of cerebral neocortex, *J. Neurosci.,* 5, 2597, 1985.
76. **Tong, J., Harrison, G., and Curthoys, N. P.,** The effect of metabolic acidosis on the synthesis and turnover of rat renal phosphate-dependent glutaminase, *Biochem. J.,* 233, 139, 1986.

77. **Shapiro, R. A., Haser, W. G., and Curthoys, N. P.,** The orientation of phosphate-dependent glutaminase on the inner membrane of rat renal mitochondria, *Arch. Biochem. Biophys.,* 243, 1, 1985.

78. **Gaudemer, Y. and Latruffe, N.,** Evidence for penetrant and non-penetrant thiol reagents and their use in the location of rat liver mitochondrial D(−)-beta-hydroxybutyrate dehydrogenase, *FEBS Lett.,* 54, 30, 1975.

79. **McIntyre, J. O., Bock, H.-G. O., and Fleischer, S.,** The orientation of D-beta-hydroxybutyrate dehydrogenase in the mitochondrial inner membrane, *Biochim. Biophys. Acta,* 513, 255, 1978.

80. **Tietze, R.,** Enzymic method for quantitative determinations of nanogram amounts of total and oxidized glutathione: applications to mammalian blood and other tissues, *Anal. Biochem.,* 27, 502, 1969.

81. **Kvamme, E., Johansen, L., Roberg, B., and Torgner, I. Aa.,** unpublished results.

82. **Kvamme, E.,** Enzymes of cerebral glutamine metabolism, in *Glutamine Metabolism in Mammalian Tissues,* Häussinger, D. and Sies, H., Eds., Springer-Verlag, Berlin, 1984, 32.

83. **Waksman, A., Rendon, A., Cremel, G., Pellicone, C., and Goubault de Brugiere, J.-F.,** Intramitochondrial intermembranal reversible translocation of aspartate aminotransferase and malate dehydrogenase through the inner mitochondrial membrane, *Biochemistry,* 16, 4703, 1977.

84. **Johnson, J. L.,** Glutamine in the dorsal sensory neuron, *Brain Res.,* 69, 366, 1974.

85. **Waelsch, H.,** Glutamic acid and cerebral function, *Adv. Protein Chem.,* 6, 299, 1951.

86. **Kvamme, E. and Lenda, K.,** Evidence for compartmentalization of glutamate in rat brain synaptosomes using the glutamate sensitivity of phosphate activated glutaminase as a functional test, *Neurosci. Lett.,* 25, 193, 1981.

87. **Kvamme, E.,** Ammonia metabolism in the CNS, *Prog. Neurobiol.,* 20, 109, 1983.

88. **Benjamin, A. M., Okamoto, K., and Quastel, J. H.,** Effects of ammonium ions on spontaneous action potentials and on contents of sodium, potassium, ammonium and chloride ions in brain *in vitro, J. Neurochem.,* 30, 131, 1978.

89. **Sandberg, M., Bradford, H. F., and Richards, C. D.,** Effect of lesions of the olfactory bulb on the levels of amino acids and related enzymes in the olfactory cortex of the guinea pig, *J. Neurochem.,* 43, 276, 1984.

90. **Sherman, A. D. and Mott, J.,** Amphetamine stimulation of glutaminase is blocked by neuroleptics, *Life Sci.,* 36, 1163, 1985.

91. **Butterworth, J., Yates, C. M., and Simpson, J.,** Phosphate-activated glutaminase in relation to Huntington's disease and agonal state, *J. Neurochem.,* 41, 440, 1983.

92. **Nasreen, Z. and Sadasivudu, B.,** Glutaminase and glutamine synthetase in rat brain in electroshock convulsions, *IRCS Med. Sci.,* 12, 214, 1984.

93. **Sadasivudu, B., Nasreen, Z., and Swamy, M.,** Functional significance of the activities of glutaminase and ornithine-(1)-aminotransferase in rat brain, *Neurochem. Int.,* 7, 449, 1985.

94. **Goodman, A. D., Fuisz, R. E., and Cahill, G. F.,** Renal Gluconeogenesis in acidosis, alkalosis and potassium deficiency: its possible role in regulation of renal ammonia production, *J. Clin. Invest.,* 45, 612, 1966.

95. **Vinay, P., Mapes, J. P., and Krebs, H. A.,** Fate of glutamine carbon in renal metabolism, *Am. J. Physiol.,* 234, F123, 1978.

96. **Hems, D. A. and Brosnan, J. T.,** Effect of metabolic acidosis and starvation on the content of intermediary metabolites in rat kidney, *Biochem. J.,* 123, 391, 1971.

97. **Alleyne, G. A. O. and Scullard, G. A.,** Renal metabolic response to acid base change. I. Enzymatic control of renal ammoniagenesis in the rat, *J. Clin. Invest.,* 48, 364, 1969.

98. **Ross, B. D. and Tannen, R. L.,** Effect of decrease in bicarbonate concentration on metabolism of the isolated perfused rat kidney, *Clin. Sci.,* 57, 103, 1979.

99. **Bourke, E., Frindt, G., Schreiner, G. E., and Preuss, H. G.,** Effects of fluorocitrate on renal ammoniagenesis and glutamine metabolism in the intact dog kidney, *Kidney Int.,* 15, 255, 1979.

100. **Lemieux, G., Vinay, P., Baverel, G., Briere, R., and Gougoux, A.,** Relationship between lactate and glutamine metabolism in vitro by the kidney: differences between dog and rat and importance of alanine synthesis in the dog, *Kidney Int.,* 16, 451, 1979.

101. **Moreadith, R. W. and Lehninger, A. L.,** The pathways of glutamate and glutamine oxidation by tumor cell mitochondria, *J. Biol. Chem.,* 259, 6215, 1984.

102. **Ardawi, M. S. M. and Newsholme, E. A.,** Maximum activities of some enzymes of glycolysis, the tricarboxylic acid cycle and ketone-body and glutamine utilization pathways in lymphocytes of the rat. *Biochem. J.,* 208, 743, 1982.

103. **Brand, K., Williams, J. F., and Weidemann, M. J.,** Glucose and glutamine metabolism in rat thymocytes, *Biochem. J.,* 221, 471, 1984.

104. **Reitzer, L. J., Wice, B. M., and Kennell, D.,** Evidence that glutamine, not sugar, is the major energy source for cultured HeLa cells, *J. Biol. Chem.,* 254, 2669, 1979.

105. **Zielke, H. R., Ozand, P. T., Tildon, J. T., Sevdalian, D. A., and Cornblath, M.,** Reciprocal regulation of glucose and glutamine utilization by cultured human diploid fibroblasts, *J. Cell. Physiol.,* 95, 41, 1978.

106. **Sumbilla, C. M., Zielke, C. L., Reed, W. D., Ozand, P. T., and Zielke, H. R.,** Comparison of the oxidation of glutamine, glucose, ketone bodies, and fatty acids by human diploid fibroblasts, *Biochim. Biophys. Acta,* 675, 301, 1981.
107. **Wice, B. M., Reitzer, L. J., and Kennell, D.,** The continuous growth of vertebrate cells in the absence of sugar, *J. Biol. Chem.,* 256, 7812, 1981.
108. **Zielke, H. R., Zielke, C. L., and Ozand, P. T.,** Glutamine: a major energy source for cultured mammalian cells, *Fed. Proc., Fed. Am. Soc. Exp. Biol.,* 43, 121, 1984.
109. **Kvamme, E. and Svenneby, G.,** The effect of glucose on glutamine utilization of Ehrlich ascites tumor cells, *Cancer Res.,* 21, 92, 1961.
110. **Brand, K.,** Glutamine and glucose metabolism during thymocyte proliferation. Pathways of glutamine and glutamate metabolism, *Biochem. J.,* 228, 353, 1985.
111. **Linder-Horowitz, M., Knox, W. E., and Morris, H. P.,** Glutaminase activities and growth rates of rat hepatomas, *Cancer Res.,* 29, 1195, 1969.
112. **Ardawi, M. S. M. and Newsholme, E. A.,** Glutamine metabolism in lymphocytes of the rat, *Biochem. J.,* 212, 835, 1983.
113. **Newsholme, E. A., Crabtree, B., and Ardawi, M. S. M.** Glutamine metabolism in lymphocytes: its biochemical, physiological and clinical importance, *Q. J. Exp. Physiol.,* 70, 473, 1985.
114. **Kvamme, E. and Svenneby, G.,** The effect of anaerobiosis on glutamine utilization by Ehrlich ascites tumor cells, *Cancer Res.,* 23, 291, 1963.

Chapter 5

TRANSGLUTAMINASES

Elling Kvamme

TABLE OF CONTENTS

I. INTRODUCTION

Transglutaminases (TGs) catalyze the following reactions: (R-glutaminyl-peptide: -amine-γ-glutamyltransferase EC 2.3.2.13)

$$(1)\ P_1-CH_2\overset{\gamma}{C}H_2CNH_2\ +\ H_2N\overset{\epsilon}{C}H_2CH_2CH_2CH_2-P_2\ \rightarrow$$
$$\underset{O}{\overset{\|}{}}$$

$$P_1-CH_2\overset{\gamma}{C}H_2CN\overset{\epsilon}{C}H_2CH_2CH_2CH_2-P_2\ +\ NH_3$$
$$\underset{O}{\overset{\|\,H}{}}$$

$$(2)\ P_1-CH_2\overset{\gamma}{C}H_2CNH_2\ +\ H_2NA\ \rightarrow\ P_1-CH_2\overset{\gamma}{C}H_2CNHA\ +\ NH_3$$
$$\underset{O}{\overset{\|}{}}\qquad\qquad\qquad\qquad\underset{O}{\overset{\|}{}}$$

$$(3)\ P_1-CH_2\overset{\gamma}{C}H_2CNH_2\ +\ H_2O\ \rightarrow\ P_1-CH_2\overset{\gamma}{C}H_2COH\ +\ NH_3$$
$$\underset{O}{\overset{\|}{}}\qquad\qquad\qquad\qquad\underset{O}{\overset{\|}{}}$$

$$NH_3\ +\ H_2O\ \rightarrow\ NH_4^+\ +\ OH^-$$

TGs catalyze (1) cross-linking of proteins (P_1 and P_2) by creating γ-glutamyl-ϵ-lysine peptides (side-chain), (2) incorporation of amines (A) of low molecular weight into proteins, and (3) hydrolysis of protein-bound glutamine with the formation of protein-bound glutamate. It is of interest that Reactions 1 and 2 compete with each other and that Reaction 3 only occurs at relatively low levels of primary amines.[1,2] For further details the reader is referred to several review articles which have been published.[3-9] In this review, recent findings will be particularly dealt with.

II. HISTORICAL BACKGROUND

Previously, the historical background has been extensively reviewed[3,8] and only some main points will be mentioned here.

The designation "transglutaminase" was first used by Waelsch and co-workers in 1959.[10] They described a Ca^{2+}-dependent transamidation reaction followed by ammonia liberation and incorporation of amines such as histamine or putrescine into proteins (e.g., casein) in the guinea pig liver and other tissues.

Rogers and Springell[11] first reported transpeptidation and transamination reactions in wool and in 1962 Rogers [12] found a citrulline- and glutamate-rich protein located in the inner root sheath of hair follicles, medulla from hair, and related structures. Pisano and Peyton[13] demonstrated in 1969 that the cross-linking of glutamine and lysine in the fibrinogen-fibrin transformation was catalyzed by coagulation factor XIII. Asquith et al.[14] reported in 1970 ϵ-(γ-glutamyl)-lysine bonds in digests of wool keratin and Harding and Rogers[15] in 1971 reported ϵ-lysine cross-links in the citrulline-containing protein of medulla cells from hair and quills. Labeled antisera against tryptic peptides stained the inner root sheath and medulla cells coincidental with the keratohyalin-equivalent trichohyalin.[16]

TG was purified from the guinea pig liver in 1971,[17] and from the guinea pig hair follicle in 1972.[18] The latter structure contained two enzymes, one of which being indistinguishable from the liver enzyme on the basis of chemical, physical, enzymological, and immunological properties. Later, TG has been purified and characterized from the cow snout and hair follicle free epidermes.[19,20] Factor XIII preparation from platelets, blood plasma, and other human and guinea pig tissues were shown to be proenzymes (zymogenes) that were converted to active TG (factor XIIIa) upon incubation with thrombin.[3]

III. PURIFICATION AND ASSAY

In principle, guinea pig liver TG is purified to apparent homogeneity by diethylaminoethyl (DEAE)-cellulose chromatography of the 105,000 g supernatant of homogenate in sucrose, followed by protamine precipitation. The extract of the precipitate is subject to exclusion chromatography as the final step.[17] Human plasma factor XIII is purified by treatment of human plasma in acid citrate dextrose with $BaCl_2$ and glycine, followed by exposure to heat and exclusion chromatography, whereas platelet factor XIII undergoes steps involving DEAE cellulose and hydroxyapatite chromatography.[21-23] TGs from the human epidermis and guinea pig hair follicle are purified by modification of these methods.[20] Recently improved methods for purification of guinea pig[24] and rat liver TG[25] using Sepharose® affinity columns have been described.

Most TGs are assayed by measurement of incorporation of radiolabeled putrescine into casein. However, the activity of, for example, liver TG has also been assayed by determining the incorporation of other radiolabeled primary amines such as methylamine or glycine ethyl ester into various proteins (mixed or pure caseins and acetylated B chain of oxidized insulin) or synthetic substrate peptide derivatives (e.g., benzyloxycarbonyl (Z) — glutaminylglycine).[9]

Recently, a cellular enzyme-linked immunoabsorbent assay has been developed for estimating cellular TG *in situ* using a monoclonal antibody produced against tissue TG.[26]

IV. MOLECULAR PROPERTIES

The molecular weight of the monomeric form of guinea pig liver TG is about 75 kdaltons.[17,27] It contains 16 to 18 SH groups and no disulfide bonds. One of the SH groups is essential for catalytic activity and the sequence around this cystein residue is Tyr-Gly-Gln-Cys-Trp.[28] Ca^{2+} is also essential for catalytic activity by inducing conformational changes in the enzyme protein. Ca^{2+} probably activates the enzyme by binding to the monomeric form.[17]

The plasma factor XIII (zymogen) is a tetramer and has a molecular weight of about 300 kdaltons. It contains two pairs of subunits, one pair containing two identical a-chains and another pair containing two identical b-chains. The a-chains are catalytically active and have molecular weights of about 75 kdaltons, whereas the noncatalytical b-chains have molecular weights of 80 kdaltons.[21] It should be noted that the platelet factor XIII (zymogen) with a molecular weight of about 150 kdaltons only contains two a-chains.[21,29] Thrombin catalyzes limited proteolysis of the zymogen in vitro in the absence of Ca^{2+},[30,31] whereby the a-chain becomes modified and reduced in molecular weight to about 71 kdaltons. Ca^{2+} is necessary for catalytic activity. With Ca^{2+} present the active form of the plasma enzyme is reversibly dissociated to modified a-dimers and b-dimers,[23] whereas the active platelet enzyme will consist of modified a-dimers only. The active enzyme factor XIIIa contains six SH groups per modified a-subunit, one of which being essential for catalytic activity. This essential cystein is surrounded by the same sequence of amino acids as that of the guinea pig liver enzyme.[32] Human epidermal (callus) TG has a molecular weight of about 55 kdaltons that is unaffected by denaturing agents. Recently a high molecular weight form of 72 kdaltons of human epidermal TG has been described.[33] Ca^{2+} is also essential here for catalytic activity. The activity is greatly increased by treatment with trypsin, chaotropic salts, certain organic solvents,[34] and heat[20] in the presence of Ca^{2+}. Antiserum against the enzyme did not cross-react with bovine or human factor XIII and epidermal TG was found to be immunochemically distinct from other TGs.[19,35]

In contrast to the epidermal enzyme, guinea pig hair follicle TG has an apparent molecular weight of only about 27 kdaltons in sodium dodecyl sulfate.[18] Moreover, it has been found that the rat hair follicle TG and epidermal TG show similar differences as these TGs of the guinea pig.[36]

V. CATALYTIC PROPERTIES

The purified TGs are generally rather stable enzymes when stored frozen at $-20°C$ and the specificity of each of the enzymes toward acceptor substrate is broad with the exception of factor XIIIa.

Guinea pig liver TG (called tissue Tg because of its general occurrence) catalyzes not only intermolecular ε-(γ-glutamyl)-lysine cross-linking, but also hydrolysis and aminolysis of some aliphatic amides and of esters such as p-nitrophenyl esters.[37-40] A covalent trimethylacetyl enzyme has been isolated suggesting formation of a stable enzyme-substrate intermediate.[41] This is in accordance with the kinetics which have been found to follow a modified ping-pong mechanism for all of these reactions.

The specificities of factor XIIIa and guinea pig liver TG toward peptide-bound lysine residues and other amines are rather similar,[42] but the specificities of these enzymes toward peptide-bound glutamine differ markedly. Thus, secondary interactions of enzymes with amino acid residues surrounding glutamine influences the specificity.[43,44]

The catalytical mechanisms for hair follicle and liver TG are probably identical, although these enzymes are different in other respects.[22] Generalized models for the mechanism and specificity of the ε-(γ-glutamyl)-lysine-bound formation as catalyzed by TG have been proposed.[5,8]

Ca^{2+} appears to be a universal activator for all known latent intracellular TGs and 10^{-4} to 5×10^{-4} M Ca^{2+} is apparently required for half maximal activation. Zn^{2+} ions compete with Ca^{2+} and inhibit TG with a K_i of about 10^{-7} M.[8] The great sensitivity of tissue TG to Ca^{2+} suggests that this enzyme may function as a receptor protein for Ca^{2+} during stimulus-response coupling as mediated by Ca^{2+}.[45] TGs are in general insensitive to calmoduline. However, two newly described TGs from human platelets and chicken gizzard are activated by 10 to 200 nM calmoduline in the presence of Ca^{2+} and inhibited at concentrations higher than 300 nM.[46]

Physiologically important regulators of active TGs are largely unknown, but the enzyme in the pancreatic islet may be inhibited in vitro by disulfide containing metabolites such as cystamine (by an exchange reaction), by alkylamines, bacitrasin, and monodansylcadaverine.[47] Phenylthiourea derivatives which have been synthesized also act as selective inhibitors of tissue TG.[48] Guinea pig liver TG has been reported to be competitively inhibited by α-difluoromethylornithine,[49] an irreversible inhibitor of ornithine decarboxylase.

Certain TGs are activated by heating and by solutes.[20] Thus human epidermal TG (see above) and the nonsecretory TG of the guinea pig prostate gland are activated a hundredfold in the presence of the organic solute dimethylsulfoxide. In addition, TGs may be regulated at the substrate level by limited proteolytic degradation or modification of substrate protein. In this way, by conversion of fibrinogen to fibrin, a much better substrate is produced for factor XIIIa. Phosphorylation, methylation, or acetylation of side chains may also alter the substrate reactivity towards TGs. Moreover, amines (e.g., spermidine, spermine and putrescine, and histamine) may compete against the cross-linking of protein (see Section I) and act as inhibitors. Purified guinea pig liver TG can incorporate amines into its own structure, whereby the activity towards some protein substrate may possibly be altered.[50]

The consequences of posttranslational modification of proteins by small molecular weight primary amines (e.g., drugs) are unknown. Thus, enzymes may become activated or inhibited by incorporation of a drug amine into its structure. This may alter its antigenic properties whereby an autoimmune response could be precipitated.[8]

VI. STRUCTURAL LOCALIZATION

TGs are located either extracellularly, such as plasma factor XIIIa and the rodent seminal plasma TG, or intracellularly. The following different intracellular TGs have been characterized: tissue TG (identifiable with the well-known liver TG) which is found in the cell cytosol of all tissues and organs,[51] epidermal TG,[19,20] hair follicle TG,[18] prostate TG, and factor XIIIa (in the zymogen form, factor XIII) in human platelets, placenta,[52] monocytes, and macrophages.[53] Guinea pig liver TG is mainly present in the unsedimentable fraction of the homogenate, but appears also to be localized in lysosomes.[54] However, Slife et al.[55] found that 83% of rat liver TG was present in the cytosol and 17% associated with plasma membranes. Recently, a novel form of TG has been detected in the rat lung matrix. Since this TG is predominantly found in a particulate fraction,[56] it is distinct from the liver TG.

VII. FUNCTIONAL PROPERTIES

A. General Function

In spite of the general broad specificity of most TGs toward acceptor substrates, the intermolecular ϵ-(γ-glutamyl)-lysine cross-linking is particularly important from a physiological point of view. Thus the ϵ-amino group of a lysine residue in one molecule of protein exchanges with ammonia at the amide group of a glutamine residue of another protein molecule. This causes, for example, polymerization of fibrin during blood clotting, the formation of the chemically resistant envelope stratum corneum, and production of the vaginal postejaculatory plug derived from the seminal fluid in rodents. It should be noted that an interaction between TG and phospholipid vesicles has been reported, resulting in a modulation of the TG activity.[57]

TGs may be engaged in surface-related immunological reactions, cell proliferation,[58] and receptor-mediated endocytosis[59-61] with regard to the internalization of certain ligands (e.g., the epidermal growth factor, α-macroglobulin, and insulin).[62-64] Mouse mast cells show increase in TG activity, release of histamine, and a marked increase in the level of protein-bound γ-glutamyl histamine[65] on stimulation by an IgE-dependent mechanism or by exposure to certain ionophores. This suggests that TG may have a function in the metabolic regulation of the biologically important compound histamine. It is also possible that activation of TG may be important in the process of egg fertilization in the sea urchin.[8,66] The binding of spermidine to rat sperm has been reported to be TG-mediated. The enzyme can modify one of the major proteins secreted by the rat seminal vesicle epithelium whereby it obtains the capability of binding to the sperm cells.[67]

Human phagocytosis suppresses the induction and expression of TG in cultured peritoneal macrophages.[68] Furthermore, human mononuclear leukocyte TG activity is reported to be enhanced after incubation with certain bacterial toxins or concanavalin A.[69]

The activation of macrophages in vivo is associated with large increases in TG activity,[70] and the enzyme activity of cultured peritoneal macrophages increases markedly in serum-containing media.[71] Based on the finding of Yuspa et al.[72] in 1982 that transretinoic acid, a natural metabolite of vitamin A (retinol), increases TG activity in cultured mouse keratinocytes, the serum activation of TG was found to be caused by serum transretinoic acid.

I. REACTION CATALYZED

The enzyme glutamate dehydrogenase [L-glutamate:NAD(P) oxidoreductase (deaminating)] catalyzes the reversible oxidative deamination of L-glutamate according to the overall reaction:

L-Glutamate + NAD(P)$^+$ + H$_2$O $\rightleftharpoons$ 2-oxoglutarate + NAD(P)H + H$^+$ + NH$_4^+$

Plants and microorganisms contain enzymes that are essentially specific for NAD(H) (EC 1.4.1.2) or NADP(H) (EC 1.4.1.4) but in vertebrates the enzyme (EC 1.4.1.3) can use either of these coenzymes.[1-3] This review will be restricted to the properties and behavior of mammalian glutamate dehydrogenase.

The equilibrium of the reaction is very much in favor of glutamate formation. The equilibrium constant (K$_{eq}$) may be determined from the equation:

$$K_{eq} = \frac{[\text{2-oxoglutarate}][\text{NAD(P)H}][\text{NH}_4^+][\text{H}^+]}{[\text{glutamate}][\text{NAD(P)}^+][\text{H}_2\text{O}]}$$

At 38°C and 0.25 ionic strength, conditions which are believed to approximate those in the liver,[4] the K$_{eq}$ has been determined as 6.97 × 10^{-15} M with NAD(H) and 4.48 × 10^{-15} M with NADP(H).[5] The K$_{eq}$ is, however, dependent on ionic strength and temperature and at 25°C and an ionic strength of 0.1 the values with NAD(H) and NADP(H) were found to be 1.54 × 10^{-15} M and 0.86 × 10^{-15} M, respectively.[5]

At higher values the effects of ionic strength (I) on the K$_{eq}$ are complex but below 0.1 they follow the relationship:

$$\log K_{eq} = \log K_0 + AI$$

where the values of the constant A are 1.4 for NAD$^+$ and 2.4 for NADP$^+$ at 27°C. The value of the K$_{eq}$ at zero ionic strength (K$_0$) has been calculated at 27°C to be 0.64 × 10^{-15} M for NAD$^+$ and 0.193 × 10^{-15} M for NADP$^+$. The heat of reaction (ΔH) was determined to be 70.73 kJ mol^{-1} (16.9 kcal mol^{-1}) for the reaction involving NAD$^+$ and 73.3 kJ mol^{-1} (17.5 kcal mol^{-1}) for that with NADP$^+$. The standard free energy changes (ΔG$_0$) for the oxidation of glutamate by NAD$^+$ and NADP$^+$ were determined to be 77.24 kJ mol^{-1} (18.45 kcal mol^{-1}) and 80.22 kJ mol^{-1} (19.16 kcal mol^{-1}), respectively.[5]

II. TISSUE AND CELLULAR DISTRIBUTION

The enzyme is present in most mammalian tissues with the liver being the richest source. The activity per gram of tissue in the kidney cortex is about one fifth of that in the liver and relatively lower amounts of activity are present in the pancreas, brain, intestinal and gastric mucosa, heart, spleen, skeletal muscle, and lung.[6,7] Immunological studies have suggested the enzymes in the ox spleen, brain, heart, and liver to be closely similar or identical[8] and this is supported by their similar kinetic properties.[9] Although it has been shown possible to separate glutamate dehydrogenase preparations into several fractions by chromatographic and electrophoretic procedures these fractions appear to represent different aggregation states of the enzyme rather than true isoenzymes.[10]

Despite this evidence for the close similarity of glutamate dehydrogenase from the different tissues of the same organism Plaitakis and Berl[11] have suggested that there are two isoenzymes of glutamate dehydrogenase in human leukocytes. One form of the enzyme, which was shown to be associated with particulate material, was thermo-labile whereas the other was soluble and relatively heat-stable. It appears that these two forms of the enzyme might be under separate genetic control since the heat-labile form is deficient in individuals with recessive olivopontocerebellar atrophy.[11,12] In the rat heart only 18% of the glutamate dehydrogenase activity was found to be mitochondrial, whereas the remainder of the activity was found to be cytosolic and also to be more heat-stable than the mitochondrial activity.[13]

Earlier work suggested that, in the brain, glutamate dehydrogenase was low in synaptosomes[14,15] and nerve cell bodies.[17] However, the enzyme has been shown to be present in primary cultures of cerebral neurones,[18] cerebellar granule cells,[18,19] and astrocytes.[19-23] Examination of synaptic and nonsynaptic (free) mitochondria prepared from different regions of the rat brain showed the glutamate dehydrogenase activities to be similar in synaptic mitochondria from the cortex, striatum, and medullar oblongata and also in nonsynaptic mitochondria derived from the first two of these regions.[24] However, the activity in nonsynaptic mitochondria from the medullar oblongata was about twice that observed in the other mitochondrial preparations. These results would suggest that the higher glutamate dehydrogenase activities observed in brain regions with higher glutamatergic innervation may be due to mitochondria derived from nonsynaptic regions rather than those in neurones.[24] A rather even distribution of glutamate dehydrogenase between neuronal and extraneuronal structures in the brain would be consistent with the observation that lesions of the auditory nerve resulted in no change in the activity of glutamate dehydrogenase in the cochlear nucleus whereas the activities of the neuronally located enzymes aspartate aminotransferase and glutaminase decreased and that of glutamine synthetase, which is located in glial cells, increased as a result of proliferation of those cells.[25]

Within liver and brain cells glutamate dehydrogenase is localized in the mitochondrial matrix[26,27] and is frequently used as a marker enzyme for mitochondria in cellular fractionation studies. However, there have been conflicting reports of relatively small amounts of the enzyme in nuclei.[28] The yield of glutamate dehydrogenase associated with the nuclear fraction has been found to depend on the ionic strength of the extraction medium used which suggests that the enzyme might adsorb nonspecifically to nuclear membranes.[29] That such binding can indeed occur has been demonstrated by experiments in which purified rat liver glutamate dehydrogenase was added to homogenates of that tissue before subcellular fractionation.[30]

No kinetic differences could be detected between the enzyme preparations obtained from the nuclear and mitochondrial fractions of the rat liver.[31] However, the enzyme purified from the nuclear fraction of the ox liver was reported to have a higher anodic mobility on cellulose acetate electrophoresis and to be more strongly activated by phosphate ions than the corresponding mitochondrial enzyme.[29,32] Differential centrifugation of homogenates of human leukocytes has allowed the separation of the mitochondrial form of the enzyme from a component that did not sediment at $100,000 \times g$. This latter form was found to be more stable to incubation at 47.5°C than the activity associated with the mitochondrial fraction.[11] A greater thermal stability of the activity associated with the cytosolic fraction in the rat heart as compared with the mitochondrial activity has also been reported.[13] The relative molecular mass and kinetic properties of the cytosolic and mitochondrial forms of glutamate dehydrogenase from the rat heart have been reported to differ.[13] A modified form of the enzyme, with a greater sensitivity to inhibition by GTP, has also been reported to occur in the serum of patients with Reye's syndrome.[33] In the brain the kinetic properties of the enzyme in synaptic and nonsynaptic mitochondria have also been reported to differ.[34] Further work will be necessary to define the differences that lead to these changed properties. However, some caution is necessary in comparing the behavior of the mitochondrial enzyme with that of isolated preparations since its sensitivity to activation by L-leucine has been reported to be greater in ultrasonically disrupted mitochondria than in purified preparations.[35]

Earlier work had suggested that glutamate dehydrogenase was synthesized outside the mitochondrion and then transported into it.[30,36] Evidence was also presented to indicate that some posttranslational modification of the enzyme was associated with this process.[36] More recently Mihara et al.[37] have shown the rat liver enzyme to be synthesized as a larger molecular-weight precursor by cytoplasmic free polysomes and this precursor has also been shown to be enzymically active.[38] It is, however, unclear whether this precursor form corresponds to that detected in the high-speed supernatant fraction from rat hearts[13] and human leukocytes.[11]

The process whereby glutamate dehydrogenase is transported into the mitochondrion remains to be elucidated. The enzyme has been shown to bind to phospholipids such as cardiolipin, a constituent of mitochondrial membranes, and phosphatidylserine and it is possible that such phospholipid interactions may be involved in the transport process.[30,39] However, it is also possible that interactions between the enzyme and the mitochondrial inner membrane[40,41] may play a part in the regulation of its activity. The observation that posttranslational modification is associated with the transport of the enzyme into the mitochondrion may explain why it has not proved possible to demonstrate reversible denaturation of the purified mitochondrial enzyme.[42-44]

III. MOLECULAR PROPERTIES

A. Relative Molecular Mass and Aggregation

Glutamate dehydrogenase has an oligomeric structure. Polyacrylamide gel electrophoresis in the presence of sodium dodecyl sulfate,[45] sedimentation-equilibrium studies in the presence of 6 M guanidinium chloride,[46] and amino acid sequence analysis[47] have established the existence of only one type of subunit with a relative molecular mass of about 56,000. Studies on the oligomeric structure of the ox liver enzyme were hindered by its tendency to aggregate at higher protein concentrations. (For a review see Reference 48.) At concentrations less than 1 mg mℓ^{-1} a relative molecular mass of about 320,000 has been determined under nondenaturing conditions by quasi-elastic light scattering,[49] intensity light scattering and velocity sedimentation,[50] and by equilibrium sedimentation.[51]

Thus, under these conditions the enzyme has a hexameric structure and this has been confirmed by electron microscopic examination[52] which indicated the subunits to be arranged in two layers of trimers in the form of a triangular antiprism.[48,52] The hexameric structure has also been confirmed by cross-linking studies.[53] Studies on the denaturation of the enzyme in the presence of guanidinium chloride have shown that dissociation into trimers first occurs in a process that involves little loss of conformation, as assessed by circular dichroism, followed by complete dissociation into monomers associated with unfolding of the polypeptide chains.[54,55] Studies on the effects of dilution of the guanidinium chloride-treated enzyme have shown that the trimers are without catalytic activity but they can reassociate to form the active hexamer. In contrast the monomeric form produced at higher guanidinium chloride concentrations cannot be renatured.[44] The technique of irradiation-inactivation has also indicated the smallest enzymically active form of glutamate dehydrogenase to be the hexamer.[56,57]

At protein concentrations above about 1.0 mg mℓ^{-1} ox liver glutamate dehydrogenase forms higher polymers. This has been demonstrated by sedimentation equilibrium,[46] sedimentation velocity,[50] and light-scattering[49,50] techniques. Analysis of such data has shown that the relative molecular mass of the enzyme increases continuously with increasing concentration.[48,51] Studies on the effects of temperature on the association process have indicated it to be entropy driven at lower temperatures (below about 20°C in the buffer system used) but enthalpy driven at higher temperatures.

Light-scattering,[58] low-angle X-ray scattering,[59] and sedimentation and viscosity[60-63] measurements have shown that the aggregation process involves the association of glutamate dehydrogenase oligomers to form rods that continuously increase in size as the protein concentration is increased. The formation of these linear polymers has been confirmed by electron microscopic examination.[52,64] However, under appropriate conditions higher-order structures can be seen in which the linear polymers associate side-by-side to form two-dimensional sheets[64] or in which four polymer chains fold into helical tubular structures.[64,65] The features of these structures have been discussed in detail by Eisenberg et al.[48] but their biological significance is unknown.

Glutamate dehydrogenase preparations from different mammalian sources may differ in their abilities to associate in solution. The enzymes from pig[66] and human[67] livers and from the ox brain[68] appear to behave similarly to that from the ox liver but that from the rat liver has been reported only to polymerize to a small extent[31] or not at all.[69] The reasons for this difference are unclear since the amino acid sequences of the rat liver and ox liver enzymes have been found to be very similar.[1]

A number of compounds can influence the polymerization equilibrium of glutamate dehydrogenase. Since these include allosteric effectors, these effects will be discussed later (Section IV.D).

B. Structure

Determination of the amino acid sequences of glutamate dehydrogenases from different sources has indicated the structure to be remarkably conserved. The sequences of the enzymes from the ox[47] and chicken[70,71] liver, for example, differ in only 27 of the 500 residues that overlap with 17 of these differences being conservative substitutions.[1] Comparison of sequence data for the enzymes from the ox and human liver showed them only to differ in 24 of the 454 residues that have been identified in the latter enzyme.[72] The incomplete sequence that has been published for the enzyme from the rat liver also indicates extensive homology with ox liver glutamate dehydrogenase.[1] Peptide-mapping studies[73] as well as immunological cross-reactivity[73a] have confirmed earlier suggestions[8,9,74] that the enzymes purified from the ox liver and brain are identical or at least very similar. In contrast, the enzymes from the rat liver and brain may not be identical, since they have been reported to have different properties.[75] Although the sequence of the NADP-dependent enzyme from *Neurospora* shows considerable differences from those of the mammalian enzymes there is still a significant degree of homology.[1]

Alignment of the published amino acid sequences of glutamate dehydrogenase preparations from ox, rat, human, and chicken livers[1] has shown the latter two enzymes to possess three or four additional residues at the amino-terminal end. In the case of the chicken liver enzyme these residues were cysteine or cysteic acid, glutamic acid, and alanine[71] whereas in the case of the human liver enzyme the sequence was Ser-Glu-Ala-Val.[72] It has recently been shown that when prepared by conventional purification procedures[76,77] the enzyme from the ox liver suffers limited proteolysis in which a tetrapeptide is removed from the amino-terminal end. The sequence of this peptide was shown to be X-Asp-Ala-Ala.[73] Our recent, unpublished work with the enzyme purified from the ox brain has indicated the amino-terminal residue, X, which was unidentified in the earlier studies,[73] to be cysteine.

This limited proteolysis has been shown to affect the aggregation[68] and kinetic[78,79] properties of the enzyme (see Section IV.D). Such proteolysis has been shown to have occurred in a number of the glutamate dehydrogenase preparations obtained from commercial suppliers.[68,73] As preparations from such suppliers have been used in many published studies on behavior of the enzyme, some caution in the interpretation of the results obtained may be necessary. The use of purification procedures involving affinity chromatography on GTP-Sepharose®[73,80] or affinity precipitation with a bifunctional NAD+-derivative[43,81] appears to avoid this problem of limited proteolysis occurring during the purification process.

The high degree of structural conservation in glutamate dehydrogenase from different species together with its normal presence in human serum[7] and that of laboratory animals,[7,82] as a result of cellular degradation and its elevation in a number of disease states,[83-85] have resulted in the purified enzyme being a relatively poor antigen in a number of animal systems. Although antibodies have been raised to glutamate dehydrogenase (see References 8, 86, and 87), large amounts of immunogen have been required and the titers obtained have often been rather low. The production of monoclonal antibodies to the enzyme may thus be of particular value.[88] However, the aggregation of the enzyme at higher concentrations may result in anomolous antigen-antibody interaction.[86,87]

Although crystalline preparations of mammalian glutamate dehydrogenase have been available for many years (see References 76 and 89) it has not, so far, been shown possible to grow single crystals of sufficient size for detailed structural studies by X-ray diffraction. It has been suggested that the difficulties encountered in obtaining such crystals may be related to its association properties in solution.[48] Comparison of the sequences of glutamate dehydrogenases with those of other dehydrogenases for which X-ray structures are known indicates the presence of the characteristic NAD(P)-binding region.[1]

IV. CATALYTIC PROPERTIES

A. Specificity

Ox liver glutamate dehydrogenase has been shown to be capable of catalyzing the oxidation of glutamate analogues such as L-homocysteine sulfinic acid[90] and a number of monocarboxylic amino acids. Of the latter, L-norvaline has been shown to be the best alternative substrate with a rate of oxidation 17% of that of glutamate at pH 9.0.[91] The rates of oxidation of the monocarboxylic amino acids leucine, valine, norleucine, isoleucine, methionine, alanine, and α-aminobutyrate were all less than 3% of the initial rate of glutamate oxidation under these conditions. The optimal pH values for the oxidation of monocarboxylic α-amino acids have been shown to be rather higher than that for the oxidation of glutamate.[91,92]

The use of different reaction conditions by different research workers makes a direct comparison between the kinetic parameters for the oxidation of different amino acid substrates difficult. At pH 7.6 and 25°C with NAD^+ as the coenzyme K_m values of 1.1, 404, and 111 mM have been reported for L-glutamate, L-alanine, and L-leucine, respectively, and the corresponding maximum velocities were 0.77, 0.29, and 0.00094 μmol min^{-1} per μg enzyme.[93]

Studies on the effects of monocarboxylic L-amino acids as substrates have been complicated by the observation that several, including alanine, leucine, and methionine, are also activators of the enzyme.[93-97] L-Leucine appears to activate the oxidation of glutamate and the reduction of 2-oxoglutarate equally well[94] and it has frequently been used as a component in the assay mixture for determination of glutamate dehydrogenase activity.[7] It has been suggested that leucine and alanine occupy different catalytic sites on the enzyme from that occupied by glutamate.[72] However, that would not be in accord with the observation that leucine can competitively inhibit the oxidation of glutamate.[96] Studies on the effects of chemical modification of glutamate dehydrogenase by pyridoxal 5'-phosphate have, indeed, shown alanine, leucine, and glutamate to share the same active site on the enzyme, although they also indicated the presence of a separate regulatory site to which leucine was able to bind.[93]

Ox liver glutamate dehydrogenase has been reported to be capable of using glutamine, but not asparagine, as an alternative to ammonia in the reductive amination of 2-oxoglutarate.[98]

Although the enzyme can use either NAD(H) or NADP(H) its behavior differs depending on the coenzyme used (see Section IV.C). Studies on the stereospecificity of hydrogen transfer indicate that the hydrogen is removed from the pro-S-position of the pro-chiral C-4 position, the B-face, of NAD(P)H.[99]

B. Assay

Because of the potential clinical importance of serum glutamate dehydrogenase determinations, standardized conditions have been recommended for the assay of the enzyme in the direction of glutamate formation.[7] In order to optimize the activity ADP[100] or ADP plus L-leucine[101] have been included in some, but not all,[102] of such assay mixtures. The enzyme from most mammalian sources is unstable at low ionic strengths, particularly in Tris buffer[31,103-105] and this has led to inaccuracies in attempts to determine the activity of the enzyme. The loss of activity under these conditions appears to be associated with extensive conformational changes which may be monitored by the loss of fluorescence or the appearance of sulfhydryl groups that are normally inaccessible. NAD(P)H stabilizes the enzyme at high concentrations but at lower concentrations (less than 10 μM) inactivation is promoted.[103] GTP also enhances inactivation[105] whereas ADP has a protecting effect.[31,104] Heavy metals such as zinc also promote inactivation.[105] Buffers containing a polyvalent anion, such as phosphate, also stabilize the enzyme and ox liver glutamate dehydrogenase has been shown to be stable for 60 min at 41°C in 0.2 M phosphate buffer, pH 7.6.[104] Because of this the enzyme is frequently assayed in phosphate buffer.

The concentration of homogeneous preparations of ox liver glutamate dehydrogenase may be conveniently determined from the absorbance at 280 nmol using an absorption coefficient of 0.93 cmol^{-1} for a 1 mgmℓ^{-1} solution,[106] a value somewhat lower than that reported earlier.[76]

C. Kinetic Behavior

Most studies on the kinetics of mammalian glutamate dehydrogenase have been carried out with the enzyme from the ox liver. The kinetic mechanism in the direction of glutamate oxidation has been difficult to deduce because the variation of initial rate with increasing concentrations of NAD(P)$^+$ is complex. In double-reciprocal form the data describe a series of straight lines with fairly abrupt discontinuities between them.[107,108] Although this behavior was initially interpreted in terms of negative cooperativity, a detailed analysis suggested that the interactions must involve a mixture of negative and positive cooperativity and that the binding isotherms were also distorted by the catalytic activity of the enzyme.[109] Alternative explanations for this behavior proposed that a random-order steady-state mechanism, without the involvement of site-site cooperative interactions, was involved[110] or that binding of NAD(P)$^+$ to a second, noncatalytic, site on each subunit was involved.[111]

That complexities of the steady-state kinetic mechanism obeyed are not sufficient alone to explain this complex behavior has been demonstrated by direct studies on the binding of NAD$^+$ to the enzyme in the presence of the substrate analogue glutarate.[112] These showed that NAD(P)$^+$ bound more strongly to the enzyme in the presence of glutarate and it was proposed that the binding curves obtained could be explained on the basis of negative interactions between subunits within the hexameric enzyme in the formation of the unreactive enzyme-NAD(P)-glutarate ternary complex.[111] Studies on the inhibition of the oxidation of glutamate by 2-oxoglutarate also indicated that negative interactions could occur in the formation of the unreactive ternary complex with that substrate.[113]

The existence of a second site that can bind NAD(P)$^+$ and the corresponding reduced coenzymes has been demonstrated in a number of studies. Failure of the NAD$^+$ analogue 1-N^6-etheno-NAD$^+$ to bind to this second site has been advanced as an explanation for the noncooperative binding curves given by this analogue.[114] However, this site has a very much lower affinity for NADP$^+$ than NAD^{+}[115,116] and thus might not account for the complex behavior seen with the former coenzyme. This view has been confirmed by a detailed kinetic analysis of the effects of glutamate analogues on the oxidation of that substrate.[113] Those studies have also indicated that glutamate, or an analogue of it, was necessary for the induction of the conformational changes leading to negative cooperativity and that a substituent in the L-configuration at the C-2 position was necessary for this to occur.

At relatively low concentrations of glutamate the complex behavior of NAD(P)$^+$ is not evident and it is also not observed with monocarboxylic L-amino acid substrates.[107,113] Taking advantage of these observations, steady-state kinetic studies were carried out which indicated that the enzyme bound its two substrates randomly to form a ternary complex under conditions of thermodynamic equilibrium.[107] Such a mechanism was also consistent with the results of stopped-flow experiments,[117] the observation that either substrate or coenzyme can form a binary complex with the enzyme[112,118] and the results of isotope exchange measurements at pH 8.0,[119] although at pH 8.8 application of the last of these methods suggested that a compulsory mechanism was obeyed.[120]

In the presence of ADP at concentrations greater than 0.2 mM the primary double-reciprocal plots with respect to the coenzyme were found to be linear and under these conditions the results were consistent with a compulsory-order mechanism being obeyed with glutamate as the first substrate to bind.[121]

Studies on the effects of isotope substitution on the kinetics of norvaline oxidation, however, led to the proposal that a random-order mechanism operated under steady-state conditions.[122] Departure from strict Michaelis-Menten behavior with norvaline as the substrate was also interpreted in terms of such a mechanism.[123] Transient kinetic studies[124,125] with glutamate as the substrate and investigations of the deuterium isotope effect on the transient[126] were also consistent with a random-order steady-state mechanism.

In the direction of NAD(P)H oxidation kinetic studies have been hampered by both NADH and 2-oxoglutarate acting as inhibitors at high concentrations.[122,127,128] The inhibition by NADH is believed to be due to a second noncatalytic binding site on each subunit with a lower affinity for this coenzyme.[129] Direct evidence for the existence of this second binding site, which has a considerably lower affinity for NADPH,[130,131] has been obtained by following the changes in absorbance,[132] fluorescence,[133] or circular dichroism[131,132,134] as the enzyme was titrated with NADH. The limited proteolysis that can occur during the purification of the enzyme from the ox liver and brain[73] has been found to decrease the sensitivity of the enzyme to inhibition by NADH.[79] The high substrate inhibition by NADH has been reported to be abolished at high enzyme concentrations.[135] (However, see Reference 144.)

Because of these complications most studies on the kinetics of 2-oxoglutarate amination have been carried out with NADPH as the coenzyme. Earlier studies were interpreted in terms of a compulsory order mechanism although with different orders of substrate addition[127,136] which may have reflected differences in the assay conditions used.[136] However, these results did not exclude a random-order mechanism and more detailed studies by Engel and Dalziel[128] suggested that such a mechanism was obeyed. This was also supported by the results of the product inhibition studied[136] and by isotope exchange studies at equilibrium.[119] Spectrophotometric, fluorescence,[124,137] and NMR[138] studies also provided evidence for the existence of some of the binary and ternary complexes that would occur in such a mechanism.

However, Rife and Cleland[122] proposed that an ordered kinetic mechanism was followed with NADPH binding to the free enzyme, followed by the α-keto acid, and then ammonia. The evidence for this was more convincing with the artificial substrates 2-oxovalerate and 2-oxobutyrate and the substrate inhibition patterns observed with 2-oxoglutarate would indicate random-order binding to be possible with this substrate. Comparison between the kinetic data obtained by different groups, is however, difficult because of the different assay buffers that were used. Studies on the behavior of the enzyme have shown the kinetic properties to differ in different buffers.[107]

An explanation for these apparently contradictory results might be that the mechanism obeyed is essentially random-order but that under different conditions pathways involving the prior binding of either glutamate or coenzyme can become preferred.

D. Regulatory Properties

Any discussion on the regulatory properties of glutamate dehydrogenase is complicated by the large number of ligands that affect its activity and by the observation that several of these affect the aggregation of the enzyme hexamers that occurs at higher concentrations.

1. Enzyme Association

Although there have been a number of proposals that the aggregation of the enzyme and its allosteric properties may be intimately linked (see References 49 and 139), it is, at least to some extent, possible to separate them.[140,141] The specific activity of the ox liver enzyme remains constant with increasing enzyme concentration indicating that aggregation does not affect its activity.[142] Aromatic compounds, such as toluene and benzene, also induce polymerization without affecting activity.[143] Preparations of the enzyme from the rat liver, which apparently do not aggregate, show similar allosteric properties to those of the ox liver enzyme.[1,31] Chemical cross-linking with glutaraldehyde has been used to produce aggregates that were unable to dissociate.[144] These retained about 80% of the activity of the untreated enzyme and showed rather similar kinetic parameters. K_m values for NAD^+ were unchanged as was the response to low concentrations of NADH suggesting that the coenzyme binding active site was unaffected. However, the sensitivity to inhibition by NADH was reduced, but not abolished (see Reference 135), as was the sensitivity to GTP inhibition.[144] Since these two compounds promote dissociation of the aggregated enzyme,[145] the results with the cross-linked preparations would suggest that the association/dissociation of the enzyme is not essential for allosteric regulation, although other effects resulting from the chemical modification of the enzyme cannot be ruled out. Detailed studies on the kinetics of the aggregation/disaggregation process have also indicated that it may not play a major role in the allosteric control of enzyme activity.[140,141]

Although these considerations indicate that allosteric regulation of glutamate dehydrogenase is not dependent on the polymerization process, the effects of the latter could complicate the behavior of the enzyme within the mitochondrion. The concentration of glutamate dehydrogenase in the mitochondrial matrix has been estimated to be in the range 1 to 1.25 mg/mℓ[146] which is close to the dissociation constant for the aggregation process.[49] Since the binding of substrates and allosteric effectors[49,127,139,145] to the enzyme is affected by its degree of aggregation, the behavior in vivo might be expected to differ somewhat from that observed at the considerably more dilute concentrations used in in vitro kinetic experiments. With that reservation, the remainder of this section will be largely devoted to the interaction of effectors with the disaggregated, hexameric enzyme.

2. Coenzymes and Nucleoside Phosphates

The inhibitory action of higher concentrations of NADH has already been discussed. This effect appears to be pH-dependent with inhibition being observed at pH 6.0 but not at pH 8.0.[147] Studies on the binding of this coenzyme to the active sites in the hexamer indicate that, depending on the conditions, this can be either positively or negatively cooperative. Determination of the changes in fluorescence on titration of the enzyme with either NADH or NADPH revealed that glutamate considerably enhanced the binding of coenzyme and that, in its presence, two dissociation constants were required to describe the binding curve obtained.[113] Since this behavior, resulting from the formation of an abortive enzyme-NAD(P)H-glutamate complex, was similar with both reduced coenzymes, the possibility that binding to the NADH regulatory site could be complicating the results can be excluded. In contrast, the substrate analogue glutarate did not induce cooperativity, although it did enhance coenzyme binding, albeit to a lesser extent, than glutamate. These and other similar[148] results were interpreted in terms of a nonequivalence of the identical subunits in glutamate dehydrogenase that could be induced by substrate binding. The suggestion that the enzyme may function as two interacting nonequivalent trimeric subunits is consistent with the results of chemical modification[93,149-154] and kinetic studies[113,116,155] and also with determinations of the binding of an NAD-analogue to the enzyme.[114] Half of the sites' reactivity has also been suggested to account for hysteresis[156] seen in the direction of reductive amination.[116] Evidence for conformational changes that may provide the basis for this induced cooperativity has been provided by studies showing that, in the presence of glutarate, the binding of coenzyme to half the subunits in the hexamer induced a conformational change in the other half of the oligomer.[157]

GTP inhibits the enzyme[94,137] and also promotes dissociation of the aggregates formed at higher enzyme concentrations.[50] It has been shown that GTP promotes the binding of NADH to its inhibitory site.[50,131-134] The extent of inhibition may also be dependent on the assay conditions since inorganic phosphate has been reported to decrease the binding of GTP to glutamate dehydrogenase.[158] It has also been pointed out that complex formation between GTP and magnesium ions is likely to be an important factor under cellular conditions. Studies in the presence of this ion indicated that the Mg-GTP complex had no significant effect on the activity of the enzyme.[159] Thus, the effects of Mg^{2+} would be to decrease the inhibitory effect of GTP by complex formation. The concentrations of free Mg^{2+} in mitochondria have been reported to vary from about 0.1 to 1.0 mM depending on metabolic state[160,161] and thus, regardless of any changes in the total nucleotide concentrations, they would be expected to influence the effects of GTP profoundly. GDP and, to a lesser extent, ITP, and IDP are also inhibitors of the enzyme.[94,137]

In contrast to its behavior on the interconversion of glutamate and 2-oxoglutarate, GTP has been reported to activate the activity when alanine was used as the substrate.[162] This difference has been rationalized by the proposals that the effect of GTP is to enhance the binding of NAD(H) to the enzyme[114,131-134] and that the release of the reduced coenzyme is the rate-limiting step in glutamate oxidation whereas it is not for alanine oxidation where enhanced coenzyme binding has an activatory effect.[163] Consistent with this interpretation is the observation that the effects of GTP are dependent on alanine concentration with inhibition being observed at high and activation at lower concentrations of this substrate.[96]

The effects of ADP appear to be generally reciprocal to those of GTP and it has been shown to decrease the affinity of the catalytic site for NAD(P)(H)[96,134,164] thus activating the oxidation of glutamate but inhibiting that of alanine. The behavior of this ligand is further complicated by its ability to displace NADH from its inhibitory binding site in an apparently competitive manner.[133,134] Thus, because of the much lower affinity of NADPH for that site the effects observed will be to some extent dependent on the coenzyme used and its concentration. Furthermore at pH values below 7.0 ADP has been reported to inhibit, rather than activate, glutamate oxidation.[147] ATP has similar effects on ox liver glutamate dehydrogenase although with a lower affinity than that shown with ADP.[1,137] Studies on the effects of magnesium ions have indicated the Mg-ATP complex has no direct effect on the activity of the enzyme although it appeared to be able to bind to the enzyme in competition with free ATP.[159] In contrast Mg^{2+} has been reported to have no significant effects on the interactions of ADP with the enzyme.[147]

3. Amino Acids

As discussed earlier (Section IV.A) a number of monocarboxylic L-amino acids are able to act as activators as well as poor substrates for glutamate dehydrogenase. Of these, leucine has been most extensively studied. It appears to have similar effects on enzyme-coenzyme interactions to those of ADP although the site to which it binds is distinct from that occupied by ADP.[93,97,165] Studies on the effects of chemical modification on the activation of glutamate oxidation and the inhibition of alanine oxidation by leucine provided further evidence for the kinetic nonequivalence of the subunits of glutamate dehydrogenase.[93] Neither leucine nor ADP have any direct effect on the aggregation of the enzyme but in decreasing NADH binding to its regulatory site they oppose the dissociative effect of that compound.[165,166]

4. Other Effectors

Although the effects of nucleoside phosphates and amino acids may be physiologically important, a large number of other compounds, including zinc ions,[167] thyroxine,[168] steroid derivatives,[169,170] and phosphoenolpyruvate[171] affect the activity of the enzyme. Contrary to earlier claims, the native enzyme does not contain bound zinc, but it is inhibited by this ion under which conditions one gram-atom of zinc is bound per subunit.[167] The inhibition of rabbit renal glutamate dehydrogenase by phosphoenolpyruvate has been reported to be abolished by leucine.[171] Further work will be required before the significance of these effects can be assessed.

The significance of the steroid inhibition of glutamate dehydrogenase is not clear. Studies with the alkylating analogue, bromoacetyldiethylstilbestrol, showed 1 mol of this to react irreversibly with each enzyme subunit in the presence of NADH. Diethylstilbestrol and ADP protected against this labeling and only reversible effects were seen in the absence of NADH.[172] Nemat-Gorgani and Dodd[40,41] have, however, argued that the true function of this site is the binding of cardiolipin. As steroids promote disaggregation of glutamate dehydrogenase these workers have argued that the aggregation observed in vitro may be an artefact resulting from exposure of the phospholipid binding sites on extraction of the enzyme from the mitochondrion. Some direct evidence has indeed been produced to show binding of the enzyme to the mitochondrial inner membrane.[39] The binding of phosphatidylserine and cardiolipin results in the inhibition of glutamate dehydrogenase and studies on the effects of substrates and effectors have led to the suggestion that reversible inhibition by binding to the mitochondrial membrane might constitute an important regulatory mechanisms.[39-41]

Gel-filtration,[173] fluorescence titration,[174] and cross-linking[175] experiments have shown glutamate dehydrogenase to be capable of complexing with aspartate aminotransferase (EC 2.6.1.1.). The complex formed was shown to possess aspartate dehydrogenase activity. A similar complex formed with alanine aminotransferase (EC 2.6.1.2.) was found to possess increased alanine dehydrogenase activity;[173] ADP and GTP were shown to affect the aspartate dehydrogenase activity of mixtures of aspartate aminotransferase and glutamate dehydrogenase, probably by affecting the the self-association of glutamate dehydrogenase and thus regulating the amount of disaggregated glutamate dehydrogenase available for interaction with the aminotransferase.[173] The concentrations of these two enzymes in liver and brain mitochondria were estimated to be higher than the dissociation constant for their complex.[173] However, since aggregated forms of glutamate dehydrogenase did not appear to interact with the aminotransferase, competition between these processes, and perhaps membrane binding as well, would be expected to occur and the physiological significance of the process remains unclear.

A number of studies have indicated ox brain and liver glutamate dehydrogenase to be inhibited by antipsychotic drugs such as chlorpromazine,[74] phenothiazines, and butyrophenones.[176,177] The kinetic and binding parameters for a range of phenothiazines and butyrophenones were found to correlate with their pharmacological potencies.[176,177] The significance, if any, of these observations remains unclear. Our own (unpublished) studies have indicated that phosphate ions are antagonistic to inhibition by these compounds and that their inhibitory potencies are such that these effects might be unlikely to be of importance in vivo unless the drugs were concentrated in the mitochondria.

5. Covalent Modification

Although evidence has been produced to indicate that glutamate dehydrogenase from yeast may be regulated by the action of protein kinase,[178] no convincing evidence for phosphorylation of the mammalian enzyme has been obtained.

The limited proteolysis that can occur during the preparation of the enzyme results in relatively small decreases in sensitivity to inhibition by NADH and GTP and to activation by ADP and ATP at inhibitory NADH concentration.[79] At higher protein concentrations the proteolyzed enzyme is also less readily depolymerized by NADH and GTP[68] and it is also somewhat less sensitive to inhibition by high (greater than 500 μM) concentrations of chloride ions.[79] The recoveries of enzyme activity during purification by the procedure involving affinity chromatography and the absence of any detectable amounts of proteolyzed material in preparations obtained in that way[73] make it unlikely that such limited digestion is a significant regulatory phenomenon in vivo. A substantial activation of commercially obtained preparations of glutamate dehydrogenase has, however, been observed on limited digestion with chymotrypsin[179,180] but no evidence has been produced to suggest that this has any physiological significance.

6. Models of Regulatory and Catalytic Behavior

The absence of detailed X-ray structural data on mammalian glutamate dehydrogenase has necessitated the use of indirect methods in attempts to define the numbers of binding sites involved in catalysis and regulation. Extensive chemical modification studies have been carried out in order to identify specific amino acid residues involved in these processes (see References 1, 48, 93, 149, and 150). Fisher and co-workers[137,181,182] proposed that distinct but overlapping binding sites existed on the enzyme for glutamate, NADPH, GTP, and ADP and suggested that the allosteric behavior of the enzyme might be understood in terms of the overlapping nature of these sites resulting in the binding of some ligands, excluding the binding of others. As discussed earlier such a model would need to be extended to take account of the observation that there is an NADH regulatory site distinct from the catalytic site and also to accommodate the effects of leucine.

In view of the effects of the proteolytic removal of a tetrapeptide from the amino-terminal end of each of the peptide chains[68,79] it would be tempting to ascribe a direct role for that region in the binding of nucleotides. Such a conclusion would be consistent with earlier studies suggesting the N-terminal region of the enzyme to be involved in its interactions with allosteric nucleotides.[53] However, labeling of the GTP and NADH regulatory sites with specific affinity labels implicated residues far removed from this region.[183,184] However, these studies provided no evidence that could account for the observed synergism between these two sites.[150,185]

An alternative model which is in some ways analogous to the classical model of Monod et al.[186] was suggested by several workers.[105,146,162,164] They envisaged the hexameric enzyme existing in two conformations, one of which had a higher affinity for activators such as ADP and leucine whereas the other had a higher affinity for inhibitors such as GTP and high concentrations of NADH. In its simplest form such a model could not account for the negatively cooperative interactions seen with coenzymes and the substrate-induced or preexisting inequality of subunits in the hexamer. Thus, a considerably more elaborate model would be required to take account of all the presently known interactions of glutamate dehydrogenase.

Chemical modification and isotope exchange studies have indicated that the reaction may proceed by way of an enzyme-bound imine intermediate formed by the oxidation of glutamate by $NAD(P)^+$. This would then react with a lysine residue in the enzyme, which has been identified by chemical modification studies as being essential for activity, to form a Schiff-base with the liberation of ammonia. Hydrolysis of this Schiff-base intermediate would then give rise to 2-oxoglutarate.[1,187]

V. CONCLUSIONS

The metabolic functions of glutamate dehydrogenase will be discussed in other sections of this book. However, there is still disagreement (compare References 147 and 188 to 190) about the direction of net flux through the enzyme and one of the most attractive suggestions concerning its function is that it might function in a mitochondrial ammonia-buffering system.[147] However, the complexity of its allosteric regulation is still difficult to relate fully to its proposed functions. Unfortunately, the often-quoted statement of Carl Frieden[9] in 1968, "the question is not that the enzyme is under control, or even that the control is regulated by purine nucleotides but just what function the controlling factors serve," still remains to be answered.

REFERENCES

1. **Smith, E. L., Austen, B. M., Blumenthal, K. M., and Nyc, J. F.,** Glutamate dehydrogenases, in *The Enzymes,* Vol. 11A, 3rd ed., Boyer, P. D., Ed., Academic Press, New York, 1975, 293.
2. **Fahien, L. A., Wiggert, B. O., and Cohen, P. P.,** Crystallization and kinetic properties of glutamate dehydrogenase from frog liver, *J. Biol. Chem.,* 240, 1083, 1965.
3. **Corman, L., Prescott, L. M., and Kaplan, N. O.,** Purification and properties of dogfish liver glutamate dehydrogenase, *J. Biol. Chem.,* 242, 1383, 1967.
4. **Williamson, D. H., Lund, P., and Krebs, H. A.,** The redox state of free nicotinamide-adenine dinucleotide in the cytoplasm and mitochondria of rat liver, *Biochem. J.,* 103, 514, 1967.
5. **Engel, P. C. and Dalziel, K.,** The equilibrium constant of the glutamate dehydrogenase systems, *Biochem. J.,* 105, 691, 1967.
6. **Herzfeld, A.,** The distribution of glutamate dehydrogenase in rat tissues, *Enzyme,* 13, 246, 1972.
7. **Schmidt, E. and Schmidt, F. W.,** Glutamate dehydrogenase, in *Methods of Enzymatic Analysis,* Vol. 3, 3rd ed., Bergmeyer, H. U., Ed., Verlag Chemie, Weinheim, 1983, 216.
8. **Talal, N. and Tomkins, G. M.,** Allosteric properties of glutamate dehydrogenases from different sources, *Science,* 1406, 1309, 1964.
9. **Frieden, C.,** Glutamate dehydrogenase, in *The Role of Nucleotides in the Function and Conformation of Enzymes,* Kalckar, H. M., Klenour, H., Murch-Peterson, A., Ottessen, M., and Thaysen, H. J., Eds., Munksgaard, Copenhagen, 1968, 194.
10. **Lehmann, F. G. and Pfleiderer, G.,** Glutamat-dehydrogenase aus menschlicher leber; kristallisation und biochemische eigenschaften, *Hoppe-Seyler's Z. Physiol. Chem.,* 350, 609, 1969.
11. **Plaitakis, A. and Berl, S.,** Involvement of glutamate dehydrogenase in degenerative neurological disorders, in *Glutamine, Glutamate and GABA in the Central Nervous System,* Hertz, L., Kvamme, E., McGeer, E. G., and Schousboe, A., Eds., Alan R. Liss, New York, 1983, 609.
12. **Plaitakis, A.,** Abnormal metabolism of neuroexcitatory amino acids in olivopontocerebellar atrophy, *Adv. Neurol.,* 41, 255, 1984.
13. **McDaniel, H. G., Yea, M., Jenkins, R., Freeman, B., and Simmons, J.,** Glutamic dehydrogenase activity in rat heart: demonstration of two forms of enzyme activity, *Am. J. Physiol.,* 246, H483, 1984.
14. **Neidle, A., Van den Berg, C. J., and Grynbaum, A.,** Heterogeneity of rat brain mitochondria isolated in continuous sucrose gradients, *J. Neurochem.,* 16, 225, 1969.
15. **Wilson, J. E. and Barch, D.,** Heterogeneity of rat brain mitochondria, *Fed. Proc., Fed. Am. Soc. Exp. Biol.,* 30, 1139, 1971.
16. **Reijnierse, G. L. A., Veldstra, H., and Van den Berg, C. J.,** Short-chain fatty acid synthesis in brain, *Biochem. J.,* 152, 477, 1975.
17. **Kuhlman, R. E. and Lowry, O. H.,** Quantitative histochemical changes during the development of rat cerebral cortex, *J. Neurochem.,* 1, 173, 1956.
18. **Larsson, O. M., Hertz, L., and Schousboe, A.,** Developmental profiles of glutamate and GABA metabolizing enzymes in cultured glutamatergic and GABAergic neurons, *J. Neurochem.,* 41, S85D, 1983.
19. **Patel, A. J., Hunt, A., Gordon, R. D., and Balazs, R.,** The activities in different neuronal cell types of certain enzymes associated with the metabolic compartmentation of glutamate, *Dev. Brain Res.,* 4, 3, 1982.

20. **Tardy, M., Fages, C., Rolland, B., Bardakjian, J., and Gonnard, P.,** Effect of prostaglandins and dibutyl cyclic AMP on the morphology of cells in primary astroglial cultures and of metabolic enzymes of GABA and glutamate metabolism, *Experientia,* 37, 19, 1981.

21. **Schousboe, A., Svenneby, G., and Hertz, L.,** Uptake and metabolism of glutamate in astrocytes cultured from dissociated mouse brain hemispheres, *J. Neurochem.,* 29, 999, 1977.

22. **Hertz, L., Bock, E., and Schousboe, A.,** GFA content, glutamate uptake and activity of glutamate metabolizing enzymes in differentiating astrocytes in primary cultures, *Dev. Neurosci.,* 1, 226, 1978.

23. **Roth-Schechter, B. F., Laluet, M., Tholey, G., and Mandel, P.,** The effect of pentobarbital on the carbohydrate metabolism of glial cells in culture, *Biochem. Pharmacol.,* 26, 1307, 1977.

24. **Leong, S. F. and Clark, J. B.,** Regional development of glutamate dehydrogenase in the rat brain, *J. Neurochem.,* 43, 106, 1984.

25. **Wenthold, R. J. and Altschuler, R. A.,** Immunocytochemistry of aspartate aminotransferase and glutaminase, in *Glutamine, Glutamate and GABA in the Central Nervous System,* Hertz, L., Kvamme, E., McGeer, E. G., and Schousboe, A., Eds., Alan R. Liss, New York, 1983, 33.

26. **De Duve, C., Wattiaux, R., and Baudhuin, P.,** Distribution of enzymes between subcellular fractions in animal tissues, *Adv. Enzymol.,* 24, 291, 1962.

27. **Salganicoff, L. and De Robertis, E.,** Subcellular distribution of the enzymes of the glutamic acid, glutamine and γ-aminobutyric acid cycles in rat brain, *J. Neurochem.,* 12, 287, 1965.

28. **Di Matteo, G., Di Prisco, G., and Romeo, G.,** Mitochondrial and nuclear glutamate dehydrogenase in chinese hamster ovary cells in culture, *Biochim. Biophys. Acta,* 429, 694, 1976.

29. **Di Prisco, G. and Garafano, F.,** Crystallization and partial characterization of glutamate dehydrogenase from ox liver nuclei, *Biochemistry,* 14, 4673, 1975.

30. **Godinot, C. and Lardy, H. A.,** Biosynthesis of glutamate dehydrogenase in rat liver. Demonstration of its microsomal localization and hypothetical mechanism of transfer to mitochondria, *Biochemistry,* 12, 2051, 1973.

31. **King, K. S. and Frieden, C.,** The purification and physical properties of glutamate dehydrogenase from rat liver, *J. Biol. Chem.,* 245, 4391, 1970.

32. **Di Prisco, G. and Garafano, F.,** Purification and some properties of glutamate dehydrogenase from ox liver nuclei, *Biochem. Biophys. Res. Commun.,* 58, 683, 1974.

33. **Holt, J. T., Arvan, D. A., Mayer, T., Smith, T. J., and Bell, J. E.,** Glutamate dehydrogenase in Reye's syndrome. Evidence for the presence of an altered enzyme in serum with increased susceptibility to inhibition by GTP, *Biochim. Biophys. Acta,* 749, 42, 1983.

34. **Dennis, S. C., Lai, J. C. K., and Clark, J. B.,** Comparative studies on glutamine metabolism in synaptic and non-synaptic rat brain mitochondria, *Biochem. J.,* 164, 727, 1977.

35. **McGivan, J. D., Bradford, N. M., Crompton, M., and Chappell, J. B.,** Effect of L-leucine on the nitrogen metabolism of isolated rat liver mitochondria, *Biochem. J.,* 134, 209, 1973.

36. **Kawajiri, K., Harano, T., and Omura, T.,** Biogenesis of the mitochondrial matrix enzyme glutamate dehydrogenase in rat liver cells. II. Significance of binding of glutamate dehydrogenase to microsomal membrane, *J. Biochem.,* 82, 1417, 1977.

37. **Mihara, K., Omura, T., Harano, T., Brenner, S., Fleischer, S., Rajagopalan, K. V., and Blobel, G.,** Rat liver L-glutamate dehydrogenase, D-β-hydroxybutyrate dehydrogenase, malate dehydrogenase and sulfite oxidase are each synthesized as larger precursors by cytoplasmic free polysomes, *J. Biol. Chem.,* 257, 3355, 1982.

38. **Felipo, V., Miralles, V., Knecht, E., Hernandez-Yaso, J., and Grisolia, S.,** The precursor of rat liver mitochondrial glutamate dehydrogenase has enzymatic activity, *Eur. J. Biochem.,* 133, 641, 1983.

39. **Godinot, C.,** Nature and possible functions of association between glutamate dehydrogenase and cardiolipin, *Biochemistry,* 12, 4029, 1974.

40. **Nemat-Gorgani, M. and Dodd, G.,** The interaction of phospholipid membranes and detergents with glutamate dehydrogenase. I. Kinetic studies, *Eur. J. Biochem.,* 74, 129, 1977.

41. **Nemat-Gorgani, M. and Dodd, G.,** The interaction of phospholipid membranes and detergents with glutamate dehydrogenase. II. Fluorescence and stopped-flow studies, *Eur. J. Biochem.,* 74, 139, 1977.

42. **Muller, K. and Jaenicke, R.,** Denaturation and renaturation of bovine liver glutamate dehydrogenase after dissociation in various denaturants, *Z. Naturforsch.,* 35C, 222, 1980.

43. **Graham, L. D., Griffin, T. O., Beattie, R. E., McCarthy, A. D., and Tipton, K. F.,** Purification of liver glutamate dehydrogenase by affinity precipitation and studies on its denaturation, *Biochim. Biophys. Acta,* 828, 266, 1985.

44. **Bell, E. T. and Bell, J. E.,** Catalytic activity of bovine glutamate dehydrogenase requires a hexamer structure, *Biochem. J.,* 217, 327, 1984.

45. **Weber, K. and Osborn, M.,** The reliability of molecular weight determinations by dodecyl sulphate polyacrylamide gel electrophoresis, *J. Biol. Chem.,* 244, 4406, 1969.

46. **Cassman, M. and Schachman, H. K.,** Sedimentation equilibrium studies on glutamate dehydrogenase, *Biochemistry,* 10, 1015, 1971.

47. **Moon, K. and Smith, E. L.,** Sequence of bovine liver glutamate dehydrogenase, *J. Biol. Chem.,* 248, 3082, 1973.
48. **Eisenberg, H., Josephs, R., and Reisler, E.,** Bovine liver glutamate dehydrogenase, *Adv. Protein Chem.,* 30, 101, 1976.
49. **Cohen, R. J., Jedziniak, J. A. and Benedek, G. B.,** The functional relationship between polymerisation and catalytic activity of beef liver glutamate dehydrogenase. II. Experiments, *J. Mol. Biol.,* 108, 179, 1976.
50. **Markau, K., Schneider, J., and Sund, H.,** Studies on glutamate dehydrogenase. The mechanism of the association dissociation equilibrium of beef liver glutamate dehydrogenase, *Eur. J. Biochem.,* 24, 393, 1971.
51. **Reisler, E., Pouyet, J., and Eisenberg, H.,** Molecular weights, association, and frictional resistance of bovine liver glutamate dehydrogenase at low concentrations. Equilibrium and velocity sedimentation, light-scattering studies, and settling experiments with macroscopic models of the enzyme oligomer, *Biochemistry,* 9, 3095, 1970.
52. **Josephs, R.,** Electron microscope studies on glutamic dehydrogenase subunit structure of individual molecules and linear associates, *J. Mol. Biol.,* 55, 147, 1971.
53. **Hucho, F., Rasched, I., and Sund, H.,** Studies of glutamate dehydrogenase: analysis of functional areas and functional groups, *Eur. J. Biochem.,* 52, 221, 1975.
54. **Tashiro, R., Inoue, T., and Shimozawa, R.,** Subunit dissociation and unfolding of bovine liver glutamate dehydrogenase induced by guanidine hydrochloride, *Biochim. Biophys. Acta,* 706, 129, 1982.
55. **Inoue, T., Fukushima, K., Tastumoto, T., and Shimozawa, R.,** Light-scattering study on subunit association-disassociation equilibria of bovine liver glutamate dehydrogenase, *Biochim. Biophys. Acta,* 786, 144, 1984.
56. **Blum, E. and Alper, T.,** Radiation-target molecular weights of urease and L-glutamate dehydrogenase, and their relevance to the size of the functional subunits, *Biochem. J.,* 122, 677, 1971.
57. **Kempner, E. S. and Miller, J. H.,** Radiation inactivation of glutamate dehydrogenase hexamer: lack of energy transfer between subunits, *Science,* 222, 586, 1983.
58. **Eisenberg, H. and Tomkins, G. M.,** Molecular weights of the subunits, oligomeric and associated forms of bovine liver glutamate dehydrogenase, *J. Mol. Biol.,* 31, 37, 1968.
59. **Sund, H., Pilz, I., and Herbst, M.,** Studies on glutamate dehydrogenase. V. The X-ray small angle investigation of beef liver glutamate dehydrogenase, *Eur. J. Biochem.,* 7, 517, 1969.
60. **Eisenberg, H. and Reisler, E.,** Physical model for the structure of glutamate dehydrogenase, *Biopolymers,* 9, 113, 1970.
61. **Sund, H. and Weber, K.,** The quaternary structure of proteins, *Angew. Chem. Int. Ed. Engl.,* 5, 231, 1966.
62. **Reisler, E. and Eisenberg, H.,** Studies on the viscosity of solutions of bovine liver glutamate dehydrogenase and on related hydrodynamic models; effect of toluene on enzyme association, *Biopolymers,* 9, 877, 1970.
63. **Pilz, I. and Sund, H.,** Studies of glutamate dehydrogenase. The X-ray small angle investigation of the beef liver glutamate dehydrogenase oligomer, *Eur. J. Biochem.,* 20, 561, 1971.
64. **Mann, E. A.,** Structure of oligomeric and polymeric forms of ox liver glutamate dehydrogenase examined by electron microscopy, *Biochim. Biophys. Acta,* 284, 301, 1972.
65. **Josephs, R. and Borisy, G.,** Self-assembly of glutamate dehydrogenase into ordered superstructures: multichain tubes formed by association of single molecules, *J. Mol. Biol.,* 65, 127, 1972.
66. **Dessen, P. and Pantaloni, D.,** Glutamate deshydrogenase. Structure quaternaire et proprietes rotatoires, *Eur. J. Biochem.,* 8, 292, 1969.
67. **Kubo, H., Iwatsubu, M., Watari, H., and Soyama, T.,** Polymerisation and molecular form of glutamate dehydrogenase, *J. Biochem.,* 46, 1171, 1959.
68. **McCarthy, A. D., Johnson, P., and Tipton, K. F.,** Sedimentation properties of native and proteolysed preparations of ox glutamate dehydrogenase, *Biochem. J.,* 199, 235, 1981.
69. **Ifflaender, U. and Sund, H.,** Association behaviour of rat liver glutamate dehydrogenase, *FEBS Lett.,* 20, 287, 1972.
70. **Moon, K., Piszkiewicz, D., and Smith, E. L.,** Glutamate dehydrogenase: amino-acid sequence of the bovine enzyme and comparison with that from chicken liver, *Proc. Natl. Acad. Sci. U.S.A.,* 69, 1380, 1972.
71. **Moon, K., Piszkiewicz, D., and Smith, E. L.,** Amino acid sequence of chicken liver glutamate dehydrogenase, *J. Biol. Chem.,* 248, 3093, 1973.
72. **Julliard, J. H. and Smith, E. L.,** Partial aminoacid sequence of the glutamate dehydrogenase of human liver and a revision of the sequence of the bovine enzyme, *J. Biol. Chem.,* 254, 3427, 1979.
73. **McCarthy, A. D., Walker, J. M., and Tipton, K. F.,** Purification of glutamate dehydrogenase from ox brain and liver. Evidence that commercially available preparations of the enzyme from ox liver have suffered proteolytic cleavage, *Biochem. J.,* 191, 605, 1980.
73a. **Couée, I. and Tipton, K. F.,** unpublished results.

74. **Fahien, L. A. and Shemisa, O.,** Effects of chlorpromazine on glutamate dehydrogenase, *Mol. Pharmacol.,* 6, 156, 1969.

75. **Chee, P. Y., Dahl, J. L., and Fahien, L. A.,** Purification and properties of rat brain glutamate dehydrogenase, *J. Neurochem.,* 35, 52, 1979.

76. **Olson, J. A. and Anfinsen, C. B.,** Crystallization and characterization of L-glutamic acid dehydrogenase, *J. Biol. Chem.,* 197, 67, 1959.

77. **Fahien, L. A., Strmecki, M., and Smith, S.,** Studies on gluconeogenic mitochondrial enzymes. I. A new method for preparing beef liver glutamate dehydrogenase and effects of purification methods on the properties of the enzyme, *Arch. Biochem. Biophys.,* 130, 449, 1969.

78. **McCarthy, A. D. and Tipton, K. F.,** Glutamate dehydrogenase, in *Glutamine, Glutamate and GABA in the Central Nervous System,* Hertz, L., Kvamme, E., McGeer, E. G., and Schousboe, A., Eds., Alan R. Liss, New York, 1983, 19.

79. **McCarthy, A. D. and Tipton, K. F.,** Ox glutamate dehydrogenase. Comparison of the kinetic properties of native and proteolysed preparation, *Biochem. J.,* 230, 95, 1985.

80. **Godinot, C., Julliard, J. H., and Gautheron, D. C.,** A rapid and efficient new method of purification of glutamate dehydrogenase by affinity chromatography on GTP-Sepharose, *Anal. Biochem.,* 61, 264, 1974.

81. **Beattie, R. E., Graham, L. D., Griffin, T. O., and Tipton, K. F.,** Purification of NAD + -dependent dehydrogenases by affinity precipitation with adipo-N2, N2′-dihydrazidobis- (N6-carboxymethyl-NAD +) (bis-NAD +), *Biochem. Soc. Trans.,* 12, 433, 1984.

82. **Möhr, J. R., Mattenheimer, H., Holmes, A. W., Deinhardt, F., and Schmidt, F. W.,** Enzymology of experimental liver disease in marmoset monkeys. I. Patterns of enzyme activity in liver, other organs and serum of marmosets compared to man and other mammals, *Enzyme,* 12, 99, 1971.

83. **Adolph, L. and Lorenz, R.,** *Enzyme Diagnosis in Diseases of the Heart, Liver and Pancreas,* S. Karger, Basel, 1982, 91.

84. **Weime, R. and Demeulenaere, L.,** Enzyme assays in liver disease, *J. Clin. Pathol.,* 24 (Suppl. 4), 51, 1971.

85. **Jenkins, W. J., Rosalki, S. B., Foo, Y., Scheuer, P. J., Nemesanszky, E., and Sherlock, S.,** Serum glutamate dehydrogenase is not a reliable marker of liver cell necrosis in alcoholics, *J. Clin. Pathol.,* 35, 207, 1982.

86. **Lehmann, F. G.,** Glutamate dehydrogenase from human liver. III. Antibody-binding sites and properties of the antigen-antibody complex, *Biochim. Biophys. Acta,* 235, 259, 1971.

87. **Fahien, L. A., Steinman, H. G., and McCann, R.,** Immunochemical studies of bovine and frog liver glutamate dehydrogenase, *J. Biol. Chem.,* 241, 4700, 1966.

88. **Martinez-Ramon, A. and Renau-Piqueras, J.,** Monoclonal antibody to glutamate dehydrogenase, isolation and characterization, *Cell. Biol. Int. Rep.,* 8, 665, 1984.

89. **Strecker, H. J.,** Glutamic dehydrogenase, *Arch. Biochem. Biophys.,* 46, 128, 1953.

90. **Jolles-Bergeret, B.,** Désamination oxydative de l'acide L-homocystéine-sulphinique par la L-glutamo-déshydrogénase de foie de boeuf. Inhibition de l'enzyme par l'acide L-homocystéine, *Biochim. Biophys. Acta,* 146, 45, 1967.

91. **Bassler, K. H. and Hammar, C. H.,** Reduktive aminierung von α-ketovaleriansaure an glutaminsaure-dehydrogenase, *Biochem. Z.,* 330, 446, 1958.

92. **Struck, J. and Sizer, I. W.,** The substrate specificity of glutamic acid dehydrogenase, *Arch. Biochem. Biophys.,* 86, 260, 1960.

93. **Syed, S.-E.-H. and Engel, P. C.,** Ox liver glutamate dehydrogenase: the use of chemical modification to study the relationship between catalytic sites for different amino acid substrates and the question of kinetic non-equivalence of subunits, *Biochem. J.,* 222, 621, 1964.

94. **Yielding, K. L. and Tomkins, G. M.,** An effect of L-leucine and other essential amino acids on the structure and activity of glutamic dehydrogenase, *Proc. Natl. Acad. Sci. U.S.A.,* 47, 983, 1961.

95. **Yamaguchi, T.,** Regulation of glutamate dehydrogenase by histidine, *Biochim. Biophys. Acta,* 227, 241, 1971.

96. **Markau, K. and Steinhübel, I.,** Kinetic measurements with monocarboxylic acids as substrates and effectors of glutamate dehydrogenase, *FEBS Lett.,* 28, 115, 1972.

97. **Hershko, A. and Kindler, S. H.,** Mode of interaction of purine nucleotides and amino acids with glutamate dehydrogenase, *Biochem. J.,* 101, 661, 1966.

98. **Blumenthal, K. M. and Smith, E. L.,** Alternative substrates for glutamate dehydrogenase, *Biochem. Biophys. Res. Commun.,* 62, 78, 1975.

99. **Levy, H. R. and Vennesland, B.,** The stereospecificity of enzymatic hydrogen transfer from diphospho-pyridine nucleotide, *J. Biol. Chem.,* 228, 85, 1957.

100. Recommendations of German Society for Clinical Chemistry: standardisation of methods for the estimation of enzyme activity in biological fluids. Supplement to the standard method for the determination of glutamate dehydrogenase (GLDH) activity, *J. Clin. Chem.,* 12, 392, 1974.

101. **Jung, K., Sokolowski, A., and Egger, E.,** An optimized assay of human serum glutamate dehydrogenase activity, *Enzyme,* 14, 44, 1972/73.
102. **Ellis, G. and Goldberg, D. M.,** Optimal conditions for the kinetic assay of serum glutamate dehydrogenase activity at 37°C, *Clin. Chem.,* 18, 523, 1972.
103. **Frieden, C.,** Glutamate dehydrogenase. IV. Studies on enzyme inactivation and coenzyme binding, *J. Biol. Chem.,* 238, 146, 1963.
104. **Olson, J. A. and Anfinsen, C. B.,** Kinetic and equilibrium studies on crystalline L-glutamic acid dehydrogenase, *J. Biol. Chem.,* 202, 841, 1953.
105. **Bitensky, M. W., Yielding, K. L., and Tomkins, G. M.,** The effect of allosteric modifiers on the rate of denaturation of glutamate dehydrogenase, *J. Biol. Chem.,* 240, 1077, 1965.
106. **Egan, R. R. and Dalziel, K.,** Active centre equivalent weight of glutamate dehydrogenase from dry weight determinations and spectrophotometric titrations of abortive complexes, *Biochem. J.,* 250, 47, 1971.
107. **Engel, P. C. and Dalziel, K.,** Kinetic studies of glutamic dehydrogenase with glutamate and norvaline as substrates, *Biochem. J.,* 115, 621, 1969.
108. **Dalziel, K. and Engel, P. C.,** Antagonistic homotropic interactions as a possible explanation of coenzyme activation of glutamate dehydrogenase, *FEBS Lett.,* 1, 349, 1968.
109. **Engel, P. C. and Ferdinand, W.,** The significance of abrupt transitions in Lineweaver-Burk plots with particular reference to glutamate dehydrogenase, *Biochem. J.,* 131, 97, 1973.
110. **Barton, J. S. and Fisher, J. R.,** Nonlinear kinetics of glutamate dehydrogenase. Studies with substrates — glutamate and nicotinamide-adenine dinucleotide, *Biochemistry,* 10, 577, 1971.
111. **Frieden, C.,** Glutamic dehydrogenase. III. The order of substrate addition in the enzymatic reaction, *J. Biol. Chem.,* 234, 2891, 1959.
112. **Dalziel, K. and Egan, R. R.,** The binding of oxidised coenzymes by glutamate dehydrogenase and the effects of glutamate and purine nucleotides, *Biochem. J.,* 225, 209, 1985.
113. **Bell, E. T., LiMuti, C., Renz, C. L., and Bell, J. E.,** Negative co-operativity in glutamate dehydrogenase. Involvement of the 2-position in glutamate in the induction of conformational changes, *Biochem. J.,* 225, 209, 1985.
114. **Favilla, R. and Mazzini, A.,** The binding of 1-N^6-etheno-NAD to bovine liver glutamate dehydrogenase, *Biochim. Biophys. Acta,* 788, 48, 1984.
115. **Dalziel, K.,** Kinetics and mechanism of nicotinamide-nucleotide linked dehydrogenases, in *The Enzymes,* Vol. 11, 3rd ed., Boyer, P. D., Ed., Academic Press, New York, 1975, 1.
116. **Smith, T. J. and Bell, J. E.,** Mechanism of hysteresis in bovine glutamate dehydrogenase: role of subunit interactions, *Biochemistry,* 21, 733, 1982.
117. **Colen, A. H., Prough, R. A., and Fisher, H. F.,** The mechanism of glutamate dehydrogenase reaction. IV. Evidence for random and rapid binding of substrate and coenzyme in the burst phase, *J. Biol. Chem.,* 247, 7905, 1972.
118. **Prough, R. A., Colen, A. H., and Fisher, H. F.,** Spectrophotometric observation of a glutamate dehydrogenase-L-glutamate complex, *Biochim. Biophys. Acta,* 284, 16, 1972.
119. **Silverstein, E. and Sulebele, G.,** Equilibrium kinetic study of the catalytic mechanism of bovine liver glutamate dehydrogenase, *Biochemistry,* 12, 2164, 1973.
120. **Silverstein, E.,** Equilibrium kinetic study of bovine liver glutamate dehydrogenase at high pH, *Biochemistry,* 13, 3750, 1974.
121. **Hornby, D. P., Aitchison, M. J., and Engel, P. C.,** The kinetic mechanism of ox liver glutamate dehydrogenase in the presence of the allosteric effector ADP, *Biochem. J.,* 223, 161, 1984.
122. **Rife, J. E. and Cleland, W. W.,** Kinetic mechanism of glutamate dehydrogenase, *Biochemistry,* 19, 2321, 1980.
123. **LiMuti, C. and Bell, J. E.,** A steady-state random-order mechanism for the oxidative deamination of norvaline by glutamate dehydrogenase, *Biochem. J.,* 211, 99, 1983.
124. **Di Franco, A. and Iwatsubo, M.,** Reaction mechanism of L-glutamate dehydrogenase. Characterization of optical and kinetic properties of various enzyme-reduced-coenzyme complexes, *Eur. J. Biochem.,* 30, 517, 1972.
125. **DiFranco, A.,** Reaction mechanism of L-glutamate dehydrogenase. Transient complexes in the oxidative deamination of L-glutamate catalyzed by NAD(P)-dependent L-glutamate dehydrogenase, *Eur. J. Biochem.,* 45, 407, 1974.
126. **Fisher, H. F., Bard, J. R., and Prough, R. A.,** Transient-state intermediates involved in the hydride transfer step of the glutamate dehydrogenase reaction, *Biochem. Biophys. Res. Commun.,* 41, 601, 1970.
127. **Frieden, C.,** Glutamic dehydrogenase. I. The effect of various nucleotides on the association-dissociation and kinetic properties, *J. Biol. Chem.,* 234, 809, 1959.
128. **Engel, P. C. and Dalziel, K.,** Kinetic studies of glutamate dehydrogenase, *Biochem. J.,* 118, 409, 1970.
129. **Frieden, C.,** Glutamate dehydrogenase. V. The relation of enzyme structure to the catalytic function, *J. Biol. Chem.,* 238, 3286, 1963.

130. **Krause, J., Büchner, M., and Sund, H.,** Studies of glutamate dehydrogenase. The binding of NADH and NADPH to beef liver glutamate dehydrogenase, *Eur. J. Biochem.,* 41, 593, 1974.

131. **Jallon, J. M. and Iwatsubo, M.,** Evidence for two nicotinamide binding sites on L-glutamate dehydrogenase, *Biochem. Biophys. Res. Commun.,* 45, 964, 1971.

132. **Pantaloni, D. and Dessen, P.,** Glutamate déshydrogénase. Fixations des coenzymes NAD et NADP et d'autres nucleotides dérivés de l'adénosine-5'-phosphate, *Eur. J. Biochem.,* 11, 510, 1969.

133. **Malencik, D. A. and Anderson, S. R.,** Reduced pyridine nucleotide binding to beef liver and dog fish liver glutamate dehydrogenase, *Biochemistry,* 11, 2766, 1972.

134. **Koberstein, R. and Sund, H.,** Studies of glutamate dehydrogenase. The influence of ADP, GTP, and L-glutamate on the binding of the reduced coenzyme to beef liver glutamate dehydrogenase, *Eur. J. Biochem.,* 36, 545, 1973.

135. **Goldin, B. R. and Frieden, C.,** L-glutamate dehydrogenases, *Curr. Top. Cell. Regul.,* 4, 77, 1971.

136. **Engel, P. C. and Chen, S. S.,** A product inhibition study of bovine liver glutamate dehydrogenase, *Biochem. J.,* 151, 305, 1975.

137. **Fisher, H. F.,** Glutamate dehydrogenase — ligand complexes and their relationship to the mechanism of the reaction, *Adv. Enzymol.,* 39, 369, 1973.

138. **Andrec, P. J.,** Nuclear magnetic resonance on the binding of substrate, coenzyme, and effectors to glutamate dehydrogenase, *Biochemistry,* 17, 772, 1978.

139. **Cohen, R. J. and Benedek, G. B.,** The functional relationship between the polymerization and catalytic activity of beef liver glutamate dehydrogenase. III. Analysis of Thusius's critique, *J. Mol. Biol.,* 129, 37, 1979.

140. **Thusius, D.,** Does a functional relationship exist between the polymerization and catalytic activity of glutamate dehydrogenase?, *J. Mol. Biol.,* 115, 243, 1977.

141. **Zeiri, L. and Reisler, E.,** Uncoupling of the catalytic activity and the polymerization of beef liver glutamate dehydrogenase, *J. Mol. Biol.,* 124, 291, 1978.

142. **Fisher, H. F., Cross, D. G., and McGregor, L. L.,** Catalytic activity of subunits of glutamate dehydrogenase, *Nature,* 196, 895, 1962.

143. **Reisler, E. and Eisenberg, H.,** Solubility of toluene in bovine liver glutamate dehydrogenase solutions and enhancement of enzyme association, *Biochim. Biophys. Acta,* 258, 351, 1972.

144. **Josephs, R., Eisenberg, H., and Reisler, E.,** Some properties of cross-linked polymers of glutamic dehydrogenase, *Biochemistry,* 12, 4060, 1973.

145. **Frieden, C. and Colman, R. F.,** Glutamate dehydrogenase concentration as a determinant in the effect of purine nucleotides on enzymatic activity, *J. Biol. Chem.,* 242, 1705, 1967.

146. **Tomkins, G. M., Yielding, K. L., Talal, N., and Curran, T. F.,** Protein structure and biological regulation, *Cold Spring Harbor Symp. Quant. Biol.,* 28, 461, 1963.

147. **Bailey, J., Bell, E. T., and Bell, J. E.,** Regulation of bovine glutamate dehydrogenase. The effects of pH and ADP, *J. Biol. Chem.,* 257, 5579, 1982.

148. **George, A. and Bell, J. E.,** Effects of adenosine 5'-diphosphate on bovine glutamate dehydrogenase: diethyl pyrocarbonate modification, *Biochemistry,* 19, 6057, 1980.

149. **Rasool, C. G., Nicolaidis, S., and Akhtar, M.,** The asymmetric distribution of enzymic activity between the six subunits of bovine glutamate dehydrogenase, *Biochem. J.,* 157, 675, 1976.

150. **Pal, P. K., Wechler, W. J., and Colman, R. F.,** Affinity labelling of the inhibitory DPNH site of bovine liver glutamate dehydrogenase by 5'-fluorosulfonylbenzoyl adenosine, *J. Biol. Chem.,* 250, 8140, 1975.

151. **Talbot, J. C., Gros, C., Cosson, M. P., and Pantaloni, D.,** Physicochemical evidence for the existence of two pyridoxal 5'-phosphate binding sites on glutamate dehydrogenase and characterization of their functional role, *Biochim. Biophys. Acta,* 494, 19, 1977.

152. **Freedman, R. B. and Radda, G. K.,** Chemical modification of glutamate dehydrogenase by 2,4,6-trinitrobenzenesulphonic acid, *Biochem. J.,* 114, 611, 1969.

153. **Coffee, C. J., Bradshaw, R. A., Goldin, B. R., and Frieden, C.,** Identification of the sites of modification of bovine liver glutamate dehydrogenase reacted with trinitrobenzenesulfonate, *Biochemistry,* 10, 3516, 1971.

154. **Goldin, B. R. and Frieden, C.,** Effect of trinitrophenylation of specific lysyl residues on the catalytic, regulatory, and molecular properties of bovine liver glutamate dehydrogenase, *Biochemistry,* 10, 3527, 1971.

155. **Hornby, D. P., Engel, P. C., and Hatanaka, S.,** Beef liver glutamate dehydrogenase: a study of the oxidation of various alternative amino acid substrates retaining the correct spacing of the two carboxylate groups, *Int. J. Biochem.,* 15, 495, 1983.

156. **Frieden, C.,** Glutamate dehydrogenase, in *The Behaviour of Regulatory Enzymes,* Thorne, C. J. R. and Tipton, K. F., Eds., Biochemical Society, London, 1973, 3.

157. **Bell, J. E. and Dalziel, K.,** A conformational transition of the oligomer of glutamate dehydrogenase induced by half-saturation with NAD+ or NADP+, *Biochim. Biophys. Acta,* 309, 237, 1973.

158. **Pal, P. K. and Colman, R. F.,** Affinity labelling of allosteric GTP site of bovine glutamate dehydrogenase by 5'-p-fluorosulfonylbenzoylguanosine, *Biochemistry*, 18, 838, 1979.

159. **McCarthy, A. D. and Tipton, K. F.,** The effects of magnesium ions on the interactions of ox brain and liver glutamate dehydrogenase with ATP and GTP, *Biochem. J.*, 220, 853, 1984.

160. **Veloso, D., Guynn, R. W., Oskarsson, M., and Veech, R. L.,** The concentration of free and bound magnesium in rat tissues. Relative constancy of free Mg + + concentrations, *J. Biol. Chem.*, 248, 4811, 1973.

161. **Kohn, M. C., Achs, M. J., and Garfinkel, D.,** Computer simulation of metabolism in pyruvate perfused rat heart. II. Krebs cycle, *Am. J. Physiol.*, 237, R159, 1979.

162. **Tompkins, G. M., Yielding, K. L., Curran, J. F., Summers, M. R., and Bitensky, M. W.,** The dependence of the substrate specificity on the conformation of crystalline glutamate dehydrogenase, *J. Biol. Chem.*, 240, 3793, 1965.

163. **Iwatsubo, M. and Pantaloni, D.,** Regulation of glutamate dehydrogenase activity by the effectors GTP and ADP; stopped-flow study, *Bull. Soc. Chim. Biol.*, 49, 1563, 1967.

164. **Frieden, C.,** Different structural forms of reversibly dissociated glutamic dehydrogenase: relation between enzymatic activity and molecular weight, *Biochem. Biophys. Res. Commun.*, 10, 410, 1963.

165. **Prough, R. A., Culver, J. M., and Fisher, H. F.,** Spectrophotometric evidence for a glutamate dehydrogenase-L-leucine complex, *Arch. Biochem. Biophys.*, 149, 414, 1972.

166. **Fisher, H. F., Culver, J. M., and Prough, R. A.,** The independence of adenosine-5-diphosphate binding and the state of association of L-glutamate dehydrogenase, *Biochem. Biophys. Res. Commun.*, 46, 1462, 1972.

167. **Colman, R. F. and Foster, D. S.,** The absence of zinc in bovine liver glutamate dehydrogenase, *J. Biol. Chem.*, 245, 6190, 1970.

168. **Wolff, J. and Wolff, E. C.,** The effect of thyroxine on isolated dehydrogenases, *Biochim. Biophys. Acta*, 26, 387, 1957.

169. **Pons, M., Michel, P., Descomps, B., and Crastes de Paulet, A.,** Structural requirements for maximal inhibitory allosteric effect of estrogens and estrogen analogues on glutamate dehydrogenase, *Eur. J. Biochem.*, 84, 257, 1978.

170. **Michel, F., Pons, M., Descomps, B., and Crastes de Paulet, A.,** Affinity labelling of the estrogen binding site of glutamate dehydrogenase with iodoacetyldiethylstilbestrol, *Eur. J. Biochem.*, 84, 267, 1978.

171. **Bryla, J. and Matyaszczyk, M.,** Inhibition of glutamate dehydrogenase activity in rabbit renal mitochondria by phosphoenolpyruvate, *FEBS Lett.*, 162, 244, 1983.

172. **Kallos, J. and Shaw, K. P.,** Covalent attachment of diethylstilbestrol to glutamate dehydrogenase: implications for allosteric regulation, *Proc. Natl. Acad. Sci. U.S.A.*, 68, 916, 1971.

173. **Fahien, L. A. and Smith, S. E.,** The enzyme-enzyme complex of transaminase and glutamate dehydrogenase, *J. Biol. Chem.*, 249, 2696, 1974.

174. **Churchich, J. E.,** Interaction between brain enzymes glutamate dehydrogenase and aspartate aminotransferase, *Biochem. Biophys. Res. Commun.*, 83, 1105, 1978.

175. **Fahien, L. A., Ruoho, A., and Kmiotek, E.,** A study of glutamate dehydrogenase-aminotransferase complexes with a bifunctional imidate, *J. Biol. Chem.*, 253, 5745, 1978.

176. **Shemisa, O. and Fahien, L. A.,** Modifications of glutamate dehydrogenase by various drugs which affect behaviour, *Mol. Pharmacol.*, 7, 8, 1971.

177. **Veronese, F. M., Bevilacqua, R., and Chaiken, I. M.,** Drug-protein interactions: evaluation of the binding of antipsychotic drugs to glutamate dehydrogenase by quantitative affinity chromatography, *Mol. Pharmacol.*, 15, 313, 1979.

178. **Uno, I., Matsumoto, K., Adachi, K., and Ishikawa, T.,** Regulation of NAD-dependent glutamate dehydrogenase by protein kinases in *Saccharomyces cerevisiae*, *J. Biol. Chem.*, 259, 1288, 1984.

179. **Place, G. A. and Beynon, R. J.,** The chymotrypsin-catalysed activation of bovine liver glutamate dehydrogenase, *Biochem. J.*, 205, 75, 1982.

180. **Place, G. A. and Beynon, R. J.,** Chymotryptic activation of glutamate dehydrogenase, *Biochim. Biophys. Acta*, 747, 26, 1983.

181. **Fisher, H. F., Gates, R. E., and Cross, D. G.,** Ligand exclusion theory of allosteric effects, *Nature*, 228, 247, 1970.

182. **Cross, D. G. and Fisher, H. F.,** The mechanism of glutamate dehydrogenase reaction. III. The binding of ligands at multiple subsites and resulting kinetic effects, *J. Biol. Chem.*, 245, 2612, 1970.

183. **Schmidt, J. A. and Colman, R. F.,** Identification of the lysine and tyrosine peptides labelled by 5'-p-fluorosulfonylbenzoyladenosine in the NADH inhibitory site of glutamate dehydrogenase, *J. Biol. Chem.*, 259, 14515, 1984.

184. **Jacobson, M. A. and Colman, R. F.,** Isolation and identification of a tyrosyl peptide labelled by 5'-[p-(fluorosulfonyl)-benzoyl]-1, N6-ethenoadenosine, at a GTP site of glutamate dehydrogenase, *Biochemistry*, 23, 6377, 1984.

185. **Jacobson, M. A. and Colman, R. F.,** Affinity labelling of a guanosine-5'-triphosphate site of glutamate dehydrogenase by a fluorescent nucleotide analogue, 5'-[p-(fluorosulfonyl)-benzoyl]-1-N6-ethenoadenosine, *Biochemistry,* 21, 2177, 1982.

186. **Monod, J., Wyman, J., and Changeux, J.-P.,** On the nature of allosteric transitions: a plausible model, *J. Mol. Biol.,* 12, 88, 1965.

187. **Fisher, H. F. and Viswanathan, T. S.,** Carbonyl oxygen exchange evidence of imine formation in the glutamate dehydrogenase reaction and identification of the ''occult role'' of NADPH, *Proc. Natl. Acad. Sci. U.S.A.,* 81, 2747, 1984.

188. **McGivan, J. D. and Chapell, J. B.,** On the metabolic function of glutamate dehydrogenase in rat liver, *FEBS Lett.,* 52, 1, 1975.

189. **Rognstad, R.,** Sources of ammonia for urea synthesis in isolated rat liver cells, *Biochim. Biophys. Acta,* 496, 249, 1977.

190. **Krebs, H. A., Hems, R., Lund, P., Halliday, D., and Read, W. W. C.,** Sources of ammonia for mammalian urea synthesis, *Biochem. J.,* 191, 605, 1978.

Chapter 7

GLUTAMATE DECARBOXYLASE

Jang-Yen Wu, Larry A. Denner, Chin-Tarng Lin, and Bang Hwang

TABLE OF CONTENTS

I. INTRODUCTION

L-Glutamate decarboxylase (GAD, EC4.1.1.15) which catalyzes the conversion of L-glutamate to γ-aminobutyric acid (GABA), an important inhibitory neurotransmitter, is a specific marker for GABAergic neurons and their processes.[1-4] Although GABA and GAD were originally believed to exist exclusively in the central nervous system (CNS) of the vertebrate,[5] with more sensitive methods GABA and GAD activity has been detected in glia and nonneural tissues such as the kidney, heart, liver, pancreas, adrenal medulla, and blood vessels.[6-16] However, little is known with certainty about the properties of glial or nonneural GAD. Contrary to the glial GAD, the neuronal GAD has been purified to homogeneity from several species including the mouse,[17] rat,[18,19] bovine,[20] catfish,[21] and human[22] and its properties have also been extensively characterized.[23-27] In addition, specific polyclonal and monoclonal antibodies against the neuronal GAD have also been obtained and characterized[28-31] and applied extensively for immunochemical and immunocytochemical studies of GAD in the vertebrate (for a review see References 2 to 4 and 32). In this review, the authors would like to cover the purification procedures, the criteria of purity, and the basic kinetic, physical, and immunochemical properties of GAD in addition to their application of the identification of GABAergic neurons and their projections.

II. DISTRIBUTION OF L-GLUTAMATE DECARBOXYLASE

The distribution of GAD in various tissues is summarized in Table 1. In addition to the brain, the pancreas also has high concentrations of GAD.[12] Other tissues that have been examined contain rather low concentrations of GAD activity. The function of GAD in the nonneural tissues remains unknown.

III. PURIFICATION AND CHARACTERIZATION OF L-GLUTAMATE DECARBOXYLASE

A. Purification

GAD has been purified to apparent homogeneity from the brain of the mouse,[17] rat,[18,19] bovine,[20] human,[18] and catfish.[21] The purification procedures involved the initial extraction of GAD activity from the whole brain or from the crude mitochondrial fraction, followed by ammonium sulfate fractionation or concentration by ultrafiltration and a series of column chromatographies including diethylaminoethyl (DEAE)-cellulose, hydroxylapatite, and gel filtration and finally by preparative nondenaturing polyacrylamide gel electrophoresis. The purification of GAD from 1000 rat brains or 9000 mouse brains is summarized in Table 2.

B. Criteria of Purity

The purity of the GAD preparations was established based on the following analyses: the purified GAD preparations migrated as a single protein band which comigrated with GAD activity in nondenaturing, 5% polyacrylamide gels (Figure 1A), in nondenaturing polyacrylamide gradient gels of 3.6 to 25% (Figure 1B), or 6 to 10% (data not shown) and in narrow range isoelectric focusing gels (Figure 1C). In addition, the mouse brain preparation was homogenous in size as judged from high-speed sedimentation-equilibrium experiments in both H_2O and D_2O solutions as well as in the presence of 6 M guanidine HCl and 0.1 M 2-mercaptoethanol. Under all three conditions a linear plot of the logarithm of concentrations against the squares of the distance from the center of rotation to points of interest was obtained suggesting that the GAD preparation was homogeneous in terms of size.[17,25]

TABLE 1
DISTRIBUTION OF L-GLUTAMATE DECARBOXYLASE ACTIVITY

| | Activity (units $\times$ 10³/mg protein) | | |
Tissue	CO₂ method	GABA method	%[a]
Mouse brain	4.63	4.27	100
Mouse heart	0.82	0.315	7.4
Mouse kidney	1.00	0.268	6.3
Mouse liver	0.22	0.065	1.5
Bovine cultured chromaffin cells	523[b]	769[b]	—
Bovine adrenal medulla	473[c]	345[c]	—
Rat whole pancreas			2.58[d]
Rat islets of Langerhans			66.7[d]
Rat acini			4.67[d]
Human pancreas (nontumor region)			2.01[d]
Human pancreas (tumor region, adenoma of β cells)			138.2[d]

[a]   GAD activity in brain homogenate was used as reference, 100%.
[b]   pmol/10⁶ cells per hour.[14]
[c]   nmol/g of wet weight per hour.[14]
[d]   GAD activity was assayed by enzymatic cycling method and expressed as mmol GABA/kg/hr.[12]

TABLE 2
PURIFICATION OF GAD FROM RAT BRAIN[a] AND MOUSE BRAIN[b]

| | Total activity (units)[c] | | Total protein (mg) | | Specific activity (units/mg $\times$ 10³) | |
Sample	Rat brain	Mouse brain	Rat brain	Mouse brain	Rat brain	Mouse brain
Homogenate	418	1,680	232,000	480,000	1.8	3.5
P2 Crude extract	—	429	—	16,500	—	26
Supernatant	292	—	127,000	—	2.3	—
(NH₄)₂SO₄ (27—62%)	—	300	—	6,000	—	50
DEAE-cellulose	140	—	12,100	—	11.6[d]	—
Sephadex® G-200	—	180	—	1,500	—	120[e]
Hydroxylapatite	49	88	472	195	104[f]	450[g]
DEAE-Sephadex®	—	31	—	18	—	1,720[h]
Gel filtration	20.6	—	66	—	312[f]	—
Sephadex® G-200	—	20	—	6	—	3,300
Gel electrophoresis	7.2	—	30	—	2,400	—

[a]   Purification of GAD was made from 1000 rat brains.
[b]   Purification of GAD was made from 9000 mouse brains.
[c]   One unit = 1 μmol of product formed per minute at 37°C under standard conditions.
[d-i]   The peak fraction had a specific activity of 15.1[d], 170[e], 128[f], 650[g], 2100[h], and 349[i].

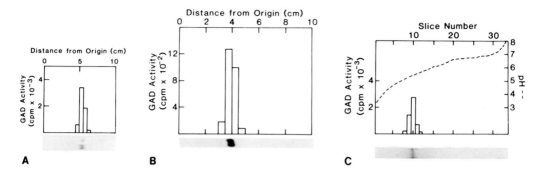

FIGURE 1.   Polyacrylamide gel electrophoresis and isoelectric focusing of purified GAD preparation. (A) Non-denaturing polyacrylamide gel electrophoresis of GAD on a 5% analytical gel. Two lanes (bottom) were silver stained for protein (upper band, 100 ng; lower band, 500 ng). A parallel lane was cut in 0.5 cm slices and assayed for GAD activity (top). (B) Nondenaturing polyacrylamide gradient gel electrophoresis of GAD on a linear 3.6 to 25% gradient gel. One land containing 1 μg of purified GAD was silver stained for protein (bottom); a parallel lane was cut in 0.5 cm slices and assayed for enzyme activity (top). (C) Isoelectric focusing of GAD in a pH 4 to 7 agarose gel. Parallel lanes were silver stained (500 ng) for protein (bottom), cut in 0.3 cm slices and assayed for GAD activity (open bars), or cut in 0.3 cm slices and macerated in water for pH determination (dashes).

C. Physical Characterization

The molecular weight of native mouse brain GAD was determined as 85,000 ± 2000 and 86,000 daltons by high-speed sedimentation equilibrium and gel filtration, respectively.[17,25] The molecular weight of native rat brain GAD was estimated as 120,000 ± 10,000 and 110,000 ± 10,000 by nondenaturing polyacrylamide gradient gel electrophoresis and gel filtration chromatography, respectively.

The mouse brain GAD appears to contain six identical subunits of a minimum molecular weight of 15,000 ± 1000 daltons. The native enzyme was dissociated into two identical trimer subunits of 42,000 ± 2000 daltons by the treatment of 6 M guanidine HCl and 0.1 M 2-mercaptoethanol whereas the treatment with sodium dodecyl sulfate (SDS) and 2-mercaptoethanol resulted in the dissociation of GAD molecule to various forms of subunit with the major species as the tetramer, 60,000-dalton subunits.[17,25,33] The rat brain GAD dissociated into two subunits of 40,000 and 80,000 daltons by SDS and 2-mercaptoethanol. Whether the 80,000-dalton subunit is the dimer fo the 40,000-dalton subunit remains to be determined.

D. Kinetic Properties

Of all the amino acids tested, only L-aspartic acid, L-cysteic acid, and L-cysteinesulfinic acid are decarboxylated by GAD at a significant rate in addition to its substrate, L-glutamate. For mouse brain GAD, L-aspartic acid is decarboxylated at 3 to 5% as that of L-glutamic acid.[17,25] Cysteinesulfinic acid is decarboxylated at about 10% of the rate of glutamate by rat brain GAD. The K_m value of L-glutamate for GAD from various species is between 0.7 to 2 mM. The K_m values of cysteic acid and cysteinesulfinic acid for bovine brain GAD is 5.4 and 5.2 mM, respectively.[20] Although GAD can use L-aspartic acid, cysteic/cysteine-sulfinic acids as the substrate, this activity is not physiologically significant because under normal conditions the concentration of L-glutamate is much higher than aspartic, cysteic, or cysteinesulfinic acids. GAD activity is inhibited by a variety of substances. The most potent inhibitors are sulfhydryl reagents and carbonyl-trapping reagents, followed by mer-capto acids and divalent cations. The K_i values of important inhibitors of mouse brain GAD are as follows: 5,5′-dithiobis(2-nitrobenzoic acid DTNB), 11 nM; 3-mercaptopropionic acid, 1.8 μM; 2-mercaptopropionic acid, 53 μM; 2-mercaptoacetic acid, 0.33 mM; D-glutamate, 0.9 mM; α-ketoglutarate (2-oxoglutarate), 1.2 mM; L-norepinephrine, 1.3 mM; fumarate,

1.8 m*M*; D,L-β-hydroxyglutamate, 2.8 m*M*; L-aspartate, 3.1 m*M*; glutarate, 3.5 m*M*; D,L-α-methylglutamate, 6.2 m*M*; oxalacetate, 6.2 m*M*; and NaCl, 17 m*M*.

Zinc acetate is the most potent inhibitor among the divalent cations tested, inhibiting to the extent of 50%, at 10 μ*M* concentration, followed by the acetates of Cd^{2+}, Hg^{2+}, and Cu^{2+}. The remaining divalent cations are far less effective as inhibitors. The percentages of inhibition by these divalent cations at 10 m*M* concentration are as follows: Ni^{2+}, 90%; Mn^{2+} and Co^{2+}, 80%; Ba^{2+}, 75%; Ca^{2+}, 50%; Mg^{2+}, 45%; and Sr^{2+}, 30%. The decreasing order of inhibitory potency is $Zn^{2+} > Cd^{2+}$, Hg^{2+}, $Cu^{2+} > Ni^{2+} > Mn^{2+}$, $Co^{2+} > Ba^{2+} > Ca^{2+} > Mg^{2+} > Sr^{2+}$. The rat brain GAD, similar to the mouse brain enzyme, is sensitive to various inhibitors. Inhibition of 50% of the rat brain GAD activity occurred at the following concentrations for each inhibitor: DTNB, 2.5 μ*M*; aminooxyacetic acid (AOAA), 1 μ*M*; 3-mercaptopropionic acid, 15 μ*M*; zinc acetate, 25 μ*M*; NaCl, 17.5 m*M*; α-ketoglutarate, 9 m*M*; and β-methylene-D,L-aspartate, 0.1 m*M*. Other physiological substances such as mono- and dicarboxylic acids, nucleotides, and biogenic amines are all moderate to weak inhibitors. However, no activator for the neuronal GAD has been found yet.

IV. PRODUCTION AND CHARACTERIZATION OF ANTIBODIES AGAINST L-GLUTAMATE DECARBOXYLASE

A. Production of Polyclonal Antibodies
Once the purity of GAD preparations was established from extensive analyses, the purified GAD preparations were used as an antigen for the production of specific antibodies. Briefly, rabbits were given seven biweekly subscapular injections of 10 to 30 μg of purified GAD each in Freund's complete adjuvant followed by intermittent monthly boosters of 10 to 30 μg as previously described.[30,31] Animals were bled from the ear vein 1 week after the fifth injection.

Serum was isolated by brief centrifugation after clotting for 1 hr at 37°C and 8 to 16 hr at 4°C. This technique has been successfully used in our laboratory for the production of antibodies against various proteins purified from the nervous system. For instance, a total of 7 to 150 μg of purified GABA-transaminase (GABA-T)[26,34] and GAD from the mouse brain,[28,30] choline acetyltransferase (CAT) from the electric organ of *Torpedo*,[35] neurofilament protein from *Myxicola*,[36] GAD, CAT, and cysteinesulfinic acid decarboxylase (CSAD) from the bovine brain,[20,37] and GAD from the rat brain[31] were able to evoke production of specific antibodies in rabbits.

B. Characterization of Polyclonal Antibodies
Anti-GAD serum was characterized extensively by various immunochemical techniques including immunodiffusion, immunoelectrophoresis, enzyme inhibition test, microcomplement fixation, immunoprecipitation, dot immunoassay, enzyme-linked immunoadsorbent assay (ELISA), and the Western immunoblotting test.[28,30,31] In both immunodiffusion and immunoelectrophoresis, a single immunoprecipitin band was obtained when a crude GAD preparation was tested against anti-GAD serum suggesting that anti-GAD serum is specific to GAD (Figures 2A and B). Furthermore, the immunoprecipitin band still retained GAD activity or corresponded to the position of GAD activity in immunoelectrophoresis.[28,30,31] In a microcomplement fixation test, 50% fixation of complement was obtained with about 6 μg of anti-GAD IgG and 40 ng of mouse brain GAD. Furthermore, the fixation curves obtained with the partially purified GAD and the purified GAD preparations became superimposable when the amount of GAD protein was estimated from the specific activities of GAD preparations, suggesting that the antiserum is specific to GAD only.[28,30] In the enzyme inhibition test, GAD activity was inhibited to a maximum of 50 to 70% by anti-GAD IgG. In the immunoprecipitation test, GAD activity was quantitatively precipitated by

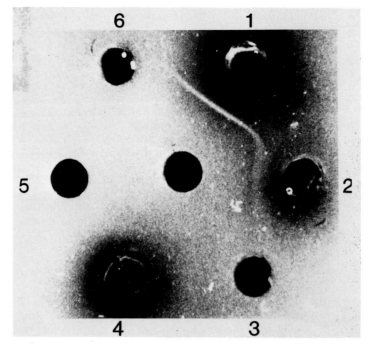

A

FIGURE 2. Immunodiffusion, immunoelectrophoresis, and Western immunoblotting tests with partially purified GAD and anti-GAD serum. (A) Immunodiffusion test: The center well contained 10 μℓ of partially purified GAD. Wells 1 and 2 contained 10 and 1 μℓ, respectively, of serum from a rabbit that had received 30 μg of purified GAD per injection. Wells 3 and 4 contained 10 and 1 μℓ, respectively, of serum from a rabbit that had received 10 μg of purified GAD per injection. Wells 5 and 6 contained preimmune serum from the respective rabbits. (B) Immunoelectrophoresis: Approximately 5 μℓ of partially purified GAD preparation (about 5% pure, 5 mg/mℓ) was applied and electrophoresed. After electrophoresis, one lane was cut into 0.5 cm per slice and assayed for GAD activity as shown at the top. GAD activity was expressed as cpm per slice per 30 min. The protein pattern of the gel after electrophoresis, immunodiffusion, and extensive washing in phosphate-saline buffer is shown at the bottom. (C) Western immunoblotting tests. After 20 μg of partially purified GAD preparation (10% pure) was applied to 10% SDS slab gel and electrophoretically transferred to the nitrocellulose sheet. Lane A: stained with polyclonal anti-GAD IgG showing two protein bands corresponding to the position of GAD subunits, namely 80,000- and 40,000-dalton. Lane B: stained with monoclonal anti-GAD IgG (#12-24) showing protein band corresponding to the position of GAD α-subunit, 80,000-dalton subunit. The numbers on the left represent the positions of standard molecular weight markers in kilodaltons.

anti-GAD directly, or by the addition of second antibodies or protein A.[28,30,31] In the ELISA and immunodot assay, as little as 50 ng of GAD either in a purified or crude preparation could be easily detected.[31] Furthermore, the intensity of reaction product is roughly proportional to the amount of antigen added for both crude and purified GAD preparations and independent of the purity of the GAD preparations suggesting the specificity of anti-GAD. In the western immunoblotting test, anti-GAD serum recognized only GAD subunits, the 40,000- and 80,000-dalton subunits in a relatively crude rat brain GAD preparation which contained many other proteins further indicating the high degree of specificity of anti-GAD serum (Figure 2C, Lane A).

C. Production of Monoclonal Antibodies

Monoclonal antibodies were prepared by procedures previously described[39,40] with some modifications.[31,41] BALB/C mice were injected intraperitoneally with 100 μg of GAD protein

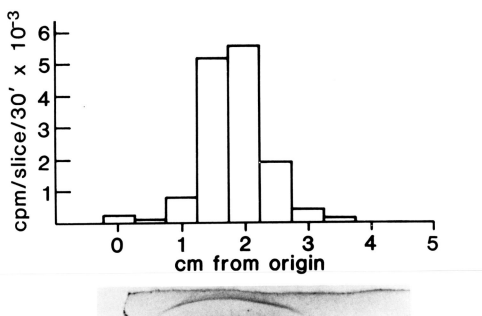

FIGURE 2B.

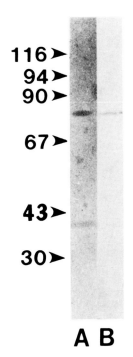

A B

FIGURE 2C.

(approximately 50% pure) emulsified in Freund's complete adjuvant. Blood was collected from the tail vein and serum analyzed for antibodies production by immunodiffusion. When an immunoprecipitin band was seen, spleen cells were harvested, incubated with 0.17 *M* ammonium chloride at 4°C for 10 min to lyse erythrocytes, and fused with a myeloma cell line (P3x63Ag3) at a ratio of 10:1 in 50% polyethylene glycol 1000 for 4 min. Cells were evenly suspended and distributed into 96 well microtiter plates (one drop per well). The next day an additional drop of 2X HAT medium (hypoxanthine, aminopterin, and thymidine)

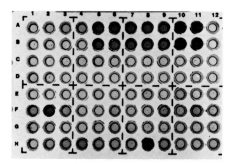

FIGURE 3. ELISA of monoclonal antibodies to GAD. All wells were coated with 200 ng of pure GAD. Screening of ascitic fluids including positive, mouse anti-GAD serum, (11A and 11B) and negative, ascitic fluids from mice received myeloma cells, (3A and 3B) controls. Ascitic fluids used in wells 5A, 5B, 6A, 6B, 7A, 7B, 8A, 8B, 9A, 9B, 10A, 10B, 2F, 4H, and 8H contained strong antibodies to GAD.

was added to each well. After 1 week, cells were fed with one drop of HT medium (hypoxanthine and thymidine, no aminopterin) to select for the growth of hybrids. Approximately 17 days after cell fusion, antibody-producing hybrids were detected by an ELISA test using pure GAD as the antigen and by an immunoprecipitation test using protein A technique with rabbit antimouse IgG as the second antibody. These hybrids were then cloned by limiting dilution into microtiter plates. After approximately 2 weeks, the culture medium was screened with the ELISA and immunoprecipitation tests. Positive wells were subcloned by limiting dilution, rescreened by ELISA and immunoprecipitation tests, and grown to confluency in 250 mℓ bottles. Clones yielding strong positive responses in both ELISA and immunoprecipitation tests were then injected into the peritoneal cavity of immunosuppressed mice. Ascites fluid was collected about 7 to 10 days later, and characterized by four different tests, namely, the ELISA test using pure GAD as the antigen, immunoprecipitation test, Western immunoblotting test, and immune complex test by gel filtration column chromatography.

D. Characterization of Monoclonal Antibodies

1. ELISA Test

Aliquots of 50 μℓ of purified GAD preparations containing 200 ng of GAD were added to microtiter wells and incubated with constant agitation at room temperature overnight. Wells were washed three times with 200 μℓ of buffer B [phosphate-saline containing 0.05% Tween®-20, 0.1% bovine serum albumin (BSA), pH 7.4]. Of either 1:100 diluted preimmune serum, or ascites fluid, 50 μℓ was added and incubated for 2 hr. The wells were washed three times. After an additional 2-hr incubation with peroxidase conjugated rabbit antimouse IgG diluted 1:200 with buffer B, wells were washed three more times and treated with 100 μℓ of substrate [0.05%, 2,2′-azino-di(3-ethylbenzothiazolinsulfonate) (ABTS), 0.1 M citric acid, pH 4.2, 0.02% hydrogen peroxide] for 15 min at room temperature. The reaction was terminated by aspirating the substrate and adding 40 μℓ 0.0006% sodium azide. Positive controls: mouse anti-GAD serum (Wells 11A and 11B). Negative controls: ascites fluids derived from mice which had been injected with myeloma cells (Wells 3A and 3B). Ascites fluids used in wells, 5A, 5B, 6A, 6B, 7A, 7B, 8A, 8B, 8H, 9A, 9B, 10A, 10B, 2F, and 4H contained strong antibodies against GAD (Figure 3).

2. Immunoprecipitation Test

In a typical experiment, 50 $\mu\ell$ of ascites fluid, 5 $\mu\ell$ GAD solution (about 30% pure, 2 mg/mℓ), and 45 $\mu\ell$ of GAD buffer [50 mM potassium phosphate, 0.2 mM pyridoxal phosphate (PLP), 1 mM 2-aminoethylisothiouronium bromide hydrobromide (AET), pH 7.2] were incubated for 4 days at 4°C. After adding 50 $\mu\ell$ of rabbit or antimouse immunoglobulin (1:10 dilution) to the above mixture, the whole mixture was further incubated for 1 hr at room temperature. To the above incubation mixture, 50 $\mu\ell$ of bead-conjugated protein A (100 mg/0.8 mℓ) was added and the incubation was continued for one additional hour. The mixture was then centrifuged and the pellet thus obtained was washed three times prior to the GAD assay. Four clones, GAD_6, GAD_{12-10}, GAD_{12-14}, and GAD_{12-33}, could remove GAD activity from the supernatant with a concomitant increase of GAD activity in the precipitate. The controls which included the substitution of testing ascites fluids with those obtained with the myeloma cells showed no GAD activity in the precipitate.

3. Western Immunoblotting Test

Briefly, 20 μg of partially purified GAD preparation (about 10% pure) was applied to a 10% SDS slab gel and electrophoresed for 4 hr at 20 mA. Proteins were then transferred from the SDS gel to a nitrocellulose sheet by electrophoretic transfer at 25 V for 16 hr. The nitrocellulose sheet was then treated with 5% skim milk at room temperature for 2 hr. After rinsing in 0.01 M phosphate-saline buffer containing 0.2% BSA and 0.05% Tween®-20, the nitrocellulose strips were immersed in 0.02 mg/mℓ of monoclonal anti-GAD IgG for 2 hr at room temperature. For the control experiments, the same amount of IgG isolated from controlled ascites fluid was used instead of anti-GAD IgG. After brief rinsing in the same buffer, the strips were further incubated with peroxidase labeled rabbit IgG antimouse IgG at 1:100 dilution for 1 hr, followed by a brief incubation with peroxidase substrate. Although many proteins were present in the partially purified GAD sample, only the 80,000-dalton subunit was stained with monoclonal anti-GAD IgG (#12-24) (Figure 2C, Lane B). No protein band was stained in the control experiments where polyclonal anti-GAD IgG and monoclonal anti-GAD IgG were replaced by the same amount of normal rabbit and mouse IgG, respectively.

4. Demonstration of GAD·Anti-GAD Complex by Gel Filtration and Sodium Dodecyl Sulfate-Polyacrylamide Gel Electrophoresis

Monoclonal antibodies against GAD were further characterized by Sephadex® G-200 gel filtration column chromatography and SDS-polyacrylamide gel electrophoresis (SDS-PAGE). Briefly, about 3.55 mg of partially purified GAD preparation (approximately 10% pure) was incubated with 4.52 mg of monoclonal anti-GAD IgG (monoclone #24-24) for 16 hr prior to the application to a Sephadex® G-200 column, 2.5 × 60 cm. The column was eluted with 50 mM phosphate buffer, pH 7.2 containing 1 mM AET, 0.2 mM PLP, and 1 mM EDTA. About 2 mℓ per fraction was collected. For the control experiments the conditions were the same as described above with the exception that monoclonal anti-GAD IgG was replaced by the same amount of normal mouse IgG. When the incubation-mixture containing GAD and monoclonal anti-GAD IgG #12-24 was applied to Sephadex® G-200 column, the elution position of GAD was found to shift from fraction 90 to fraction 82 suggesting the formation of a higher molecular weight complex, presumably GAD·anti-GAD IgG (Figures 4A and B). Similar results were obtained with monoclonal anti-GAD IgG #12-1, #12-10, and #12-33. When the peak fraction and one fraction on each side of the GAD activity peak from the Sephadex® G-200 column were analyzed in 10% SDS-PAGE, it was found that the fractions deriving from GAD and monoclonal anti-GAD IgG mixture contained much higher amounts of IgG than the comparable fractions deriving from GAD and normal mouse IgG mixture (Figure 4C) further suggesting that the complex is GAD·anti-GAD IgG complex.

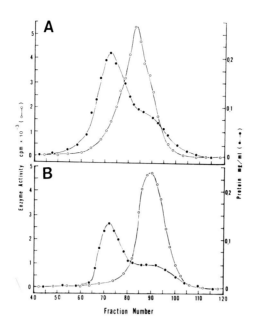

FIGURE 4.   Demonstration of GAD·anti-GAD IgG complex by Sephadex® G-200 gel filtration column chromatography and SDS-PAGE. (A) 3.55 mg of partially purified GAD was incubated with 4.52 mg of monoclonal anti-GAD Ig G (monoclone #12-24) for 16 hr prior to the application to Sephadex® G-200 column. Th epeak function was fraction 82. (B) The conditions were the same as (A) except that monoclonal anti-GAD IgG was replaced by normal mouse IgG and the amount of GAD and IgG was changed to 2.72 and 3.46 mg, respectively. The ratio of GAD to IgG was the same in (A) and (B). The peak fraction was fraction 90. A shift of elution position of GAD towards higher molecular weight (from fraction 90 to 82) is obtained in (A). (C) Further demonstration of GAD·anti-GAD complex by SDS-PAGE. Fractions from Sephadex® G-200 column (Figure 4A and B) were analyzed in SDS-PAGE for the presence of IgG molecule. Lane 1: molecular weight markers; phosphorylase b (94,000) BSA (67,000); ovalbumin (43,000); carbonic anhydrase (30,000). Lane 2: partially purified GAD sample used in the experiment. Lane 3: monoclonal anti-GAD IgG (monoclone #12-24). Lanes 4 to 6: fractions 96, 90, and 86 from Sephadex® G-200 column containing GAD and normal mouse IgG. Lanes 7 to 9: fraction 90, 82, and 76 from Sephadex® G-200 column containing GAD and anti-GAD IgG (monoclone #12-24).

V. SPECIES SPECIFICITY OF L-GLUTAMATE DECARBOXYLASE

The species-specificity of GAD was examined by the double diffusion, enzyme inhibition, and microcomplement fixation tests employing both antimouse brain GAD serum and anticatfish brain GAD serum. In immunodiffusion tests, a sharp, single precipitin band was observed with antimouse brain GAD serum and crude GAD preparations from the rat, rabbit, guinea pig, quail, pigeon, human, calf, and frog. The precipitin bands with the preparations from the quail, pigeon, and frog brain showed spurs; no precipitin band was obtained with the preparation from the trout brain.[28,30] When the crude GAD preparations were tested against anticatfish brain GAD, a single, sharp precipitin line was observed between anti-GAD serum and GAD preparations from the goldfish, chick, frog, and turtle brain. No precipitin line was obtained between anticatfish GAD serum and GAD preparations from the rat, mouse, bovine, or rabbit brain.[29]

In enzyme inhibition tests a crude GAD preparation from the mouse and rat brain was inhibited maximally to the extent of 50 and 35%, respectively, by antimouse brain GAD IgG. GAD preparations from other species were only slightly inhibited (5 to 10%) with the exception of that prepared from the pigeon, which was inhibited to an extent of 20%.[28,30] In the presence of anticatfish GAD IgG enzymes from the goldfish, frog, *Drosophila*, chick,

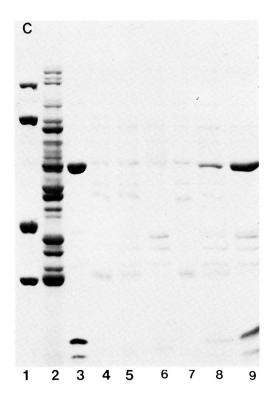

FIGURE 4C.

and crayfish were inhibited to an extent of 27, 46, 32, 38, and 57%, respectively. Enzymes from all the other species examined were not affected at all.[29]

In microcomplement fixation tests, in the presence of antimouse brain GAD IgG, the fixation curves obtained with the crude GAD preparation and purified GAD solution became superimposable when the plots were made on the basis of the amount of antigen. The complement fixation curves obtained with crude GAD preparations from the mouse, rat, and human were very similar. The maximal degree of fixation with GAD from the calf, rabbit, and guinea pig was about 40 to 65%. GAD from the quail, pigeon, frog, and trout did not react at all under these conditions.[28,30] In the presence of anticatfish GAD IgG, the fixation curves for GAD preparations from the goldfish, frog, and chick were similar.[29] From the species specificity study, it is clear that the combination of antimouse and anticatfish GAD would enable us to use immunological methods to examine the GABAergic system in almost all the vertebrate species and also some invertebrate species.

VI. IDENTIFICATION AND LOCALIZATION OF L-GLUTAMATE DECARBOXYLASE

Since GAD is a specific marker for GABAergic neurons,[1-4] the most direct means to identify GABAergic neurons and their processes is to localize GAD at precise cellular and subcellular levels using immunocytochemical methods. In the last few years, we, as well as others, have used specific and well-characterized polyclonal anti-GAD serum to localize GAD immunocytochemically in various brain regions as well as in the cultures (for a review see References 3 and 4). Recently, we have also obtained a specific monoclonal antibody against GAD and used it for immunocytochemical studies of GAD in the cerebellum and retina.[31] In summary, GAD has been localized in the cerebellum,[42-46] spinal cord,[47-49] ret-

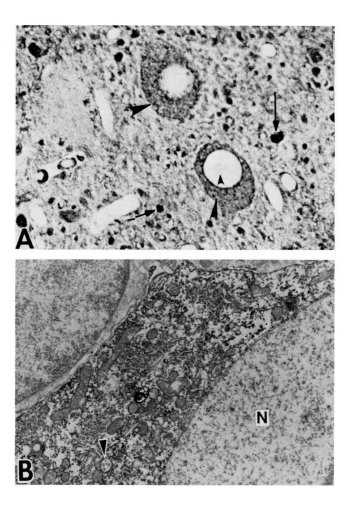

FIGURE 5. Immunocytochemical localization of GAD in rat nucleus tractus solitarius. (A) The light micrograph from a semithin section of rat NTS treated with anti-GAD serum showing two GAD-positive neurons (large arrowheads). The GAD-positive reaction product appears only in the cytoplasm. The nucleus and nucleolus (small arrowheads) are devoid of reaction product. Other GAD-positive profiles (arrows) are presumably GABA-ergic dendrites ×660. (B) This electron micrograph shows a GABAergic neuron in the NTS whose cytoplasm is GAD-positive. The mitochondria, cisternae of endoplasmic reticulum, multivesicular body (arrowheads), and the nucleus (N) are devoid of reaction product. The glial cell on the upper left is GAD-negative (×16,000). (C) Several GABAergic dendritic profiles identified by GAD-positive immunoreactive products are illustrated. There are several different axonal boutons which are GAD negative that have synaptic contacts with GABAergic dendritic profiles as indicated by arrowheads. This result shows that there are many axodendritic synapses on the GABAergic neurons (×12,500).

ina,[32,50-56] habenula,[57,58] olfactory bulb,[59,60] substantia nigra,[61,62] corpus striatum,[63] neostriatum,[64,65] red nucleus,[66-68] arcuate nucleus,[69] tuberomammillary nucleus,[70] lateral cervical nucleus,[71] cochlear nucleus,[72] vestibular nuclei,[73] dorsal column nuclei,[74] nucleus reticularis thalami,[75] globus pallidus and nucleus entopenduncularis,[76] visual cortex,[77-80] dentate gyrus,[81-84] superior colliculus,[85] sensory-motor cortex,[86,87] septal area,[88-90] hypothalamus,[91-94] hippocampus,[95-98] geniculate complex,[99,100] and nucleus tractus solitarii.[101]

In addition to the neural tissue, GAD has also been localized in nonneural tissues including

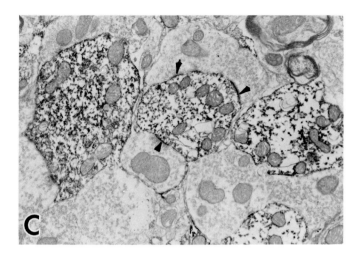

FIGURE 5C.

the pancreas,[102] pituitary gland,[91] and adrenal chromaffin cells,[103] as well as in the cultured neural cells.[104-106] Recently, GAD has been shown to coexist with other neuroactive substances or their synthetic enzymes in various parts of the mammalian nervous system such as the coexistence of GAD and tyrosine hydroxylase in the periglomerular region of the rat main olfactory bulb[60] and in neurons of the arcuate nucleus,[69] coexistence of GAD with somatostatin or cholecystokinin in the visual cortex and hippocampus of the cat,[79] and coexistence of GAD, adenosine deaminase, and histidine decarboxylase in hypothalamic neurons of the rat.[93] The details of immunocytochemical techniques[41] and immunocytochemical localization of GAD[3,4,107] will not be reviewed here since they have already been recently reviewed by the authors. The following examples of GAD immunocytochemical pictures are intended to illustrate the typical profile of GABAergic neurons and their dendrites and terminals. In addition, the immunocytochemical staining of GAD using polyclonal anti-GAD and monoclonal anti-GAD will also be compared.

A. In Rat Nucleus Tractus Solitarii

In order to determine whether GABAergic neurons may play a role in the regulation of baroreceptor reflexes, we have localized both the catecholamine (CA) and GAD in the rat nucleus tractus solitarii (NTS).[101] The GAD-positive reaction products were found in the cytoplasm of many cell bodies in the commissural NTS (Figure 5A). The nucleus, mitochondria, multivesicular bodies (MVB), and Golgi apparatus seemed to contain no reaction products (Figure 5B). In the dendritic profiles, the reaction products were around ribosome-like elements, the neurotubular structures, and membrane-bound structures such as the mitochondrial and MVB in the cytoplasm. The control sections showed no staining. Many dendritic profiles in the neurophils in the commissural NTS were labeled with GAD immunostaining. The GAD-positive dendritic profiles were most frequently seen to make axo-dendritic contacts with different axonal boutons (Figure 5C). These findings are compatible with the view of Chalmers et al.[108] that CA axon terminals in the NTS are most likely synapsing on GABA dendrites.

B. In Rat Retina

At light microscopic level, both polyclonal and monoclonal antibodies against GAD showed a similar staining pattern, namely, the staining was mainly concentrated in the inner plexiform layer (IPL) and to a lesser extent in the inner nuclear layer (INL) (Figures 6A

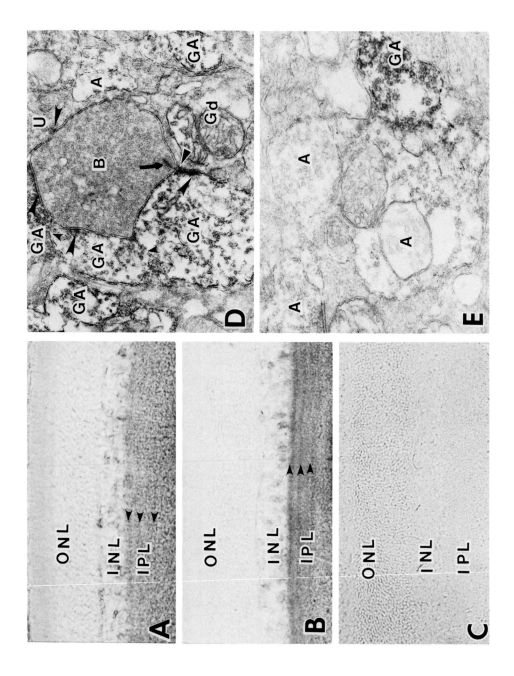

FIGURE 6. Immunocytochemical localization of GAD in rat retina. (A) The rat retinal section was stained with one of the monoclonal antibodies (#12-24). Reaction product is shown mainly in the IPL and some in the INL. Note that a clear multistriated staining pattern is seen in the IPL (arrowheads). The outer nuclear layer (ONL) is unstained ($\times$870). (B) The rat retinal section was stained with polyclonal antibodies. Reaction product is also seen in the IPL and INL but not in the ONL. Note that in the IPL the multistriated staining pattern is also found (arrowheads) ($\times$750). (C) The control section was treated either with preimmune serum or with control ascitic fluid showing no reaction product. (D) Electron microscopic immunocytochemical localization of GAD in IPL of the rat retina. An unstained bipolar terminal (B) (at the center) makes synapse to three stained amacrine (GA) terminals, one unstained possible bipolar terminal, and one ganglion cell dendrite. A typical bipolar dyad containing the synaptic ribbon (arrowhead) and its postsynaptic, stained amacrine terminal (GA) and ganglion cell dendrite (GD) is clearly discernible. Those three stained amacrine terminals (GA) also make direct contact to each other although there are no visible synapses. Reaction product in each stained terminal is seen mainly to be associated with synaptic vesicles and synaptic membrane ($\times$34,000). (E) Another electron micrograph showing some GAD-positive (GA) and GAD-negative (A) amacrine terminals in the IPL of the rat retina ($\times$33,000).

and B). Note that a clear multistriated staining pattern is seen in the IPL. Control sections which were treated with preimmune serum or control ascites fluid showed no specific staining (Figure 6C). At the ultrastructural level, the GAD-positive reaction product was observed around the synaptic vesicles in some amacrine terminals which are synapsed to other GAD-positive as well as GAD-negative amacrine terminals, and to GAD-negative bipolar terminals and ganglion dendrites (Figures 6D and E), a pattern similar to our previous observation with rabbit retina.[32]

C. In Rat Cerebellum

In the cerebellum, discrete, punctate deposits of GAD-positive reaction product were seen surrounding Purkinje cell bodies (P) in sections treated with anti-GAD serum (Figure 7A). Sections treated with GAD monoclonal antibodies from ascites fluid exhibited small punctate reaction product similar to those stained with the polyclonal antibodies (Figure 7B). Sections treated with preimmune serum or control ascites fluid derived from myeloma cells showed no staining or only diffuse background staining (Figures 7C and D). In addition to the punctate staining around Purkinje cell bodies, numerous GAD-positive staining were seen in the molecular as well as granual layer corresponding to the innervations of stellate cells on the dendritic processes of Purkinje cells in the molecular layer and the Golgi cells and their processes in the granual layer, respectively.

VII. CONCLUSION

In this review, the authors have summarized the recent progress in various aspects of GAD including the purification of GAD to homogeneity, production, and characterization of polyclonal as well as monoclonal antibodies against GAD, and identification of GABAergic neurons and their connectivities by means of immunocytochemical localization of GAD at cellular and subcellular levels. Earlier works on GAD and GABA-T have also been reviewed by one of the authors.[4,19,25,26,30] For those who are interested in this subject, those earlier review articles should be consulted and used as supplementary materials to the current one.

ACKNOWLEDGMENT

This work was supported by Grant NS20978 from the National Institute of Neurology and Communicative Disorders and Stroke, National Institutes of Health. We thank Pat Gering for her secretarial assistance.

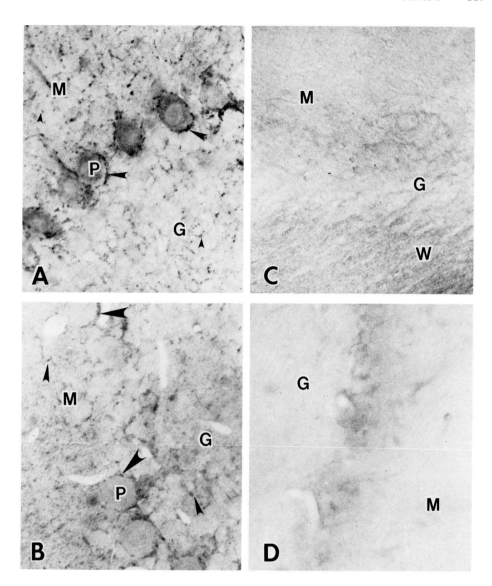

FIGURE 7. Immunocytochemical localization of GAD in rat cerebellum. (A) The rat cerebellar section was stained with polyclonal antibodies. The punctate reaction product of anti-GAD is found surrounding Purkinje cell bodies (large arrowheads), and in the molecular and granular layers (small arrowheads) ($\times$ 1200). (B) The rat cerebellar section was stained with one of the monoclonal antibodies (#12-24). The punctate reaction product is also seen surrounding the Purkinje cell bodies (large arrowheads) and in the molecular and granular layers (small arrowheads) ($\times$ 940). (C) and (D) A control section taken from the rat cerebellum and stained with either preimmune rabbit serum (C) or control ascites (D) shows no reaction product ($\times$ 1200).

REFERENCES

1. **Roberts, E. and Kuriyama, K.,** Biochemical-physiological correlations in studies of the γ-aminobutyric acid system, *Brain Res.,* 8, 1, 1968.
2. **Roberts, E.,** New directions in GABA research. I. Immunocytochemical studies of GABA neurons, in *GABA-Neurotransmitters: Pharmacochemical, Biochemical, and Pharmacological Aspects,* Korgsgaard-Larson, P., Scheel-Kruger, J., and Koford, H., Eds., Munksgaard, Copenhagen, 1979, 28.

3. **Wu, J.-Y., Lin, C.-T., Brandon, C., Chan, D.-S., Möhler, H., and Richards, J. G.,** Regulation and immunocytochemical characterization of GAD, in *Cytochemical Methods in Neuroanatomy,* Palay, S. and Palay, V., Eds., Alan R. Liss, New York, 1982, 279.

4. **Wu, J.-Y.,** Immunocytochemical identification of GABAergic neurons and pathways, in *Glutamine Glutamate and GABA in the Central Nervous System,* Hertz, L., Ed., Alan R. Liss, New York, 1983, 161.

5. **Roberts, E. and Frankel, S.,** γ-Aminobutyric acid in brain, *Fed. Proc., Fed. Am. Soc. Exp. Biol.,* 9, 219, 1950.

6. **Haber, B., Kuriyama, K., and Roberts, E.,** Decarboxylation of glutamate by tissues other than brain, non-identity with CNS GAD, *Fed. Proc., Fed. Am. Soc. Exp. Biol.,* 28, 577, 1969.

7. **Haber, B., Kuriyama, K., and Roberts, E.,** L-Glutamic acid decarboxylase: a new type in glial cells and human brain gliomas, *Science,* 168, 598, 1970a.

8. **Haber, B., Kuriyama, K., and Roberts, E.,** An anion stimulated L-glutamic acid decarboxylase in non-neural tissues: occurrence and subcellular localization in mouse kidney and developing chick embryo brain, *Biochem. Pharmacol.,* 19, 1119, 1970b.

9. **Wu, J.-Y.,** Comparative study of L-glutamate decarboxylase from brain and heart with purified preparations, *J. Neurochem.,* 28, 1359, 1977.

10. **Wu, J.-Y.,** Properties of L-glutamate decarboxylase from non-neuronal tissues, *Brain Res. Bull.,* 5 (Suppl. 2), 31, 1980.

11. **Wu, J.-Y., Chude, O., Wein, J., and Roberts, E.,** Glutamate decarboxylase from neural and non-neural tissues, *J. Neurochem.,* 30, 849, 1978a.

12. **Okada, Y., Taniguchi, H., and Shimada, C.,** High concentration of GABA and high glutamate decarboxylase activity in rat pancreatic islets and human insulinoma, *Science,* 194, 620, 1976.

13. **Okada, Y., Taniguchi, H., and Baba, S.,** High concentration of GABA in the pancreatic islets with special emphasis on B cells, in *Problems in GABA Research from Brain to Bacteria,* Okada, Y. and Roberts, E., Eds., Excerpta Medica, Amsterdam, 1982, 379.

14. **Kataoka, Y., Gutman, Y., Guidotti, A., Panula, P., Wroblewski, Y., Cosenza-Murphy, D., Wu, J.-Y., and Costa, E.,** The intrinsic GABAergic system of adrenal chromaffin cells, *Proc. Natl. Acad. Sci. U.S.A.,* 81, 3218, 1984.

15. **Kuriyama, K., Haber, K., and Roberts, E.,** Occurrence of a new L-glutamate acid decarboxylase in several blood vessels of the rabbit, *Brain Res.,* 23, 121, 1970.

16. **Zachmann, M. P., Tocci, P., and Nyhan, W. L.,** The occurrence of γ-aminobutyric acid in human tissues other than brain, *J. Biol. Chem.,* 241, 1355, 1966.

17. **Wu, J.-Y., Matsuda, T., and Roberts, E.,** Purification and characterization of glutamate decarboxylase from mouse brain, *J. Biol. Chem.,* 248, 3029, 1973.

18. **Maitre, M., Blinderman, J.-M., Ossola, L., and Mandel, P.,** Comparison of the structures of L-glutamate decarboxylase from human and rat brains, *Biochem. Biophys. Res. Commun.,* 85, 885, 1978.

19. **Wu, J.-Y., Denner, L., Lin, C.-T., and Song, G.-X.,** L-Glutamate decarboxylase from brain, in *Methods in Enzymology,* Vol. 113, Meister, A., Ed., Academic Press, New York, 1985, 3.

20. **Wu, J.-Y.,** Purification and characterization of cysteic/cysteine sulfinic acids decarboxylase and L-glutamate decarboxylase in bovine brain, *Proc. Natl. Acad. Sci. U.S.A.,* 79, 4270, 1982.

21. **Su, Y. Y. T., Wu, J-Y., and Lam, D. M. K.,** Purification of L-glutamic acid decarboxylase from catfish brain, *J. Neurochem.,* 33, 169, 1979.

22. **Blinderman, J.-M., Maitre, M., Ossola, L., and Mandel, P.,** Purification and some properties of L-glutamate decarboxylase from human brain, *Eur. J. Biochem.,* 86, 143, 1978.

23. **Wu, J.-Y. and Roberts, E.,** Properties of brain L-glutamate decarboxylase: inhibition studies, *J. Neurochem.,* 23, 759, 1974.

24. **Wu, J.-Y., Saito, K., Wong, E., Roberts, E., and Schousboe, A.,** Properties of L-glutamate decarboxylase from brains of adult and newborn mice, *J. Neurochem.,* 27, 653, 1976.

25. **Wu, J.-Y.,** Purification, characterization, and kinetic studies of GAD and GABA-T from mouse brain of L-glutamate decarboxylase (GAD) and GABA-aminotransferase (GABA-T), in *GABA in Nervous System Function,* Roberts, E., Chase, T., and Tower, D., Eds., Raven Press, New York, 1976, 7.

26. **Wu, J.-Y., Su, Y. Y. T., Lam, D. M. K., Schousboe, A., and Chude, O.,** Assay methods, purification and characterization of L-glutamate decarboxylase and GABA-transaminase, *Res. Methods Neurochem.,* 5, 129, 1981.

27. **Denner, L. A. and Wu, J.-Y.,** Two forms of rat brain glutamic acid decarboxylase differ in their dependence on free pyridoxal phosphate, *J. Neurochem.,* 44, 957, 1985.

28. **Saito, K., Wu, J.-Y., and Roberts, E.,** Immunochemical comparisons of vertebrate glutamate acid decarboxylase, *Brain Res.,* 65, 277, 1974.

29. **Su, Y. Y. T., Wu, J.-Y., and Lam, D. M. K.,** Species specificities of L-glutamate acid decarboxylase: immunochemical comparisons, *Neurochem. Int.,* 5, 587, 1983.

30. **Wu, J.-Y.**, Preparation of glutamic acid decarboxylase as immunogen for immunocytochemistry, in *Methods in the Neurosciences*, Cuello, A. C., Ed., Neuroimmunocytochemistry (IBRO) Handbook Series, John Wiley & Sons, Sussex, 1983, 159.

31. **Wu, J.-Y., Denner, L. A., Wei, S. C., Lin, C.-T., Song, G. X., Xu, Y. F., Liu, J. W., and Lin, H. S.**, Production and characterization of polyclonal and monoclonal antibodies to rat brain L-glutamate decarboxylase, *Brain Res.*, 373, 1, 1986.

32. **Wu, J.-Y., Brandon, C., Su, Y. Y. T., and Lam, D. M. K.**, Immunocytochemical and autoradiographic localization of GABA system in the vertebrate retina, *Mol. Cell. Biochem.*, 39, 229, 1981.

33. **Matsuda, T., Wu, J.-Y., and Roberts, E.**, Electrophoresis of glutamic acid decarboxylase (EC 4.1.1.15) from mouse brain in sodium-dodecyl sulphate polyacrylamide gels, *J. Neurochem.*, 21, 167, 1973.

34. **Saito, K., Schousboe, A., Wu, J.-Y., and Roberts, E.**, Some immunochemical properties and species specificity of GABA-α-ketoglutarate transaminase from mouse brain, *Brain Res.*, 65, 287, 1974.

35. **Brandon, C. and Wu, J.-Y.**, Electrophoretic and immunochemical characterization of choline acetyltransferase from *Torpedo*, *Soc. Neurosci.*, 3 (Abstr.), 404, 1977.

36. **Lasek, R. J. and Wu, J.-Y.**, Immunochemical analysis of the proteins comprising myxicola (10 nm) neurofilaments, in Abstr. 6th Annu. Meet. Soc. Neurosci., 40, 1976.

37. **Wu. J.-Y., Su, Y. Y. T., Brandon, C., Lam, D. M. K., Chen, M. S., and Huang, W. M.**, Purification and immunochemical studies of GABA-, acetylcholine-, and taurine-synthesizing enzymes from bovine and fish brains, 7th Int. Meet. of the ISN, 662, 1979.

38. **Su, Y. Y. T., Wu, J.-Y., and Lam, D. M. K.**, Purification and some properties of choline acetyltransferase from catfish brain, *J. Neurochem.*, 34, 438, 1980.

39. **Köhler, G. and Milstein, C.**, Continuous cultures of fused-cells secreting antibody of predefined specificity, *Nature*, 256, 495, 1975.

40. **Galfre, G., Howe, S. C., Milstein, C., Butcher, G. W., and Howard, J. C.**, Antibodies to major histocompatability antigens produced by hybrid cell lines, *Nature*, 266, 550, 1977.

41. **Wu, J.-Y. and Lin, C.-T.**, Immunocytochemical techniques, in *Neuromethods*, Vol. 3, Boulton, A. A., Baker, G. B., and Wood, J. D., Eds., The Humana Press, Clifton, N.J., 1985, 155.

42. **Saito, K., Barber, R., Wu, J.-Y., Matsuda, T., Roberts, E., and Vaughn, J. E.**, Immunohistochemical localization of glutamic acid decarboxylase in rat cerebellum, *Proc. Natl. Acad. Sci. U.S.A.*, 71, 269, 1974.

43. **McLaughlin, B. J., Wood, J. G., Saito, K., Barber, R., Vaughn, J. E., Roberts, E., and Wu, J.-Y.**, The fine structural localization of glutamate decarboxylase in synaptic terminals of rodent cerebellum, *Brain Res.*, 76, 377, 1974.

44. **McLaughlin, B. J., Wood, J. G., Saito, K., Roberts, E., and Wu, J.-Y.**, The fine structural localization of glutamate decarboxylase in developing axonal processes and presynaptic terminals of rodent cerebellum, *Brain Res.*, 85, 355, 1975.

45. **Chan-Palay, V., Palay, S. L., and Wu, J.-Y.**, Gamma-aminobutyric acid pathways in the cerebellum studied by retrograde and anterograde transport of glutamic acid decarboxylase antibody after *in vivo* injections, *J. Anat. Embryol.*, 157, 1, 1979.

46. **Chan-Palay, V., Nilaver, G., Palay, S. L., Beinfeld, M. C., Zimmerman, E. E., Wu, J.-Y., and O'Donohue, T. L.**, Chemical heterogeneity in cerebellar Purkinje cells: existence and coexistence of glutamic acid decarboxylase-like and motilin-like immunoreactivities, *Proc. Natl. Acad. Sci. U.S.A.*, 78, 7787, 1981.

47. **McLaughlin, B. J., Barber, R., Saito, K., Roberts, E., and Wu, J.-Y.**, Immunocytochemical localization of glutamate decarboxylase in rat spinal cord, *J. Comp. Neurol.*, 164, 305, 1975.

48. **Hunt, S. P., Kelly, J. S., Emson, P. C., Kimmel, J. R., Miller, R. J., and Wu, J.-Y.**, An immunohistochemical study of neuronal populations containing neuropeptides or GABA within the superficial layers of the rat dorsal horn, *Neuroscience*, 6, 1883, 1981.

49. **Fuji, K., Senba, E., Fujii, S., Nomura, I., Wu, J.-Y., Ueda, Y., and Tohyama, M.**, Distribution, ontogeny and projections of cholecystokinin-8, vasoactive intestinal polypeptide and gamma-aminobutyrate-containing neuron systems in the rat spinal cord: an immunohistochemical analysis, *Neuroscience*, 14, 881, 1985.

50. **Lam, D. M. K., Su, Y. Y. T., Swain, L., Marc, R. E., Brandon, C., and Wu, J.-Y.**, Immunocytochemical localization of L-glutamic acid decarboxylase in goldfish retina, *Nature*, 278, 565, 1979.

51. **Brandon, C., Lam, D. M. K., and Wu, J.-Y.**, The γ-aminobutyric acid system in rabbit retina: localization by immunocytochemistry and autoradiography, *Proc. Natl. Acad. Sci. U.S.A.*, 76, 3557, 1979.

52. **Lin, C.-T., Li, H.-Z., and Wu, J.-Y.**, Immunocytochemical localization of L-glutamate decarboxylase, gamma aminobutyric acid transaminase, cysteine-sulfinic acid decarboxylase, aspartate, aminotransferase and somatostatin in rat retina, *Brain Res.*, 270, 273, 1983.

53. **Zucker, C., Wu, J.-Y., and Yazulla, S.**, Non-correspondence of [^{3}H]-GABA uptake and GAD localization: two potential markers of GABAergic neurons, *Brain Res.*, 298, 154, 1984.

54. **Lin, C.-T., Song, G.-X., and Wu, J.-Y.,** Ultrastructural demonstration of L-glutamate decarboxylase and cysteinesulfinic acid decarboxylase in rat retina by immunocytochemistry, *Brain Res., 331*, 71, 1985.

55. **Yazulla, S., Studholme, K., and Wu, J.-Y.,** Comparative distribution of [³H]-GABA uptake and GAD-immunoreactivity in goldfish retinal amacrine cells: a double-label analysis, *J. Comp. Neurol., 244,* 149, 1986.

56. **Hendrickson, A., Ryan, M., Noble, B., and Wu, J.-Y.,** Colocalization of [³H]-muscimol and antisera to GABA and glutamic acid decarboxylase within the same neurons in monkey retina, *Brain Res., 348,* 391, 1985.

57. **Gottesfeld, Z., Brandon, C., Jacobowitz, D. M., and Wu, J.-Y.,** The GABA ststem in the mammalian habenula, *Brain Res. Bull., 5* (Suppl. 2), 1, 1980.

58. **Gottesfeld, Z., Brandon, C., and Wu, J.-Y.,** Immunochemistry of glutamate decarboxylase in the deafferented habenula, *Brain Res., 208,* 181, 1981.

59. **Ribak, C. E., Vaughn, J. E., Saito, K., Barber, R., and Roberts, E.,** Glutamate decarboxylase localization in neurons of the olfactory bulb, *Brain Res., 126,* 1, 1977.

60. **Kosaka, T., Hataguchi, Y., Hama, K., Nagatsu, I., and Wu, J.-Y.,** Coexistence of immunoreactivities of glutamate decarboxylase and tyrosine hydroxylase in some neurons in the periglomerular region of the rat main olfactory bulb: possible coexistence of GABA and dopamine, *Brain Res., 343,* 166, 1985.

61. **Ribak, C. E., Vaughn, J. E., and Roberts, E.,** GABAergic nerve terminals decrease in the substantia nigra following hemitransections of the striatonigral and pallidonigral pathways, *Brain Res., 192,* 413, 1980.

62. **Oertel, W. H., Tappaz, M. L., Berod, A., and Mugnaini, E.,** Two-color immunohistochemistry for dopamine and GABA neurons in rat substantia nigra and zona incertia, *Brain Res. Bull., 9,* 463, 1982.

63. **Ribak, C. E., Vaughn, J. E., and Roberts, E.,** The GABA neurons and their axon terminals in rat corpus striatum as demonstrated by GAD immunocytochemistry, *J. Comp. Neurol., 187,* 261, 1979.

64. **Bradley, R. H., Kita, S. T., and Wu, J.-Y.,** An immunocytochemical analysis of methionine enkephalin, substance P and glutamic acid decarboxylase within neostriatal neurons, *J. Am. Osteopath. Assoc., 84*(1), 98, 1984.

65. **Bolam, J. P., Powell, J. F., Wu, J.-Y., and Smith, A. D.,** Glutamate decarboxylase-immunoreactive structure in the rat neostriatum. A correlated light and electron microscopic study including a combination of Golgi-impregnation with immunocytochemistry, *J. Comp. Neurol., 237,* 1, 1985.

66. **Murakami, F., Katsumaru, H., Wu, J.-Y., Matsuda, T., and Tsukahara, N.,** Immunocytochemical demonstration of GABAergic synapses on identified rubrospinal neurons, *Brain Res., 267,* 357, 1983.

67. **Katsumaru, H., Murakami, F., Wu, J.-Y., and Tsukahara, N.,** GABAergic intrinsic interneurons in cat red nucleus demonstrated with combined immunocytochemistry and anterograde degeneration method, *Neurosci. Res., 1,* 35, 1984.

68. **Katsumuru, H., Murakami, F., Wu, J.-Y., and Tsukahara, N.,** Sprouting of GABAergic synapses in the red nucleus after lesion of the nucleus interpositus of the cat, *J. Neurosci., 6,* 2864, 1986.

69. **Everitt, B. J., Hökfelt, T., Wu, J.-Y., and Goldstein, M.,** Coexistence of tyrosine hydroxylase-like and gamma-aminobutyric acid-like immunoreactivities in neurons of the arcuate nucleus, *Neuroendocrinology, 39,* 189, 1984.

70. **Köhler, C., Swanson, L. W., Haglund, L., and Wu, J.-Y.,** The cytoarchitecture, histochemistry and projections of the tuberomammillary nucleus in the rat, *Neuroscience, 16,* 85, 1985.

71. **Blomquist, A., Westman, J., Köhler, C., and Wu, J.-Y.,** Immunocytochemical localization of glutamic acid decarboxylase and substance P in the lateral cervical nucleus. A light and electron microscopic study in the cat, *Neurosci. Lett., 56,* 229, 1985.

72. **Shiraishi, T., Senba, E., Tohyama, M., Wu, J.-Y., Kubo, T., and Matsunaga, T.,** Distribution and fine structure of neuronal elements containing glutamate decarboxylase in the rat cochlear nucleus, *Brain Res., 347,* 183, 1985.

73. **Nomura, I., Senba, E., Kubo, T., Shiraishi, T., Matsunaga, T., Tokyama, M., Shiotani, Y. and Wu, J.-Y.,** Neuropeptides and γ-aminobutyric acid in the vestibular nuclei of the rat: an immunohistochemical analysis. I. Distribution, *Brain Res., 311,* 109, 1984.

74. **Westman, J., Blomquist, A., Köhler, C., and Wu, J.-Y.,** Light and electron microscopic localization of glutamic acid decarboxylase and substance P in the dorsal column nuclei of the cat, *Neurosci. Lett., 51,* 347, 1984.

75. **Houser, C., Vaughn, J. E., Barber, R. P., and Roberts, E.,** GABA neurons are the major cell type of the nucleus reticularis thalami, *Brain Res., 200,* 341, 1980.

76. **Oertel, W. H., Nitsch, C., and Mugnaini, E.,** Immunocytochemical demonstration of the GABAergic neurons in rat globus pallidus and nucleus entopeduncularis and their GABAergic innervation, *Adv. Neurol., 40,* 91, 1984.

77. **Hendrickson, A. E., Hunt, S., and Wu, J.-Y.,** Immunocytochemical localization of glutamic aid decarboxylase in monkey striate cortex, *Nature, 292,* 605, 1981.

78. **Somogyi, P., Freund, T., Wu, J.-Y., and Smith, A. D.,** The section Golgi impregnation procedure. II. Immunocytochemical demonstration of glutamate decarboxylase in Golgi-impregnated neurons and in their afferent and efferent synaptic boutons in the visual cortex of the cat, *Neuroscience,* 9, 475, 1983.

79. **Somogyi, P., Hodgson, A. J., Smith, A. D., Nunzi, M. G., Gorio, A., and Wu, J.-Y.,** Different populations of GABAergic neurons in the visual cortex and hippocampus of cat contain somatostatin- or cholecystokinin-immunoreactive material, *J. Neurosci.,* 4, 2590, 1984.

80. **Freund, T. F., Martin, K. A., Smith, A. D., and Somogyi, P.,** Glutamate decarboxylase-immunoreactive terminals of Golgi-impregnated axoaxonic cells and of presumed basket cells in synaptic contact with pyramidal neurons of the cat's visual cortex, *J. Comp. Neurol.,* 221, 263, 1983.

81. **Goldowitz, D., Vincent, S. R., Wu, J.-Y., and Hökfelt, T.,** Immunohistochemical demonstration of plasticity in GABA neurons of the adult rat dentate gyrus, *Brain Res.,* 238, 413, 1982.

82. **Kosaka, T., Hama, K., and Wu, J.-Y.,** GABAergic synaptic boutons in the rat dentate gyrus, *Brain Res.,* 293(2), 353, 1984.

83. **Kosaka, T., Kosaka, K., Tateishi, K., Hamaoka, Y., Yanaihara, N., Wu, J.-Y., and Hama, K.,** GABAergic neurons containing CCK-8-like and or VIP-like immunoreactivities in the rat hippocampus and dentate gyrus, *J. Comp. Neurol.,* 239, 420, 1985.

84. **Seress, L. and Ribak, C. E.,** GABAergic cells in the dentate gyrus appear to be local circuit and projection neurons, *Exp. Brain Res.,* 50, 173, 1983.

85. **Houser, C. R., Lee, M., and Vaughn, J. E.,** Immunocytochemical localization of glutamic acid decarboxylase in normal and deafferented superior colliculus: evidence for reorganization of γ-aminobutyric acid synapses, *J. Neurosci.,* 3, 2030, 1983.

86. **Hendry, S. H., Houser, C. R., Jones, E. G., and Vaughn, J. E.,** Morphological diversity of immunocytochemistry identified GABA neurons in the monkey sensory-motor complex, *J. Neurocytol.,* 12, 639, 1983.

87. **Houser, C. R., Hendry, S. H., Jones, E. G., and Vaughn, J. E.,** Synaptic organization of immunocytochemically identified GABA neurons in the monkey sensory-motor cortex, *J. Neurocytol.,* 12, 617, 1983.

88. **Panula, P., Revuelta, A. V., Cheney, D. L., Wu, J.-Y., and Costa, E.,** An immunohistochemical study on the location of GABAergic neurons in rat septum, *J. Comp. Neurol.,* 222(1), 69, 1984.

89. **Köhler, C., Chan-Palay, V., and Wu, J.-Y.,** Septal neurons containing glutamic acid decarboxylase immunoreactivity project to the hippocampal region in the rat brain, *Anat. Embryol.,* 169, 41, 1984.

90. **Köhler, C. and Chan-Palay, V.,** Distribution of gamma aminobutyric acid containing neurons and terminals in the septal area, *Anat. Embryol.,* 167, 53, 1983.

91. **Vincent, S. R., Hökfelt, T., and Wu, J.-Y.,** GABA neuron systems in hypothalamus and the pituitary gland: immunohistochemical demonstration using antibodies against glutamate decarboxylase, *Neuroendocrinology,* 34, 117, 1982.

92. **Vincent, S. R., Hökfelt, T., Skirboll, L. R., and Wu, J.-Y.,** Hypothalamic GABA neurons project to the neocortex, *Science,* 220, 1309, 1983.

93. **Senba, E., Daddona, P. E., Watanabe, T., Wu, J.-Y., and Nagy, J. L.,** Coexistence of adenosine deaminase, histidine decarboxylase and glutamate decarboxylase in hypothalamic neurons of the rat, *J. Neurosci.,* 5, 3393, 1985.

94. **Tappaz, M. L., Wassef, M., Oertel, W. H., Paut, L., and Pujol, J. F.,** Light- and electron-microscopic immunocytochemistry of glutamic acid decarboxylase (GAD) in the basal hypothalamus: morphological evidence for neuroendocrine γ-aminobutyric (GABA), *Neuroscience,* 9, 271, 1983.

95. **Ribak, C. E., Vaughn, J. E., and Barber, R. P.,** Immunocytochemical localization of GABAergic neurons at the electron microscopical level, *Histochem. J.,* 13, 555, 1981.

96. **Somogyi, P., Smith, A. D., Nunzi, M. G., Gorio, A., Takagi, H., and Wu, J.-Y.,** Glutamate decarboxylase immunoreactivity in the hippocampus of the cat: distribution of immunoreactive synaptic terminals with special reference to the axon initial segments of pyramidal neurons, *J. Neurosci.,* 3, 1450, 1983.

97. **Kunkel, D. D., Hendrickson, A. E., Wu, J.-Y., and Schwartzkroin, P. A.,** Glutamic acid decarboxylase (GAD) immunocytochemistry of developing rabbit hippocampus, *J. Neurosci.,* 6, 541, 1986.

98. **Köhler, C., Wu, J.-Y., and Chan-Palay, V.,** Neurons and terminals in the retrohippocampal region in the rat's brain identified by anti-γ-aminobutyric acid and anti-glutamic acid decarboxylase immunocytochemistry, *Anat. Embryol.,* 173, 35, 1985.

99. **Hendrickson, A. E., Ogren, M. P., Vaughn, J. E., Barber, R. P., and Wu, J.-Y.,** Light and electron microscopic immunocytochemical localization of glutamic acid decarboxylase in monkey geniculate complex: evidence for GABAergic neurons and synapses, *J. Neurosci.,* 3, 1245, 1983.

100. **O'Hara, P. T., Lieberman, A. R., Hunt, S. P., and Wu, J.-Y.,** Neural elements containing glutamic acid decarboxylase (GAD) in the dorsal lateral geniculate nucleus of the rat: immunohistochemical studies by light and electron microscopy, *Neuroscience,* 8(2), 189, 1983.

101. **Huang, B. H. and Wu, J.-Y.,** Ultrastructural studies on catecholaminergic terminals and GABAergic neurons in nucleus tractus solitarii of the medulla oblongata of rat, *Brain Res.,* 302, 57, 1984.

102. **Vincent, S. R., Hökfelt, T., Wu, J.-Y., Elde, R. P., Morgan, L. M., and Kimmel, J. R.,** Immunohistochemical studies of the GABA system in the pancreas, *Neuroendocrinology,* 36, 197, 1983.

103. **Kataoka, Y., Gutman, Y., Guidotti, A., Panula, P., Wroblewski, Y., Cosenza-Murphy, D., Wu, J.-Y., and Costa, E.,** The intrinsic GABAergic system of adrenal chromaffin cells, *Proc. Natl. Acad. Sci. U.S.A.,* 81, 3218, 1984.

104. **Panula, P., Emson, P., and Wu, J.-Y.,** Demonstration of enkephalin-, substance P-, and glutamate decarboxylase-like immunoreactivity in cultured cell derived from newborn rat neostratium, *Histochemistry,* 69, 169, 1980.

105. **Panula, P., Wu, J.-Y., and Emson, P.,** Ultrastructure of GABA-neurons in culture of rat neostratium, *Brain Res.,* 219, 202, 1981.

106. **Panula, P., Wu, J.-Y., Emson, P., and Rechardt, L.,** Demonstration of glutamate decarboxylase-immunoreactive neurons in cultures of rat substantia nigra, *Neurosci. Lett.,* 22, 303, 1981.

107. **Wu, J.-Y.,** Immunochemical characterization and immunohistochemical localization of glutamate decarboxylase and GABA transaminase in peripheral tissues, in *GABAergic Mechanisms in Mammalian Periphery,* Bowery, N. and Erdö, S., Eds., Gedeon Richter, Budapest, 1986, 19.

108. **Chalmers, J. P., White, S. W., Geffen, J. B., and Rush, R.,** The role of central catecholamines in the control of blood pressure through the baroreceptor reflex and the nasopharyngeal reflex in the rabbit, *Prog. Brain Res.,* 47, 85, 1977.

Chapter 8

L-GLUTAMATE(2-OXOGLUTARATE) AMINOTRANSFERASES

Arthur J. L. Cooper

TABLE OF CONTENTS

I. INTRODUCTION

At the outset a brief discussion of nomenclature is in order. The older term for the class of enzymes is "transaminases". However, the term "aminotransferases" is preferred by the Nomenclature Committee of the International Union of Biochemistry. Hence, the latter term is used in the present review with the term transamination used for the actual process of amine transfer. (Some Russian workers employ the word aminopherase.) In the past, the freely reversible nature of most aminotransferases has often led to the use of several names for a given reaction. For example, the enzyme catalyzing the reversible transamination of glutamate with oxaloacetate has variously been referred to as glutamate-aspartate transaminase, glutamate-oxaloacetate transaminase, and aspartate transaminase (aminotransferase). The practice has arisen in which those aminotransferases utilizing glutamate as one of a pair of possible amino acid substrates are given the name of the *other* amino acid substrate, and are listed as such in *Chemical Abstracts*. For example, aspartate-, alanine-, tyrosine-, branched-chain amino acid-, and GABA-aminotransferases each utilize glutamate as the alternative amino donor. This practice of naming aminotransferases for the nonglutamate amino acid of the amino acid substrate pair is followed throughout the review.

For earlier reviews on the general scope of transamination see References 1 to 8. For reviews more weighted toward aspartate aminotransferase (ASPAT) see References 9 to 11. Several chapters on transamination may be found in Reference 12. More recently a book entitled *Transaminases* has been published.[13] The book covers a large number of aminotransferase reactions, the metabolic importance of such enzymes in animals, plants, and microbes, the detailed mechanism of aminotransferase reactions (particularly in reference to mitochondrial and soluble ASPATs), cellular processing of the aminotransferases, and the importance of aminotransferase determinations in human pathology and clinical chemistry. Assay procedures and some limited information on occurrence and metabolic role of the more important glutamate (α-ketoglutarate) utilizing aminotransferases have recently been compiled.[14-20] In the present review emphasis will be placed on the metabolic importance of aminotransferases in mammalian tissues.

II. HISTORICAL BACKGROUND

Several workers in Germany (e.g., Embden, Knoop, and Neubauer) in the early part of this century provided evidence that amino acids and their corresponding α-keto acids are readily interconvertible in vivo. Later Krebs (in 1935) demonstrated that the D- and L-isomers of many amino acids are enzymatically converted to ammonia and the corresponding α-keto acids. Others showed that various tissue preparations oxidized glutamate without formation of ammonia. Needham (in 1930) showed that glutamate and aspartate are converted to succinate by muscle extracts but the total amine nitrogen remained constant. Still other workers in the 1930s showed that oxaloacetate disappeared from liver extracts upon addition of glutamate. Canzanelli et al. (in 1935) found that the α-keto (2-oxo) acid analogue of thyroxine exhibited thyroxine-like activity. By the late 1930s many D-amino acids and α-keto acids had been shown to be able to replace the corresponding L-amino acid in supporting growth of the rat. Moreover, Herbst and Engel discovered nonenzymatic transamination in 1934; boiling solutions of phenylalanine and pyruvate yielded alanine, phenylacetaldehyde, and CO_2. Herbst and Engel even suggested that transamination might be of biological importance.

In retrospect, it is easy to see how the stage was set for the discovery of enzymatic transamination, but it was not until 1937 that Braunstein and co-workers in Russia discovered enzymatic transamination ("Umaminierung"). The Russian workers originally described glutamate-pyruvate and aspartate-pyruvate transaminase reactions but it was soon shown that the latter activity was due to a mixture of ASPAT and alanine aminotransferase (ALAAT). Nevertheless, for a few years it was generally thought that transamination was limited to glutamate, aspartate, alanine, and the corresponding α-keto acids.

By the early 1940s the elegant work of Schoenheimer and colleagues had shown that the amine nitrogen of amino acids is quite labile and that considerable amine transfer occurs among most of the common amino acids in vivo (with the apparent exception of lysine and threonine). At first it was not appreciated that this lability is due in part to the action of aminotransferases. However, by the early 1950s it became apparent from the work of several investigators, particularly Meister, that the scope of the transamination reaction is much wider than at first appreciated. By now more than 100 amino acids are known to participate in enzymatic transamination. It is now well established that aminotransferases (1) are important for the catabolism of certain amino acids, (2) play important roles in the input/output of carbon through the tricarboxylic acid (TCA) cycle and input of nitrogen through the urea cycle, (3) are involved in mitochondrial H shuttles, and (4) help to regulate the metabolism of certain neurotransmitters. (For a more detailed discussion of the historical background and for original references to this section consult Cooper and Meister.[21])

Herbst and Engel correctly deduced that the nonenzymatic transamination reactions involved condensation between amino acid and α-keto acid to yield a Schiff's base, followed by double-bond migration and hydrolysis. Braunstein[22] originally favored such a mechanism for enzyme-catalyzed transamination but also noted that an intermediary might be involved. Subsequently, Snell and colleagues established that vitamin B_6, in the form of pyridoxal 5'-phosphate, was the cofactor involved in all enzymatic transaminations (except in the unusual case of pyridoxamine-alanine aminotransferase). For a fascinating account of the discovery of the importance of pyridoxal 5'-phosphate in many enzyme-catalyzed reactions and a description of model reactions see Reference 23.

III. IMPORTANCE OF AMINOTRANSFERASES FOR THE CATABOLISM OF AMINO ACIDS

A. General Considerations

The custom has long been followed when considering vertebrate metabolism of categorizing amino acids as (1) glucogenic (glycogenic), (2) ketogenic, or (3) mixed glucogenic-ketogenic. The classification which is somewhat artificial depends on whether the amino acid carbon atoms can be incorporated into glucose or into ketone bodies in the liver. Carbon derived from glucogenic amino acids is ultimately converted to pyruvate or to intermediates of the TCA cycle that can act in turn as precursors of phosphoenolpyruvate (PEP). Ketogenisis results in formation of acetyl-CoA (which cannot be directly converted to pyruvate) or to acetoacetate. Alanine, glutamate, and aspartate are clearly glucogenic amino acids on this basis, giving rise by transamination to pyruvate, α-ketoglutarate, and oxaloacetate, respectively.

For many of the common amino acids the first step of catabolism is removal of the α-amine nitrogen. This removal may be brought about by (1) transamination, (2) oxidative deamination, or (3) nonoxidative deamination. The level of L-amino acid oxidase in vertebrates is very low and, except perhaps in the breakdown of lysine, is probably quantitatively unimportant. The glutamate dehydrogenase reaction is thermodynamically poised for net reductive amination of glutamate but it is probable that the reaction generally lies in the direction of net oxidative deamination of glutamate in vivo. Thus, route 2 is only important for glutamate oxidation in vertebrate metabolism. Route 3 only occurs in the special case of threonine and serine, and perhaps cysteine (in some organisms). In the case of the branched-chain amino acids, the first step of catabolism is an obligatory transamination reaction. Valine and isoleucine ultimately are degraded to succinyl-CoA and are thus glucogenic amino acids. Leucine is ultimately degraded to acetyl-CoA and is thus a ketogenic amino acid. Other amino acids are catabolized via several alternative routes, only one of which involves an initial transaminase step. This category of amino acids includes tyrosine and cysteine. In the case of cysteine, pyruvate formation may occur via several routes. In one case cysteine may be transaminated directly to β-mercaptopyruvate which is readily converted to pyruvate; in another route cysteine is converted first to cysteinesulfinate which on transamination (probably catalyzed by ASPAT) is converted to β-sulfinylpyruvate. This compound spontaneously decomposes to pyruvate. (For a review see Reference 24.) Methionine is generally considered to be metabolized largely via a transsulfuration pathway. However, Benevenga and colleagues[25,26] have argued that an alternative (i.e., transaminative) pathway may also be of importance. The product of the initial transamination reaction, α-keto-γ-methiolbutyrate, is ultimately degraded to CO_2 and sulfate. The quantitative importance of this pathway is yet to be determined. Finally, for several amino acids (phenylalanine, lysine, proline, arginine, and histidine) major catabolic routes involve a transamination step that is not the first step of the catabolic process. Lysine is converted via several steps to α-aminoadipate. This amino acid is then transaminated to yield α-ketoadipate which in turn is converted to glutaryl-CoA and finally to acetyl-CoA. Proline, arginine, and histidine carbon is incorporated into glutamate which in term is transaminated to α-ketoglutarate.

A scheme illustrating the importance of aminotransferases in the catabolism of amino acids is given in Figure 1. It may be noted that glutamine and asparagine carbon can enter the TCA cycle either by deamidation followed by transamination or by transamination followed by deamidation. The latter pathway of glutamine breakdown (glutamine transaminase-ω-amidase pathway) is discussed more fully in Chapter 3.

B. Linkage of Glutamate [α-Ketoglutarate(2-Oxoglutarate)-Utilizing] Aminotransferases with Glutamate Dehydrogenase and Purine Nucleotide Cycle

In 1957 Braunstein[27] pointed out that many glutamate-utilizing aminotransferases could be coupled, in theory, to glutamate dehydrogenase (Equations 1 to 3). Such coupled reactions might function to incorporate ammonia into amino acids or to remove ammonia from them. Braunstein coined the words "transreamination" and "transdeamination" to describe the forward and backward reactions of Equation 3, respectively.

$$\alpha\text{-Keto acid} + \text{L-glutamate} \leftrightarrows \text{L-amino acid} + \alpha\text{-ketoglutarate} \tag{1}$$

$$\alpha\text{-Ketoglutarate} + NH_3 + NAD(P)H + H^+ \leftrightarrows \text{L-glutamate} + NAD(P)^+ + H_2O \tag{2}$$

$$\text{Net: } \alpha\text{-Keto acid} + NH_3 + NAD(P)H + H^+ \leftrightarrows \text{L-amino acid} + NAD(P)^+ + H_2O \tag{3}$$

Although the terms "transdeamination" and "transreamination" have not been widely used by biochemists, the inherent ideas have led to much useful work. While there is no question that these reactions occur in vivo the relative importance of these pathways has engendered much discussion.

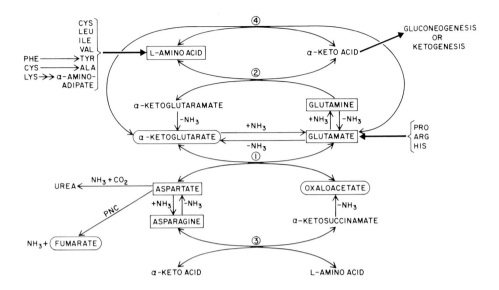

FIGURE 1. Generalized scheme for the catabolism of amino acids, emphasizing the role of transamination. Pivotal amino acids are enclosed in boxes; TCA cycle intermediates are circled. Enzymes are as follows: (1) ASPAT, (2) glutamine aminotransferases, and (3) asparagine aminotransferase. Reaction 4 represents a family of aminotransferases of which alanine-, tyrosine-, and branched-chain amino acid aminotransferases are the most thoroughly studied. PNC: purine nucleotide cycle. Note that the major route for methionine degradation is usually considered to be via the transsulfuration pathway. However, recent evidence suggests that some methionine may also be degraded via a transaminative pathway. (From Cooper, A. J. L. and Meister, A., *Transaminases,* Christen, P. and Metzler, D. E., Eds., 1985, 534. Reprinted by permission of John Wiley & Sons, Inc.©, New York.)

The free-energy change (at pH 7.0) for the NAD^+- and $NADP^+$-linked glutamate dehydrogenase reactions is large (16.5 and 16.7 kcal, respectively)[28-30] suggesting that the glutamate dehydrogenase reaction is poised for net reductive amination of α-ketoglutarate rather than for oxidative deamination. However, it must be remembered that since the reaction is reversible the overall direction of the reaction will depend heavily on the rate at which components of the reaction are removed. Second, the affinity of mammalian glutamate dehydrogenases for ammonia is low (much less than that exhibited by glutamine synthetase) and the concentration of ammonia in mammalian tissues is usually low (50 to 500 μM). Published K_m values for ammonia for rat liver and rat brain glutamate dehydrogenases are 20 and 10 mM, respectively;[31] the apparent K_m value exhibited by sheep brain glutamine synthetase has been reported to be 180 μM.[32] Thus, it is now generally considered that glutamate dehydrogenase plays a catabolic role in the metabolism of glutamate[33,34] and that glutamine synthetase is the major enzyme for the metabolism (detoxification) of extrahepatic ammonia (see Chapter 2).

The most important compound involved in the removal of waste nitrogen is urea. One nitrogen of urea is obtained from ammonia, the other from aspartate (for a comprehensive review see Reference 35). Thus, coupling of the appropriate aminotransferase (Equation 1) with glutamate dehydrogenase (Equation 2) affords a convenient means for the incorporation of amino acid nitrogen into urea. Alternatively, the amino acid nitrogen can be donated to aspartate via coupled transamination reactions to be in turn incorporated into urea. ASPAT (Equation 4) is very active in the liver.

$$\text{L-Amino acid} + \text{α-ketoglutarate} \leftrightharpoons \text{α-keto acid} + \text{L-glutamate} \tag{1}$$

$$\text{L-Glutamate} + \text{oxaloacetate} \leftrightharpoons \text{α-ketoglutarate} + \text{L-aspartate} \tag{4}$$

From the above discussion it is obvious that ASPAT plays an important role in both gluconeogenesis and ureogenesis in the liver but the flux is dependent on a number of factors. As pointed out by several workers, both gluconeogenesis and ureogenesis utilize cytosolic and mitochondrial enzymes and require transport of metabolic anions across the inner mitochondrial membrane. Important enzymes and transport systems involved directly or indirectly in both ureogenesis and gluconeogenesis include ASPAT, soluble and mitochondrial malate dehydrogenases, and the transport systems for malate, α-ketoglutarate, glutamate, and aspartate.[72] Meijer et al.[69] have suggested that perturbation of the oxidation-reduction state of the pyridine nucleotides in specific cellular compartments regulates urea synthesis by altering the concentration of cellular metabolites (e.g., malate and glutamate) and thereby their rate of translocation across mitochondrial membranes. In addition, physicochemical alterations (i.e., changes in enzyme-enzyme interactions) may also play a role in the control of ureogenesis. In liver mitochondria, carbamyl phosphate synthetase I, glutamate dehydrogenase, and mASPAT are important enzymes for the provision of carbamyl phosphate and (some) aspartate for urea synthesis[72,73] (Figure 2). It has recently been reported that mASPAT forms a complex with glutamate dehydrogenase in vitro and the strength of the interaction is affected by a number of small molecular-weight compounds and by carbamyl phosphate synthetase I.[73] Thus, in vivo certain effectors could displace ASPAT from the matrix side of the inner mitochondrial membrane (where the TCA cycle enzymes are juxtaposed) so that it can associate with glutamate dehydrogenase in the matrix. Leucine, carbamyl phosphate synthetase I, ATP, and Mg^{2+} interact synergistically to facilitate glutamate dehydrogenase activity and the interaction between this enzyme and the aminotransferase.[73] Conversely, TCA cycle intermediates, such as citrate and malate, have opposing effects. Therefore, although the components of the ASPAT reaction are in equilibrium, the metabolic fate of the individual components may vary depending on the juxtaposing of the mASPAT with different enzymes.

The redox state of the cell also is probably a controlling factor in gluconeogenesis. Thus, the observation by Cornell et al.[70] that inhibition of gluconeogenesis occurs when ASPAT is inhibited may be explained by a disruption of the malate-aspartate shuttle (see below) and an increase in the lactate/pyruvate ratio.

In conclusion, ASPAT is a key enzyme of gluconeogenesis and ureogenesis in the liver. However, it should be kept in mind that (1) since there are no known allosteric effectors (although there are certainly natural inhibitors of the enzyme) and (2) the reaction is close to equilibrium, it is likely that ASPAT acts as a conduit for the flow of carbon and nitrogen as dictated by metabolic processes that are themselves under more rigid control. Controlling factors include, among others, the redox potential, flux through membrane translocators, and physical positioning of enzymes. The process of gluconeogenesis and ureogenesis from alanine and several other amino acids is coordinated in such a way as to provide maximum conversion of excess nitrogen to nontoxic urea and at the same time to recover as much as possible of the catabolized carbon as metabolically useful glucose.

C. The Malate-Aspartate Shuttle

In 1951, Lehninger[74] showed that intact mitochondria are impermeable to externally added NADH. However, a fraction of the total NADH synthesized by the cell is manufactured in the cytoplasm during glycolysis and transport of reducing equivalents across the inner mitochondrial membrane is required for respiration and a variety of metabolic processes.[75] Various mechanisms for the transfer of reducing equivalents have been proposed (for reviews see References 76 and 77). The first shuttle was described by Estabrook and Sacktor in 1958.[78] These authors proposed that a glycerol-3-phosphate shuttle, consisting simply of cytosolic and mitochondrial forms of glycerol-3-phosphate dehydrogenase, operates in the flight muscle of the housefly, *Musca domesticus*. Apparently, the mitochondrial enzyme is

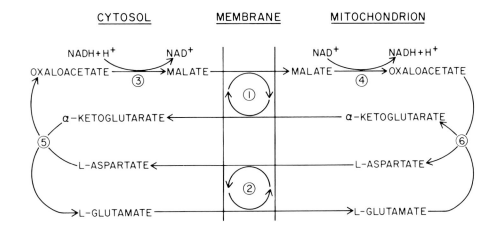

FIGURE 3.   The malate-aspartate shuttle for the transport of reducing equivalents between cytosol and mitochondrion. (1) α-Ketoglutarate-malate carrier, (2) glutamate-aspartate carrier, (3) soluble cytosolic malate dehydrogenase, (4) mitochondrial malate dehydrogenase, (5) cASPAT, and (6) mASPAT. (From Cooper, A. J. L. and Meister, A., *Transaminases,* Christen, P. and Metzler, D. E., Eds., 1985, 534. Reprinted by permission of John Wiley & Sons, Inc.©, New York.)

located on the cytoplasmic side of the inner mitochondrial membrane obviating the need for a carrier.[79] Since mitochondrial glycerol-3-phosphate dehydrogenase is flavin-linked donating electrons to the respiratory chain at the level of Coenzyme Q[79] only two molecules of ATP are potentially generated from each pair of electrons fed into the electron transport chain via this route. However, this linkage overcomes the problem of transporting NADH against a potential gradient and the transfer of reducing equivalents from cytosol to mitochondria is essentially unidirectional. In mammals, the glycerol-3-phosphate shuttle appears to predominate in the rat colon.[80] It is also possible that the shuttle plays a role in ureogenesis (from ammonia and aspartate) in the rat liver (together with mitochondrial glutamate dehydrogenase, soluble malate dehydrogenase, and cASPAT).[69]

The insect flight muscle also contains appreciable soluble and mitochondrial malate dehydrogenase activities so that at least in theory a malate-oxaloacetate shuttle could operate for the transport of reducing equivalents in the insect muscle. However, Sacktor and Dick[81] were unable to document such a shuttle. A simple malate-oxaloacetate shuttle had previously been considered by Bücher and Klingenberg[82] but it is now generally accepted (despite occasional claims to the contrary) that oxaloacetate does not readily traverse the mitochondrial membrane.[83] Later Borst[84] proposed a modification of the original malate-oxaloacetate shuttle in order to take into account the relative impermeability of the inner mitochondrial membrane to oxaloacetate. The shuttle was expanded to include c- and mASPAT and carriers for malate/α-ketoglutarate and glutamate/aspartate exchanges across the inner mitochondrial membrane.

The currently accepted malate-aspartate shuttle is shown in Figure 3. Note that gluconeogenesis in organs, such as the liver, requires a net outflow of malate from the mitochondrion to cytosol.[75] In the operation of the malate-aspartate shuttle an inflow of malate is required for the net oxidation of cytosolic NADH. The mitochondrial NAD$^+$ system is more reduced than the cytosolic system in the rat liver.[85] Efflux of aspartate from the mitochondrion is an obligatory step in the malate-aspartate shuttle, gluconeogenesis from lactate, and in urea synthesis.[86] The translocation of aspartate is by an energy-requiring process.[86] In contrast to the glycerol-3-phosphate shuttle a maximum of three ATPs are potentially available for each pair of electrons shuttled across the membrane via the malate-aspartate shuttle.

Other shuttles for the transport of reducing equivalents have been proposed, such as the fatty acid cycle and malate-citrate cycle (see Reference 76 for a review) but in general it seems that the malate-aspartate shuttle is accepted as the major route for the transport of reducing equivalents in the liver,[76,80,87] kidney,[88] pancreas,[90] and heart.[91,92] However, Hogg and Ottaway[93] suggest that in their perfused heart preparation other shuttles may operate. Rognstad and Katz[88] suggest that in the kidney the malate-aspartate shuttle may control sodium reabsorption by regulating substrate oxidation and the provision of energy.

Only limited studies have been carried out on the brain[94-97] but these studies are consistent with the presence of a malate-aspartate shuttle. More recently, we showed that β-methylene-D,L-aspartate, a suicide inhibitor of ASPAT, strongly inhibited oxygen uptake in rat cerebrocortical tissue slices respiring on glucose; on the other hand, with succinate as the substrate only a small decrease in oxygen consumption was noted.[98] The data strongly suggest that in the rat brain, oxidation of glucose is tightly coupled to transport of reducing equivalents via the malate-aspartate shuttle as previously proposed by Dennis and Clark.[97] The finding that the rate of oxygen consumption in cortical slices respiring on glucose is inhibited in a one-to-one fashion with inhibition of ASPAT[98] was initially unexpected since ASPAT activity in the brain is so high. Similarly, Cornell et al.[70] found that despite the high activity of ASPAT in hepatocytes, a 90% reduction in activity is enough to cause total cessation of glucose production from lactate. Evidence is accumulating that enzymes of the malate-aspartate shuttle and TCA cycle form complexes[98] and we have suggested that, in brain mitochondria, ASPAT is linked to citrate synthase and/or malate dehydrogenase. Such linkages may explain the apparent lack of excess ASPAT despite inherent high activity. A block of ASPAT may cause a stoichiometric block in flux through complexed enzymes.

In conclusion, soluble and mitochondrial ASPATs are crucial for the transport of reducing equivalents between cytoplasm and mitochondrion in most mammalian organs studied thus far. Coupling of mASPAT with mitochondrial malate dehydrogenase, glutamate dehydrogenase, or TCA cycle enzymes may allow for the efficient chaneling of substrates along metabolic pathways as dictated by the needs of the cell.

D. Possible Role in Amino Acid Neurotransmitter Metabolism

Several authors have speculated that ASPAT may play a role in the metabolism of the putative neurotransmitters, aspartate and glutamate. For example, Altschuler et al.[99] showed that ASPAT-like immunoreactivity is pronounced in the axons and terminals of the guinea pig auditory nerve and suggested that the enzyme may be a marker of glutamate and aspartate neurotransmitters. Wenthold[100] showed that ASPAT (and glutaminase) activity was two to five times higher in auditory nerve fibers than in other nerve fibers and suggested a role for this enzyme in the metabolism of neurotransmitter glutamate and aspartate. Recasens and Delaunoy[101] have investigated the role of soluble and mitochondrial cysteinesulfinate aminotransferases (almost certainly c- and mASPAT, respectively[101]) in the metabolism of the putative transmitter, taurine. The authors conclude that mitochondrial cysteinesulfinate aminotransferase is important in regulating taurine levels by providing the precursor, cysteinesulfinate.

Brandon and Lam[102] using an immunocytochemical technique showed that in the retina ASPAT activity is very high in cones (and in putative bipolar and amocrine cells) but much less so in rods. The authors were careful not to suggest that ASPAT was an exclusive marker but did suggest that neurotransmitter glutamate may be metabolized by ASPAT.

Since ASPAT isozymes are intimately associated with metabolic processes and the concentrations of whole brain aspartate and glutamate are high (~2.5 and 12 mM, respectively) it is difficult to assign a specialized role for ASPAT in the removal of small quantities of released neurotransmitter glutamate/aspartate. However, this does not preclude the possibility that ASPAT plays a role in the salvage of neurotransmitter carbon through the TCA cycle, but more work is needed in establishing this possibility.

V. ALANINE AMINOTRANSFERASE

A. Background

ALAAT catalyzes the following reaction:

$$\text{L-Alanine} + \alpha\text{-ketoglutarate} \leftrightarrows \text{pyruvate} + \text{L-glutamate} \tag{27}$$

ALAAT activity is widely distributed in mammalian tissues but its optimal activity tends to be lower than that of ASPAT. In the rat, activity is highest in the liver[103] with smaller amounts in the skeletal muscle,[103] heart,[103] and brain;[104] little activity is present in the rat kidney.[103] The enzyme has been obtained in highly purified form from the rat liver,[105] pig heart,[106] and beef heart[107] and the mechanism of the reaction has been extensively studied. The pig heart enzyme exhibits a single band on starch gel electrophoresis[106] whereas the rat liver enzyme exhibits two bands (possibly due to subforms) on polyacrylamide gels.[105] The rat liver enzyme is a dimer ~114,000 mol wt) and contains one pyridoxal 5′-phosphate molecule per monomer. ALAAT activity is overwhelmingly (~90%) located in the cytosol in the rat liver and pig heart.[105,106] Nevertheless, a mitochondrial ALAAT of relatively low activity appears to be present in the rat liver.[108] A distinct mitochondrial enzyme has been purified from the pig kidney.[109] Interestingly, although mitochondrial ALAAT activity is low in rat tissues, most of the total ALAAT activity of the porcine, ovine, and bovine liver and kidney is mitochondrial while in avian species it is uniquely mitochondrial.[110] The relationship of the mitochondrial enzyme to the soluble enzyme is not clear although the narrow substrate specificity of the mitochondrial enzyme would seem to suggest that it is indeed primarily concerned with catalyzing the reaction depicted by Equation 27. Swick et al.[108,110] suggest that the mitochondrial enzyme is responsible for the net conversion of alanine to pyruvate in certain gluconeogenic organs whereas the soluble enzyme is responsible for net formation of alanine (see below). Both rat liver enzymes are inducible by corticosteroids.[108,111]

The reaction catalyzed by ALAAT (Equation 27) is freely reversible. Krebs[60] reported an apparent equilibrium constant (k_{eq}) (i.e., [α-ketoglutarate][L-alanine])/[L-glutamate][pyruvate]) of 1.5 at pH 7.4, 25°C. Williamson et al.[61] report that in the rat liver K_{app} under various conditions averages 0.53 (range 0.39 to 0.64) and the reactants appear to be at steady state. Since this K_{app} value is different from the true thermodynamic equilibrium position it is possible that the reactants in the rat liver (unlike those of ASPAT) are not in thermodynamic equilibrium. However, the authors consider it more likely that the discrepancy betweeen the two values is due to compartmentation of components of ALAAT in vivo.

B. Metabolic Importance

As indicated above, alanine has long been recognized as a major gluconeogenic and ureogenic substrate in the rat liver. Obviously, ALAAT activity will provide pyruvate for the sequence: pyruvate → oxaloacetate → phosphoenolpyruvate → glucose. The details deserve some comment. DeRosa and Swick[110] have pointed out that PEP carboxykinase is present in cytosol and mitochondrial in varying ratios depending on the organ and species; cALAAT appears to be present only in those gluconeogenic organs in which PEP carboxykinase is also present in the same compartment. According to DeRosa and Swick,[110] (1) mALAAT is important for the net conversion of alanine to pyruvate when PEP carboxykinase is either soluble or mitochondrial, (2) neither cALAAT nor mALAAT is involved in gluconeogenesis from lactate when PEP carboxykinase is mitochondrial, and (3) both c- and mALAAT are important for gluconeogenesis from lactate when PEP carboxykinase is cytosolic. According to DeRosa and Swick, the components of the ALAAT reaction are such

$$\text{Oxaloacetate} + \text{acetyl-CoA} + H_2O \leftrightarrows \text{citrate} + \text{CoASH} + H^+ \tag{31}$$

$$\text{Citrate} (\rightarrow\text{isocitrate}) + \text{NAD}^+ \rightarrow \alpha\text{-ketoglutarate} + CO_2 + \text{NADH} + H^+ \tag{32}$$

Net: $2\ \text{L-Alanine} + 3\ \text{NAD}^+ + 2\ \text{ATP} + 2\ H_2O \rightarrow$

$$\text{L-glutamine} + 3\ \text{NADH} + CO_2 + 2\ \text{ADP} + 2\ P_i + 6\ H^+ \tag{33}$$

The interactions between glutamine and alanine metabolism are clearly complex but the above discussion provides ample evidence for the crucial roles of aminotransferases. It is interesting that waste nitrogen from the breakdown of amino acids in the muscle or from ammonia produced during vigorous exercise is transported as nontoxic glutamine and alanine to other organs where they are made use of for gluconeogenesis or for other reactions.

VI. BRANCHED-CHAIN AMINO ACID AMINOTRANSFERASES

A. Background
BCAAT enzymes catalyze the following reactions (Equations 34 to 36):

$$\text{L-Leucine} + \alpha\text{-ketoglutarate} \leftrightarrows \alpha\text{-ketoisocaproate} + \text{L-glutamate} \tag{34}$$

$$\text{L-Valine} + \alpha\text{-ketoglutarate} \leftrightarrows \alpha\text{-ketoisovalerate} + \text{L-glutamate} \tag{35}$$

$$\text{L-Isoleucine} + \alpha\text{-ketoglutarate} \leftrightarrows \alpha\text{-keto-}\beta\text{-methylvalerate} + \text{L-glutamate} \tag{36}$$

The activities are well represented in most mammalian tissues although the activity in the rat liver is somewhat low. There are at least two types of BCAATs in rat tissues each present in distinct cytosolic and mitochondrial forms. In addition, there appear to be several other enzymes capable of transaminating the branched-chain amino acids with various α-keto acid acceptors. Since many of these enzymes possess a broad specificity, it is not certain what their role is in branched-chain amino acid metabolism.[17,133]

Pig heart BCAAT was independently purified by Ichihara and Koyama[134] and Taylor and Jenkins[135] in 1966. It has a molecular weight of 75,000 and contains 1 mol of bound pyridoxal 5′-phosphate per 75,000 g.[135] The enzyme contains eight cysteines and is activated by 2-mercaptoethanol.[136] The enzyme is most active with valine, leucine, and isoleucine and only slightly active with methionine, norleucine, and norvaline. It utilizes α-ketoglutarate but not pyruvate as an α-keto acid acceptor.

B. Metabolic Importance
The importance of BCAATs for the net synthesis of alanine and glutamine in the muscle has already been discussed. A few other points concerning interorgan cooperativity of branched-chain amino acids are in order. In the muscle, following transamination of the branched-chain amino acids with α-ketoglutarate the corresponding α-keto acids are released in part to be reaminated in the kidney and other organs. Tracer studies have shown considerable recycling of carbon skeletons between branched-chain amino acids and the corresponding α-keto acids in vivo both in the rat and in man.[128] As Harper et al.[128] point out, reamination of branched-chain α-keto acids with transport of both substrate and product among tissues can serve as a mechanism for conservation of nutritionally indispensable branched-chain amino acid carbon skeletons.

VII. TYROSINE AMINOTRANSFERASE

A. Background

Tyrosine aminotransferase (TYRAT) catalyzes the following reaction (Equation 37):

$$\text{L-Tyrosine} + \alpha\text{-ketoglutarate} \leftrightarrows p\text{-hydroxyphenylpyruvate} + \text{L-glutamate} \qquad (37)$$

The enzyme is confined largely to the cytoplasm of liver cells. Although mTYRATs have been reported, the best evidence suggests that this activity is largely due to mASPAT (see above and References 54 and 137). Other reported cytoplasmic TYRATs are also probably largely due to cASPAT.[137]

The K_{eq} for Equation 37, i.e., ([p-hydroxyphenylpyruvate][L-glutamate])/([L-tyrosine][α-ketoglutarate]), has been reported as 0.73.[138] Jacoby and La Du[139] studied the specificity of a 6500-fold purified TYRAT from the rat liver. The activity toward L-aromatic amino acids was found to be in the order: tyrosine > 3 -iodotyrosine > 3,4-dihydroxyphenylalanine > phenylalanine > tryptophan. Rat liver TYRAT has been purified to homogeneity[140] and contains three subforms (I to III). Each of these subforms is immunologically and kinetically indistinguishable. Subform I (native enzyme) is a dimer with a subunit molecular weight of 53,000; subform III is a dimer with a subform molecular weight of 49,000; subform II is comprised of one subunit of molecular weight 53,000 and one of molecular weight 49,000. Apparently, 4000 mol wt fragments can successively be cleaved during initial fractionation of the enzyme.

B. Metabolic Importance

This aspect has been extensively reviewed by Hargrove and Granner.[141] A brief summary follows: TYRAT is the first enzyme of the major catabolic pathway of tyrosine, ultimately leading to the glucogenic and ketogenic compounds, fumarate and acetoacetate, respectively. Since the K_{eq} is close to unity, the enzyme can in theory synthesize or degrade tyrosine. However, concentrations of substrates in the liver are such that the enzyme degrades tyrosine. Under normal conditions TYRAT activity appears to be rate limiting in the pathway for tyrosine breakdown. This limitation is compounded by the rather weak binding of pyridoxal 5'-phosphate; estimates of inactive apoenzyme in vivo range from 20 to 60%. Interestingly, TYRAT is greatly inducible. On induction by hydrocortisone TYRAT activity is no longer rate limiting for tyrosine breakdown. TYRAT activity is also increased by feeding rats high protein diets; activity is very low in the liver of low-protein fed rats or rats administered glucose. In addition TYRAT activity exhibits a diurnal rhythm that coincides with feeding.

As Granner and Hargrove further point out, since the changes in TYRAT activity in the adult rat liver all follow changes in nutritional or related hormonal status, it is likely that the hormonal regulation evolved in response to nutritional needs. Although tyrosine is one of the nine amino acids taken up from the blood by the liver during postabsorptive gluco-neogenesis, it is not a major gluconeogenic precursor since it is of relatively low concentration in the liver, plasma, and muscle. A possible explanation for the induction of TYRAT in the liver is to prevent a build-up of tyrosine which, at elevated concentrations, is known to be toxic in the adult and neonate. Tyrosine is also a precursor of catecholamines in the brain and it may be disadvantageous to the animal to allow an excessive influx of tyrosine into the brain.

Finally, Hargrove and Granner discuss factors that promote an increase in and regulation of TYRAT activity in vivo. The interested reader is referred to Reference 141.

reaction. In this sense, the ASPATs will play a role, albeit a passive one, in this recycling of neurotransmitter carbon; this role is probably subordinate to the metabolic roles of c- and mASPAT. GABAAT also plays a link in this recycling process but, in this case, a directionality is imposed by the conversion of succinic semialdehyde to succinate. Thus, unlike the ASPATs the major metabolic function of GABAAT in the brain is probably to promote recycling of neurotransmitter carbon.

X. OTHER MAMMALIAN GLUTAMATE-LINKED AMINOTRANSFERASES

Just how many discrete glutamate (α-ketoglutarate)-linked aminotransferases there are in mammalian organs remains unknown. This confusion is a result of overlap in specificities of several aminotransferases and the failure of several authors to fully test the specificity of their preparations. For the most up-to-date classification of aminotransferases see References 13 and 14. A few points concerning the mammalian glutamate aminotransferases will be noted here. As noted earlier in the text, m- and cASPAT are active with the aromatic amino acids. These enzymes are also apparently identical to mitochondrial and cytosolic cysteinesulfinate aminotransferases. Mitochondrial cysteine aminotransferase (Equation 47) is identical to mASPAT.[195] However, a cysteine aminotransferase apparently distinct from ASPAT has been purified from the rat liver.[196]

$$\text{L-Cysteine} + \alpha\text{-ketoglutarate} \rightleftarrows \beta\text{-mercaptopyruvate} + \text{L-glutamate} \qquad (47)$$

L-Methionine aminotransferase activity is well represented in rat liver extracts but the activity seems to be closely associated with leucine aminotransferases. Ikeda et al.[197] have isolated leucine (methionine) aminotransferases from the cytosolic and mitochondrial fractions of the rat liver.

An unusual aminotransferase present in many rabbit organs was purified from the liver and characterized by Soffer et al.[198] This enzyme was found to catalyze transamination between α-ketoglutarate and a number of thyronine analogues. Curiously *both* the K_m and V_{max} for the substrates increased in the following order: L-triiodothyronine > L-thyroxine > 3,5-diiodo-L-tyrosine > 3-iodo-L-tyrosine > 3,5-dinitro-L-tyrosine. To some extent α-ketoglutarate could by replaced by oxaloacetate or pyruvate, except curiously in the case of 3,5-dinitro-L-tyrosine where they were ineffective. Somewhat earlier, Nakano[199] had purified a hologenated TYRAT from sonicated rat kidney mitochondria and confirmed its identity with thyroid hormone aminotransferase. Tyrosine analogues with halogen (I, Br, and Cl) substituents in both the 3 and 5 position of the ring were found to be the most active substrates. Later Tobes and Mason[200] purified an α-aminoadipate aminotransferase (Equation 48) from the soluble fraction of rat kidneys and showed that the enzyme also catalyzes a kynurenine aminotransferase reaction (Equations 49 and 50).

$$\text{L-}\alpha\text{-Aminoadipate} + \alpha\text{-ketoglutarate} \rightleftarrows \alpha\text{-ketoadipate} + \text{L-glutamate} \qquad (48)$$

$$\text{L-Kynurenine} + \alpha\text{-ketoglutarate} \rightleftarrows O\text{-aminobenzoylpyruvate} + \text{L-glutamate} \qquad (49)$$

$$O\text{-Aminobenzoylpyruvate} \xrightarrow{\text{spontaneous}} \text{kynurenic acid} \qquad (50)$$

The authors later showed that this enzyme, purified from the soluble fraction of the rat kidney, was also almost certainly identical to the halogenated TYRAT purified by Nakano. Kynurenine (α-aminoadipate, halogenated tyrosine) aminotransferase activity was also shown to be present in the mitochondria.[201] The identification of mitochondrial α-aminoadipate with kynurenine aminotransferase has been confirmed by Takeuchi et al.[202]

A hypotaurine aminotransferase has been shown to be present in the mouse liver.[203] (Equations 51 and 52); activity with pyruvate was reported to be greater than that with α-ketoglutarate.

$$\text{Hypotaurine } + \text{ pyruvate } (\alpha\text{-ketoglutarate}) \; \rightleftarrows$$

$$\text{sulfinoacetaldehyde } + \text{ L-alanine (L-glutamate)} \qquad (51)$$

$$\text{Sulfinoacetaldehyde } \xrightarrow{\text{spontaneous}} \text{acetaldehyde } + \text{ sulfite} \qquad (52)$$

Fellman and Roth[204] later reported hypotaurine aminotransferase activity to be present in the heavy mitochondrial fraction of both the rat liver and brain. Unlike the liver enzyme the brain enzyme is only active with α-ketoglutarate as an amine acceptor. Whether the hypotaurine aminotransferases are distinct enzymes remains to be determined.

XI. CONCLUSIONS

Transaminase activity is widespread in all mammalian organs. In many cases catabolism of amino acids is linked to glutamate (α-ketoglutarate) aminotransferases. The α-keto acid thus generated can often be further processed to provide metabolically useful fuel. At the same time the nitrogen can be linked to the glutamate dehydrogenase reaction or ASPAT reaction in the liver to generate precursors of urea nitrogen. Alternatively, the ammonia generated from the linked aminotransferase-glutamate dehydrogenase reaction can serve as a source of glutamine (amide) nitrogen. Glutamine nitrogen in turn is used for the biosynthesis of many useful metabolites and the carbon backbone is a fuel in some organs. Glutamine is also a temporary store of nitrogen that is eventually incorporated into urea. Thus, the transaminases are important for the maintenance of whole body nitrogen homeostasis and various interorgan nutritional cycles. In addition, aminotransferases have more specialized roles in (1) amino acid neurotransmitter metabolism and (2) the transport of reducing equivalents across the inner mitochondrial membrane.

ACKNOWLEDGMENTS

Some of the work cited from the author's laboratory was supported by U.S. Public Health Service Grant DK-16739. I thank Carol Hopkins for preparing the manuscript and Dr. James C. K. Lai for his helpful suggestions.

REFERENCES

1. **Herbst, R. M.,** The transamination reaction, *Adv. Enzymol.,* 4, 75, 1944.
2. **Braunstein, A. E.,** Transamination and the integrative functions of the dicarboxylic acids in nitrogen metabolism, *Adv. Protein Chem.,* 3, 1, 1947.
3. **Heyns, K.,** The importance of transamination in metabolic processes (in German), *Angew. Chem.,* 61, 474, 1949.
4. **Cohen, P. P.,** Transaminases, in *The Enzymes,* Vol. 1, 1st ed., Sumner, J. B. and Myrback, K., Eds., Academic Press, New York, 1951, 1040.
5. **Meister, A.,** Transamination in amino acid metabolism, *Fed. Proc., Fed. Am. Soc. Exp. Biol.,* 14, 683, 1955.
6. **Meister, A.,** Transamination, *Adv. Enzymol.,* 16, 185, 1955.

7. **Meister, A.,** *The Biochemistry of the Amino Acids,* 2nd ed., Academic Press, New York, 1965, 338.
8. **Braunstein, A. E.,** Milestones in studies of transaminase functions, structure and catalytic functions (in Russian), *Mol. Biol. (USSR),* 11, 1238, 1977.
9. **Ivanov, V. I. and Karpiesky, M. Ya.,** Dynamic three-dimensional model for enzymic transamination, *Adv. Enzymol.,* 32, 21, 1969.
10. **Braunstein, A. E.,** Binding and reactions of the vitamin B_6 coenzyme in the catalytic center of aspartate aminotransferase, *Vit. Horm.,* 22, 451, 1964.
11. **Braunstein, A. E.,** Amino group transfer, in *The Enzymes,* Vol. 9, 3rd ed., Boyer, P. D., Ed., Academic Press, New York, 1973, 379.
12. **Snell, E. E., Braunstein, A. E., Severin, E. S., and Torchinsky, Yu. M., Eds.,** Pyridoxal catalysis: enzymes and model systems, in *Proc. 2nd Int. Symp. Chem. Biol. Aspects of Pyridoxal Catalysis,* Interscience, New York, 1968.
13. **Christen, P. and Metzler, D. E., Eds.,** *Transaminases,* John Wiley & Sons, New York, 1985.
14. **Cooper, A. J. L.,** L-Glutamate-L-amino acid transaminases, *Methods Enzymol.,* 113, 63, 1985.
15. **Cooper, A. J. L.,** Glutamate-aspartate transaminase, *Methods Enzymol.,* 113, 66, 1985.
16. **Cooper, A. J. L.,** Glutamate-alanine transaminase, *Methods Enzymol.,* 113, 69, 1985.
17. **Cooper, A. J. L.,** Glutamate-branched chain amino acid transaminases, *Methods Enzymol.,* 113, 71, 1985.
18. **Cooper, A. J. L.,** Glutamate-aromatic amino acid transaminase, *Methods Enzymol.,* 113, 73, 1985.
19. **Cooper, A. J. L.,** Glutamate-ornithine transaminases, *Methods Enzymol.,* 113, 76, 1985.
20. **Cooper, A. J. L.,** Glutamate-γ-aminobutyrate transaminase, *Methods Enzymol.,* 113, 80, 1985.
21. **Cooper, A. J. L. and Meister, A.,** Metabolic significance of transamination, in *Transaminases,* Christen, P. and Metzler, D. E., Eds., John Wiley & Sons, New York, 1985, 534.
22. **Braunstein, A. E.,** Transamination and transaminases, in *Transaminases,* Christen, P. and Metzler, D. E., Eds., John Wiley & Sons, New York, 1985, 1.
23. **Snell, E. E.,** Pyridoxal phosphate in nonenzymic and enzymic reactions, in *Transaminases,* Christen, P. and Metzler, D. E., Eds., John Wiley & Sons, New York, 1985, 19.
24. **Cooper, A. J. L.,** Biochemistry of sulfur-containing amino acids, *Annu. Rev. Biochem.,* 52, 187, 1983.
25. **Case, G. L. and Benevenga, N. J.,** Significance of formate as an intermediate in the oxidation of the methionine, S-methyl-L-cysteine and sarcosine methyl carbons to CO_2 in the rat, *J. Nutr.,* 107, 1665, 1977.
26. **Steele, R. D. and Benevenga, N. J.,** Identification of 3-methylthiopropionic acid as an intermediate in mammalian methionine metabolism *in vitro, J. Biol. Chem.,* 253, 7844, 1978.
27. **Braunstein, A. E.,** Les voies principales de l'assimilation et dissimilation de l'azote chez les animaux, *Adv. Enzymol.,* 19, 335, 1957.
28. **Strecker, H. J.,** Glutamic dehydrogenase, *Arch. Biochem. Biophys.,* 46, 128, 1953.
29. **Burton, K. and Krebs, M. A.,** The tricarboxylic acid cycle. XII. The free energy changes associated with individual steps of the cycle, in *Metabolic Pathways,* Vol. 1, Greenberg, D. M., Ed., Academic Press, New York, 1960, 187.
30. **Lowenstein, J. M.,** The tricarboxylic acid cycle, in *Metabolic Pathways,* Vol. 1, 3rd ed., Greenberg, D. M., Ed., Academic Press, New York, 1967, 146.
31. **Chee, P. Y., Dahl, J. L., and Fahien, L. A.,** The purification and properties of rat brain glutamate dehydrogenase, *J. Neurochem.,* 33, 53, 1979.
32. **Pamiljans, V., Krishnaswamy, P. R., Dumville, G., and Meister, A.,** Studies on the mechanism of glutamine synthesis; isolation and properties of the enzyme from sheep brain, *Biochemistry,* 1, 153, 1962.
33. **Krebs, H. A. and Lund, P.,** Aspects of the regulation of the metabolism of branched-chain amino acids, *Adv. Enzyme Regul.,* 15, 375, 1977.
34. **Krebs, H. A., Hems, R., Lund, P., Halliday, D., and Read, W. W. C.,** Sources of ammonia for mammalian urea synthesis, *Biochem. J.,* 176, 733, 1978.
35. **Ratner, S.,** Enzymes of arginine and urea synthesis, *Adv. Enzymol.,* 39, 1, 1972.
36. **Lowenstein, J. M.,** Ammonia production in muscle and other tissues: the purine nucleotide cycle, *Physiol. Rev.,* 52, 382, 1972.
37. **Lowenstein, J. M. and Goodman, M. N.,** The purine nucleotide cycle in skeletal muscle, *Fed. Proc., Fed. Am. Soc. Exp. Biol.,* 37, 2308, 1978.
38. **Martinez-Carrion, M., Turano, C., Chiancone, E., Bossa, F., Giartosio, A., Riva, F., and Fasella, P.,** Isolation and characterization of multiple forms of glutamate-aspartate aminotransferase from pig heart, *J. Biol. Chem.,* 242, 2397, 1967.
39. **Shrawder, E. and Martinez-Carrion, M.,** Evidence of phenylalanine transaminase activity in the isoenzymes of aspartate transaminase, *J. Biol. Chem.,* 247, 2486, 1972.
40. **Wada, H. and Morino, Y.,** Comparative studies on glutamic-oxalacetic transaminases from mitochondrial and soluble fractions of mammalian tissues, *Vit. Horm. (N.Y.),* 22, 411, 1964.
41. **Marino, G., Greco, A. M., Scardi, V., and Zito, R.,** Purification and general properties of aspartate aminotransferase of ox heart, *Biochem. J.,* 99, 589, 1966.

42. **Krista, M. L. and Fonda, M. L.,** Beef brain cytoplasmic aspartate aminotransferase. Purification, kinetics and physical properties, *Biochim. Biophys. Acta,* 309, 83, 1973.

43. **Teranishi, H., Kagamiyama, H., Teranishi, K., Wada, H., Yamano, T., and Morino, Y.,** Cytosolic and mitochondrial isoenzymes of glutamic-oxaloacetic transaminase from human heart. Structural comparison with the isoenzymes from pig heart, *J. Biol. Chem.,* 253, 8842, 1978.

44. **Campos-Cavieres, M. and Munn, E. A.,** Purification and some properties of cytoplasmic aspartate aminotransferase from sheep liver, *Biochem. J.,* 135, 683, 1973.

45. **Magee, S. C. and Phillips, A. T.,** Molecular properties of the multiple aspartate aminotransferases purified from rat brain, *Biochemistry,* 10, 3397, 191.

46. **Huynh, Q. H., Sakakibara, R., Watanabe, T., and Wada, H.,** Glutamic oxaloacetic transaminase isozymes from rat liver. Purification and physiochemical characterization, *J. Biochem. (Tokyo),* 88, 231, 1980.

47. **Michuda, C. M. and Martinez-Carrion, M.,** Mitochondrial aspartate transaminase. II. Isolation and characterization of the multiple forms, *Biochemistry,* 8, 1095, 1969.

48. **Orlacchio, A., Campos-Cavieres, M., Pashev, I., and Munn, E. A.,** Some kinetic and other properties of the isoenzymes of aspartate aminotransferase isolated from sheep liver, *Biochem. J.,* 177, 583, 1979.

49. **Ovchinnikov, Yu. A., Egorov, C. A., Aldanova, N. A., Feigina, M. Yu., Lipkin, V. M., Abdulaev, N. G., Grishin, E. V., Kiselev, A. P., Modyanov, N. N., Braunstein, A. E., Polyanovsky, O. L., and Nosikov, V. V.,** The complete amino acid sequence of cytoplasmic aspartate aminotransferase from pig heart, *FEBS Lett.,* 29, 31, 1973.

50. **Barra, D., Bossa, F., Doonan, S., Fahmy, H. M. A., Hughes, G. J., Kakoz, K. Y., Martini, F., and Petruzzeli, R.,** The structure of mitochondrial aspartate aminotransferase from pig heart and comparison with that of the cytoplasmic isozyme, *FEBS Lett.,* 83, 24, 1977.

51. **Kagamiyama, H., Sakakibara, R., Wada, H., Tanase, S., and Morino, Y.,** The complete amino acid sequence of mitochondrial aspartate aminotransferase from pig heart, *J. Biochem. (Tokyo),* 82, 291, 1977.

52. **Huynh, Q. K., Sakakibara, R., Watanabe, T., and Wada, H.,** Primary structure of mitochondrial glutamic oxaloacetic transaminase from rat liver: comparison with that of the pig heart isozyme, *Biochem. Biophys. Res. Commun.,* 97, 474, 1980.

53. **Novogrodsky, A. and Meister, A.,** Specificity and resolution of glutamate-aspartate transaminase, *Biochim. Biophys. Acta,* 81, 605, 1964.

54. **Miller, J. E. and Litwack, G.,** Purification, properties, and identity of liver mitochondrial tyrosine aminotransferase, *J. Biol. Chem.,* 246, 3234, 1971.

55. **Noguchi, T., Nakatani, M., Minatogawa, Y., Okuno, E., and Kido, R.,** Cerebral aromatic aminotransferase, *J. Neurochem.,* 25, 579, 1975.

56. **Minatogawa, Y., Noguchi, T., and Kido, R.,** Purification, characterization and identification of tryptophan aminotransferase from rat brain, *J. Neurochem.,* 27, 1097, 1976.

57. **King, S. and Phillips, A. T.,** Aromatic aminotransferase activity of rat brain cytoplasmic and mitochondrial aspartate aminotransferases, *J. Neurochem.,* 30, 1399, 1978.

58. **Herzfeld, A. and Greengard, O.,** Aspartate aminotransferase in rat tissues: changes with growth and hormones, *Biochim. Biophys. Acta,* 237, 88, 1971.

59. **Henson, C. P. and Cleland, W. W.,** Kinetic studies of glutamic oxaloacetic transaminase isozymes, *Biochemistry,* 3, 338, 1964.

60. **Krebs, H. A.,** Equilibria in transamination systems, *Biochem. J.,* 54, 82, 1953.

61. **Williamson, D. H., Lopes-Vieira, O., and Walker, B.,** Concentration of free glucogenic amino acids in livers of rats subjected to various metabolic stresses, *Biochem. J.,* 104, 497, 1967.

62. **Howse, D. C. and Duffy, T. E.,** Control of the redox state of the pyridine nucleotides in the rat cerebral cortex. Effect of electroshock-induced seizures, *J. Neurochem.,* 24, 935, 1975.

62a. **Cooper, A. J. L., Nieves, E., and Gelbard, A. S., Coleman, A. E., Filc-DeRicco, S., and Gelbard, A. S.,** Short-term metabolic fate of [^{13}N]ammonia in rat liver *in vivo, J. Biol. Chem.,* 262, 1073, 1987.

63. **Müller, A. E. and Leuthardt, F.,** Conversion of glutamic acid to aspartic acid in the mitochondria of the liver, *Helv. Chim. Acta,* 33, 268, 1950.

64. **Krebs, H. A. and Bellamy, D.,** The interconversion of glutamic acid and aspartic acid in respiring tissues, *Biochem. J.,* 75, 523, 1950.

65. **De Haan, E. J., Tager, J. M., and Slater, E. C.,** Factors affecting the pathway of glutamate oxidation in rat-liver mitochondria, *Biochim. Biophys. Acta,* 131, 1, 1967.

66. **Papa, S., Tager, J. M., Francavilla, A., DeHaan, E. J., and Quagliarello, E.,** Control of glutamate dehydrogenase activity during glutamate oxidation in isolated rat-liver mitochondria, *Biochim. Biophys. Acta,* 131, 14, 1967.

67. **Ratner, S.,** Urea synthesis and metabolism of arginine and citrulline, *Adv. Enzymol.,* 15, 319, 1954.

68. **Krebs, H. A., Hems, R., and Lund, P.,** Some regulatory mechanisms in the synthesis of urea in the mammalian liver, *Adv. Enzyme Regul.,* 11, 361, 1973.

69. **Meijer, A. J., Gimpel, J. A., DeLeeuw, G. A., Tager, J. M., and Williamson, J. R.,** Role of anion translocation across the mitochondrial membrane in the regulation of urea synthesis from ammonia in isolated rat hepatocytes, *J. Biol. Chem.,* 250, 7728, 1975.

70. **Cornell, N. W., Zuurendonk, P. F., Kerich, M. J., and Straight, C. B.,** Selective inhibition of alanine aminotransferase and aspartate aminotransferase in rat hepatocytes, *Biochem. J.,* 220, 707, 1984.

71. **Smith, S. B. and Freedland, R. A.,** Functional inhibition of cytosolic and mitochondrial aspartate aminotransferase by L-2-amino-4-methoxy-*trans*-3-butenoic acid in isolated rat hepatocytes and mitochondria, *Arch. Biochem. Biophys.,* 209, 335, 1981.

72. **Meijer, A. J., Gimpel, J.A., DeLeeuw, G., Tischler, M.E., Tager, J.M., and Williamson, J.R.,** Interrelationships between gluconeogenesis and ureogenesis in isolated hepatocytes, *J. Biol. Chem.,* 253, 2308, 1978.

73. **Fahien, L. A., Kmiotek, E. H., Woldegiorgis, G., Evenson, M., Shrago, E., and Marshall, M.,** Regulation of aminotransferase-glutamate dehydrogenase interactions by carbamyl phosphate synthase-I, Mg^{2+} plus leucine *versus* citrate and malate, *J. Biol. Chem.,* 260, 6069, 1985.

74. **Lehninger, A. L.,** Phosphorylation coupled to oxidation of dihydrodiphosphopyridine nucleotide, *J. Biol. Chem.,* 190, 345, 1951.

75. **Krebs, H. A.,** Mitochondrial generation of reducing power, in *Biochemistry of Mitochondria,* Slater, E. C., Kaniuga, Z., and Wajtczak, L., Eds., Academic Press, London, 1967, 105.

76. **Meijer, A. J. and Van Dam, K.,** The metabolic significance of anion transport in mitochondria, *Biochim. Biophys. Acta,* 346, 213, 1974.

77. **Dawson, A. G.,** Oxidation of cytosolic NADH formed during aerobic metabolism in mammalian cells, *TIBS,* 4, 171, 1979.

78. **Estabrook, R. W. and Sacktor, B.,** α-Glycerophosphate oxidase of flight muscle mitochondria, *J. Biol. Chem.,* 233, 1014, 1958.

79. **Klingenberg, M.,** Localization of the glycerol-phosphate dehydrogenase in the outer phase of the mitochondrial inner membrane, *Eur. J. Biochem.,* 13, 247, 1970.

80. **Alderman, J. A. and Schiller, C. M.,** Reducing equivalent transport by substrate shuttles in rat liver and colon, *Comp. Biochem. Physiol. B,* 70, 209, 1981.

81. **Sacktor, B. and Dick, A.,** Pathways of hydrogen transport in the oxidation of extramitochondrial reduced diphosphopyridine nucleotide in flight muscle, *J. Biol. Chem.,* 237, 3259, 1962.

82. **Bücher, Th. and Klingenberger, M.,** Wege des wasserstoffs in der lebendigen organisation, *Angew. Chem.,* 70, 552, 1958.

83. **Haslam, J. M. and Krebs, H. A.,** The permeability of mitochondria to oxaloacetate and malate, *Biochem. J.,* 107, 659, 1968.

84. **Borst, P.,** Hydrogen transport and transport metabolites, in *Functionelle und Morphologische Organisation der Zelle,* Karlson, P., Ed., Springer-Verlag, Berlin, 1963, 137.

85. **Williamson, D. H., Lund, P., and Krebs, H. A.,** The redox state of free nicotinamide-adenine dinucleotide in the cytoplasm and mitochondria of rat liver, *Biochem. J.,* 103, 514, 1967.

86. **Murphy, E., Coll, K. E., Viale, R. O., Tischler, M. E., and Williamson, J. R.,** Kinetics and regulation of the glutamate-aspartate translocator in rat liver mitochondria, *J. Biol. Chem.,* 254, 8369, 1979.

87. **Williamson, J. R., Jakob, A., and Refino, C.,** Control of the removal of reducing equivalents from the cytosol in perfused rat liver, *J. Biol. Chem.,* 246, 7632, 1971.

88. **Rognstad, R. and Katz, J.,** Gluconeogenesis in the kidney cortex. Effects of D-malate and amino-oxyacetate, *Biochem. J.,* 116, 483, 1970.

89. **Ross, B., Silva, P., and Bullock, S.,** Role of malate-aspartate shuttle in renal sodium transport in the rat, *Clin. Sci.,* 60, 419, 1981.

90. **MacDonald, M. J.,** Evidence for the malate-aspartate shuttle in pancreatic islets, *Arch. Biochem. Biophys.,* 213, 643, 1982.

91. **LaNoue, K. F., Nicklas, W. J., and Williamson, J. R.,** Control of citric acid cycle activity in rat heart mitochondria, *J. Biol. Chem.,* 245, 102, 1970.

92. **LaNoue, K. F. and Williamson, J. R.,** Interrelationships between malate-aspartate shuttle and citric acid cycle in rat heart mitochondria, *Metabolism,* 20, 119, 1971.

93. **Hogg, H. R. and Ottaway, J. H.,** Flux through the malate-aspartate shuttle in perfused rat heart, *Biochem. Soc. Trans.,* 5, 709, 1977.

94. **Brand, M. D. and Chappell, J. B.,** Glutamate and aspartate transport in rat brain mitochondria, *Biochem. J.,* 140, 205, 1974.

95. **Minn, A. and Gayet, J.,** Kinetic study of glutamate transport in rat brain mitochondria, *J. Neurochem.,* 29, 873, 1977.

96. **Dennis, S. C., Lai, J. C. K., and Clark, J. B.,** Comparative studies on glutamate metabolism in synaptic and non-synaptic rat brain mitochondria, *Biochem. J.,* 164, 727, 1977.

97. **Dennis, S. C. and Clark, J. B.,** The regulation of glutamate metabolism by tricarboxylic acid-cycle activity in rat brain mitochondria, *Biochem. J.,* 172, 155, 1978.

98. **Fitzpatrick, S. M., Cooper, A. J. L., and Duffy, T. E.,** Use of β-methylene-D,L-aspartate to assess the role of aspartate aminotransferase in cerebral oxidative metabolism, *J. Neurochem.,* 41, 1370, 1983.

99. **Altschuler, R. A., Neises, G. R., Harmison, G.-C., Wenthold, R. J., and Fex, J.,** Immunocytochemical localization of aspartate aminotransferase immunoreactivity in cochlear nucleus of the guinea pig, *Proc. Natl. Acad. Sci. U.S.A.,* 78, 6553, 1981.

100. **Wenthold, R. J.,** Glutaminase and aspartate aminotransferase decrease in the cochlear nucleus after lesion of the auditory nerve, *Brain Res.,* 190, 293, 1980.

101. **Recasens, M. and Delaunoy, J. P.,** Immunological properties and immunohistochemical localization of cysteine sulfinate or aspartate aminotransferase in rat CNS, *Brain Res.,* 205, 351, 1981.

102. **Brandon, C. and Lam, D. M.-K.,** L-Glutamic acid: a neurotransmitter for cone receptors in human and rat retina, *Proc. Natl. Acad. Sci. U.S.A.,* 80, 5117, 1983.

103. **Hopper, S. and Segal, H. L.,** Comparative properties of glutamic-alanine transaminase from several sources, *Arch. Biochem. Biophys.,* 105, 501, 1964.

104. **Benuck, M., Stern, F., and Lajtha, A.,** Transamination of amino acids in homogenates of rat brain, *J. Neurochem.,* 18, 1555, 1971.

105. **Matsuzawa, T. and Segal, H. L.,** Rat liver alanine aminotransferase. Crystalization, composition and role of sulfhydryl groups, *J. Biol. Chem.,* 243, 5929, 1968.

106. **Saier, M. H., Jr. and Jenkins, W. T.,** Alanine aminotransferase. I. Purification and properties, *J. Biol. Chem.,* 242, 91, 1967.

107. **Bulos, B. and Handler, P.,** Kinetics of beef heart glutamic-alanine transaminase, *J. Biol. Chem.,* 240, 3283, 1965.

108. **Swick, R. W., Barnstein, P. L., and Stange, J. L.,** The metabolism of mitochondrial proteins. I. Distribution and characterization of the isozymes of alanine aminotransferase in rat liver, *J. Biol. Chem.,* 240, 3334, 1965.

109. **De Rosa, G., Burk, T. L., and Swick, R. W.,** Isolation and characterization of mitochondrial alanine aminotransferase from porcine tissue, *Biochim. Biophys. Acta,* 567, 116, 1979.

110. **De Rosa, G. and Swick, R. W.,** Metabolic implications of the distribution of the alanine aminotransferase isoenzyme, *J. Biol. Chem.,* 250, 7961, 1975.

111. **Segal, H. L., Beattie, D. S., and Hopper, S.,** Purification and properties of liver glutamic-alanine transaminase from normal and corticoid-treated rats, *J. Biol. Chem.,* 237, 1914, 1962.

112. **Felig, P.,** The glucose-alanine cycle, *Metabolism,* 22, 179, 1973.

113. **Mallette, L. E., Exton, J. H., and Park, C. R.,** Control of gluconeogenesis from amino acids in the perfused rat liver, *J. Biol. Chem.,* 244, 5713, 1969.

114. **Goldberg, A. L. and Chang, T. W.,** Regulation and significance of amino acid metabolism in skeletal muscle, *Fed. Proc., Fed. Am. Soc. Exp. Biol.,* 37, 2301, 1978.

115. **Goldstein, L. and Newsholme, E. A.,** The formation of alanine from amino acids in diaphragm muscle of the rat, *Biochem. J.,* 154, 555, 1976.

116. **Garber, A. J., Karl, I. E., and Kipnis, D. M.,** Alanine and glutamine synthesis and release from skeletal muscle. I. Glycolysis and amino acid release, *J. Biol. Chem.,* 251, 826, 1976.

117. **Garber, A. J., Karl, I. E., and Kipnis, D. M.,** Alanine and glutamine synthesis and release from skeletal muscle. II. The precursor role of amino acids in alanine and glutamine synthesis, *J. Biol. Chem.,* 251, 836, 1976.

118. **Pardridge, W. M. and Davidson, M. B.,** Alanine metabolism in skeletal muscle in tissue culture, *Biochim. Biophys. Acta,* 585, 34, 1979.

119. **Krebs, H. A.,** The role of chemical equilibria in organ functions, *Adv. Enzyme Regul.,* 13, 449, 1975.

120. **Marliss, E. B., Aoki, T. T., Pozefsky, T., Most, A. S., and Cahill, G. F., Jr.,** Muscle and splanchnic glutamine and glutamate metabolism in postabsorptive and starved man, *J. Clin. Invest.,* 50, 814, 1971.

121. **Ruderman, N. B. and Lund, P.,** Amino acid metabolism in skeletal muscle. Regulation of glutamine and alanine release in the perfused rat hindquarter, *Isr. J. Med. Sci.,* 8, 295, 1972.

122. **Abdul-Ghani, A.-S., Marton, M., and Dobkin, J.,** Studies on the transport of glutamine *in vivo* between the brain and blood in the resting state and during afferent electrical stimulation, *J. Neurochem.,* 31, 541, 1978.

123. **Gjedde, A., Lockwood, A. H., Duffy, T. E., and Plum, F.,** Cerebral blood flow and metabolism in chronically hyperammonemic rats: effect of an acute ammonia challenge, *Anal. Neurol.,* 3, 325, 1978.

124. **Tischler, M. E. and Goldberg, A. L.,** Leucine degradation and release of glutamine and alanine by adipose tissue, *J. Biol. Chem.,* 255, 8074, 1980.

125. **Manchester, K. L. and Young, F. G.,** Location of ^{14}C in protein from isolated rat diaphragm incubated *in vitro* with [^{14}C]amino acids and with $^{14}CO_2$, *Biochem. J.,* 72, 136, 1959.

126. **Chang, T. W. and Goldberg, A. L.,** The metabolic fates of amino acids and the formation of glutamine in skeletal muscle, *J. Biol. Chem.,* 253, 3685, 1978.

127. **Golden, M. H. N.,** Metabolism of branched-chain amino acids, in *Nitrogen Metabolism in Man,* Waterlow, J. C. and Stephen, J. M. L., Eds., Applied Science, London, 1981, 109.

128. **Harper, A. E., Miller, R. H., and Block, K. P.,** Branched-chain amino acid metabolism, *Annu. Rev. Nutr.,* 4, 409, 1984.
129. **Windmueller, H. G. and Spaeth, A. E.,** Respiratory fuels and nitrogen metabolism *in vivo* in small intestine of fed rats, *J. Biol. Chem.,* 255, 107, 1980.
130. **Pitts, R. F.,** Production of CO_2 by the intact functioning kidney of the dog, in *Medical Clinics of North America,* Vol. 59, 3rd ed., Symp. on Renal Metabolism, Baruch, S., Ed., W. B. Saunders, Philadelphia, 1975, 507.
131. **Hems, D. A.,** Metabolism of glutamine and glutamic acid by isolated perfused kidneys of normal and acidotic rats, *Biochem. J.,* 130, 671, 1972.
132. **Forissier, M. and Baverel, G.,** The conversion of alanine into glutamine in guinea-pig renal cortex. Essential role of pyruvate carboxylase, *Biochem. J.,* 200, 27, 1981.
133. **Ichihara, A.,** Aminotransferases of branched-chain amino acids, in *Transaminases,* Christen, P. and Metzler, D. E., Eds., John Wiley & Sons, New York, 1985, 430.
134. **Ichihara, A. and Koyama, E.,** Transaminase of branched chain amino acids. I. Branched chain-amino acids-α-ketoglutarate transaminase, *J. Biochem.,* 59, 160, 1966.
135. **Taylor, R. T. and Jenkins, W. T.,** Leucine aminotransferase. II. Purification and characterization, *J. Biol. Chem.,* 241, 4396, 1966.
136. **Taylor, R. T. and Jenkins, W. T.,** Leucine aminotransferase. III. Activation by β-mercaptoethanol, *J. Biol. Chem.,* 241, 4406, 1966.
137. **Hargrove, J. L. and Mackin, R. B.,** Organ specificity of glucocorticoid-sensitive tyrosine aminotransferase. Separation from aspartate aminotransferase isoenzymes, *J. Biol. Chem.,* 259, 386, 1984.
138. **Kenney, F. T.,** Properties of partially purified tyrosine-α-ketoglutarate transaminase from rat liver, *J. Biol. Chem.,* 234, 2707, 1959.
139. **Jacoby, G. A. and La Du, B. N.,** Studies on the specificity of tyrosine-α-ketoglutarate transaminase, *J. Biol. Chem.,* 239, 419, 1964.
140. **Hargrove, J. L., Diesterhaft, M., Noguchi, T., and Granner, D. K.,** Identification of native tyrosine aminotransferase and an explanation for the multiple forms, *J. Biol. Chem.,* 255, 71, 1980.
141. **Hargrove, J. L. and Granner, D. K.,** Biosynthesis and intracellular processing of tyrosine aminotransferase, in *Transaminases,* Christen, P. and Metzler, D. E., Eds., John Wiley & Sons, New York, 1985, 511.
142. **Meister, A., Radhakrishnan, A. N., and Buckley, S. D.,** Enzymatic synthesis of L-pipecolic acid and L-proline, *J. Biol. Chem.,* 229, 789, 1957.
143. **Meister, A.,** Enzymatic transamination reactions involving arginine and ornithine, *J. Biol. Chem.,* 206, 587, 1953.
144. **Peraino, C. and Pitot, H. C.,** Ornithine transaminase in rat. I. Assay and some general properties, *Biochim. Biophys. Acta,* 73, 222, 1963.
145. **Matsuzawa, T., Katsunuma, T., and Katunuma, N.,** Crystallization of ornithine transaminase and its properties, *Biochem. Biophys. Res. Commun.,* 32, 161, 1968.
146. **Jenkins, W. T. and Tsai, H.,** Ornithine aminotransferase (pig kidney), *Methods Enzymol.,* 17A, 281, 1970.
147. **John, R. A. and Fowler, L. T.,** Mammalian ω-amino acid transaminases, in *Transaminases,* Christen, P. and Metzler, D. E., Eds., John Wiley & Sons, New York, 1985, 413.
148. **Pitot, H. C. and Peraino, C.,** Studies on the induction and repression of enzymes in rat liver. I. Induction of threonine dehydrase and ornithine-δ-transaminase by oral intubation of casein hydrolysate, *J. Biol. Chem.,* 239, 1783, 1964.
149. **Katunuma, N., Okada, M., Matsuzawa, T., and Otsuka, Y.,** Studies on ornithine ketoacid transaminase. II. Role in metabolic pathway, *J. Biochem.,* 57, 445, 1965.
150. **Peraino, C.,** Interactions of diet and cortisone in the regulation of adaptive enzymes in rat liver, *J. Biol. Chem.,* 242, 3860, 1967.
151. **Peraino, C., Blake, R. L., and Pitot, H. C.,** Studies on the induction and repression of enzymes in rat liver. III. Induction of ornithine δ-transaminase and threonine dehydrase by oral intubation of free amino acids, *J. Biol. Chem.,* 240, 3039, 1965.
152. **Peraino, C. and Pitot, H. C.,** Studies on the induction and repression of enzymes in rat liver. II. Carbohydrate repression of dietary and hormonal induction of threonine deaminase and ornithine δ-transaminase, *J. Biol. Chem.,* 239, 4308, 1964.
153. **Yanagi, S., Campbell, H. A., and Potter, V. R.,** Diurnal variations in activity of four pyridoxal enzymes in rat liver during metabolic transition from high carbohydrate to high protein diet, *Life Sci.,* 17, 1411, 1976.
154. **Morris, J. E. and Peraino, C.,** Immunochemical studies of serine dehydratase and ornithine aminotransferase regulation in rat liver *in vivo, J. Biol. Chem.,* 251, 2571, 1976.
155. **Chee, P. Y. and Swick, R. W.,** Effect of dietary protein and tryptophan on the turnover of rat liver ornithine aminotransferase, *J. Biol. Chem.,* 251, 1029, 1976.

156. **Lyons, R. T. and Pitot, H. C.,** The regulation of ornithine aminotransferase synthesis by glucagon in the rat, *Arch. Biochem. Biophys.,* 174, 262, 1976.
157. **Volpe, B., Sawamura, R., and Strecker, H. J.,** Control of ornithine δ-transaminase in rat liver and kidney, *J. Biol. Chem.,* 244, 719, 1969.
158. **Herzfeld, A. and Knox, W. E.,** The properties, developmental formation, and estrogen induction of ornithine aminotransferase in rat tissues, *J. Biol. Chem.,* 243, 3327, 1968.
159. **Lyons, R. T. and Pitot, H. C.,** Hormonal regulation of ornithine aminotransferase biosynthesis in rat liver and kidney, *Arch. Biochem. Biophys.,* 180, 472, 1977.
160. **Trijbels, J. M. F., Sengers, R. C. A., Bakkeren, J. A. J. M., DeKort, A. F. M., and Deutman, A. F.,** L-Ornithine-keto acid-transaminase deficiency in cultured fibroblasts of a patient with hyperornithinaemia and gyrate atrophy of the choroid and retina, *Clin. Chim. Acta,* 79, 371, 1977.
161. **Jung, M. J. and Seiler, N.,** Enzyme-activated irreversible inhibitors of L-ornithine: 2-oxoacid aminotransferase. Demonstration of mechanistic features of the inhibition of ornithine aminotransferase by 4-aminohex-5-ynoic acid and gabaculine and correlation with *in vivo* activity, *J. Biol. Chem.,* 253, 7431, 1978.
162. **Matsuzawa, T. and Ishiguro, I.,** Ornithine metabolism in relation to stimulation of urea cycle, induced by high protein diet, *Arch. Biochem. Biophys.,* 208, 101, 1981.
163. **McGivan, J. D., Bradford, N. M., and Beavis, A. D.,** Factors influencing the activity of ornithine aminotransferase in isolated rat mitochondria, *Biochem. J.,* 162, 147, 1977.
164. **Strecker, H. J.,** Purification and properties of rat liver ornithine δ-transaminase, *J. Biol. Chem.,* 240, 1225, 1965.
165. **Katunuma, N., Matsuda, Y., and Tomino, I.,** Studies on ornithine-ketoacid transaminase. I. Purification and properties, *J. Biochem.,* 56, 499, 1964.
166. **Roberts, E. and Frankel, S.,** γ-Aminobutyric acid in brain, *Fed. Proc., Fed. Am. Soc. Exp. Biol.,* 9, 219, 1950.
167. **Roberts, E., Chase, T. N., and Tower, D. B., Eds.,** *GABA in Nervous System Function,* Raven Press, New York, 1976.
168. **Balázs, R., Machiyama, Y., Hammon, B. J., Julian, T., and Richter, D.,** The operation of the γ-aminobutyrate bypath of the tricarboxylic acid cycle in brain tissue *in vitro, Biochem. J.,* 116, 445, 1970.
169. **Martin del Rio, R.,** γ-Aminobutyric acid system in rat oviduct, *J. Biol. Chem.,* 256, 9816, 1981.
170. **Buzenet, A. M., Fages, C., Bloch-Tardy, M., and Gonnard, P.,** Purification and properties of 4-aminobutyrate 2-ketoglutarate aminotransferase from pig liver, *Biochim. Biophys. Acta,* 522, 400, 1978.
171. **Tokunaga, M., Nakano, Y., and Kitaoka, S.,** Subcellular localization of the GABA-shunt enzymes in *Euglena gracilis* Strain Z, *J. Protozool.,* 26, 471, 1979.
172. **Yonaha, K. and Toyama, S.,** γ-Aminobutyrate: α-ketoglutarate aminotransferase from *Pseudomonas* sp. F-126: purification, crystalization and enzymologic properties, *Arch. Biochem. Biophys.,* 200, 156, 1980.
173. **Schousboe, A., Wu, J.-Y., and Roberts, E.,** Purification and characterization of the 4-aminobutyrate-2-ketoglutarate transaminase from mouse brain, *Biochemistry,* 12, 2868, 1973.
174. **John, R. A. and Fowler, L. J.,** Kinetic and spectral properties of rabbit brain 4-aminobutyrate aminotransferase, *Biochem. J.,* 155, 645, 1976.
175. **Beeler, T. and Churchich, J. E.,** 4-Aminobutyrate aminotransferase fluorescence studies, *Eur. J. Biochem.,* 85, 365, 1978.
176. **Maitre, M., Ciesielski, L., Cash, C., and Mandel, P.,** Purification and studies on some properties of the 4-aminobutyrate 2-oxoglutarate transaminase from rat brain, *Eur. J. Biochem.,* 52, 157, 1975.
177. **Maitre, M., Cieselski, L., Cash, C., and Mandel, P.,** Comparison of the structural characteristics of the 4-aminobutyrate: 2-oxoglutarate transaminases from rat and human brain and their affinities for certain inhibitors, *Biochim. Biophys. Acta,* 522, 385, 1978.
178. **Nikolaeva, Z. K. and Vasil'ev, V. Yu.,** Mechanism of action of pig kidney γ-aminobutyrate-glutamate transaminase, *Biokhimiya,* 37, 469, 1972.
179. **Churchich, J. E. and Moses, U.,** 4-Aminobutyrate aminotransferase. The presence of nonequivalent binding sites, *J. Biol. Chem.,* 256, 1101, 1981.
180. **Hertz, L.,** Functional interactions between neurons and astrocytes. I. Turnover and metabolism of putative amino acid transmitters, *Progr. Neurobiol.,* 13, 277, 1979.
181. **Turner, A. J. and Whittle, S. R.,** Biochemical dissection of the γ-aminobutyrate synapse, *Biochem. J.,* 209, 29, 1983.
182. **Hearl, W. G. and Churchich, J. E.,** Interactions between 4-aminobutyrate aminotransferase and succinic semialdehyde dehydrogenase, two mitochondrial enzymes, *J. Biol. Chem.,* 259, 11459, 1984.
183. **Benavides, J., Rumigny, J. F., Bourguignon, J. J., Cash, C., Wermuth, C. G., Mandel, P., Vincendon, G., and Maitre, M.,** High affinity binding site for γ-hydroxybutyric acid in rat brain, *Life Sci.,* 30, 953, 1982.
184. **Hearl, W. G. and Churchich, J. E.,** A mitochondrial NADP+-dependent reductase related to the 4-aminobutyrate shunt. Purification, characterization, and mechanism, *J. Biol. Chem.,* 260, 16361, 1985.

185. **Berl, S., Lajtha, A., and Waelsch, H.,** Amino acid and protein metabolism. VI. Cerebral compartments of glutamic acid metabolism, *J. Neurochem.,* 7, 186, 1961.
186. **Berl, S., Takagaki, G., Clarke, D. D., and Waelsch, H.,** Metabolic compartments *in vivo.* Ammonia and glutamic acid metabolism in brain and liver, *J. Biol. Chem.,* 237, 2562, 1962.
187. **Cooper, A. J. L. and Plum, F.,** Biochemistry and physiology of brain ammonia, *Physiol. Rev.,* 67, 440, 1987.
188. **Benjamin, A M. and Quastel, J. H.,** Locations of amino acids in brain cortex slices from the rat. Tetrodotoxin-sensitive release of amino acids, *Biochem. J.,* 128, 631, 1972.
189. **Benjamin, A. M. and Quastel, J. H.,** Fate of L-glutamate in the brain, *J. Neurochem.,* 23, 457, 1974.
190. **Shank, R. P. and Campbell, G. LeM.,** α-Ketoglutarate and malate uptake and metabolism by synaptosomes: further evidence for an astrocyte-to-neuron metabolic shuttle, *J. Neurochem.,* 42, 1153, 1984.
191. **Van Den Berg, C. J. and Garfinkel, D.,** A simulation study of brain compartments. Metabolism of glutamate and related substances in mouse brain, *Biochem. J.,* 123, 211, 1971.
192. **Van Den Berg, C. J.,** A model of compartmentation in mouse brain based on glucose and acetate metabolism, in *Metabolic Compartmentation in the Brain,* Balázs, R. and Cremer, J. E., Eds., MacMillan, London, 1973, 137.
193. **Van Den Berg, C. J., Matheson, D. F., Ronda, G., Reijnierse, G. L. A., Blokhuis, G. G. D., Kroon, M. C., Clarke, D. D., and Garfinkel, D.,** A model of glutamate metabolism in brain: a biochemical analysis of a heterogeneous structure, in *Metabolic Compartmentation and Neurotransmission,* Berl, S., Clarke, D. D., and Schneider, D., Eds., Plenum Press, New York, 1974, 515.
194. **Yu, A. C. H., Drejer, J., Hertz, L., and Schousboe, A.,** Pyruvate carboxylase activity in primary cultures of astrocytes and neurons, *J. Neurochem.,* 41, 1484, 1983.
195. **Ubuka, T., Umemura, S., Ishimoto, Y., and Shimomura, M.,** Transamination of L-cysteine in rat liver mitochondria, *Physiol. Chem. Phys.,* 9, 91, 1977.
196. **Ip, M. P. C., Thibert, R. J., and Schmidt, D. E., Jr.,** Purification and partial characterization of cysteine-glutamate transaminase from rat liver, *Can. J. Biochem.,* 55, 958, 1977.
197. **Ikeda, T., Konishi, Y., and Ichihara, A.,** Transaminase of branched chain amino acids. XI. Leucine (methionine) transaminase of rat liver mitochondria, *Biochim. Biophys. Acta,* 445, 622, 1976.
198. **Soffer, R. L., Hechtman, P., and Savage, M.,** L-Triiodothyronine aminotransferase, *J. Biol. Chem.,* 248, 1224, 1973.
199. **Nakano, M.,** Purification and properties of halogenated tyrosine and thyroid hormone transaminase from rat kidney mitochondria, *J. Biol. Chem.,* 242, 73, 1967.
200. **Tobes, M. C. and Mason, M.,** α-Aminoadipate aminotransferase and kynurenine aminotransferase. Purification, characterization, and further evidence for identity, *J. Biol. Chem.,* 252, 4591, 1977.
201. **Tobes, M. C. and Mason, M.,** Kynurenine aminotransferase and α-aminoadipate aminotransferase. III. Evidence for identity with halogenerated tyrosine aminotransferase, *Life Sci.,* 22, 793, 1978.
202. **Takeuchi, F., Otsuka, H., and Shibata, Y.,** Purification, characterization and identification of rat liver mitochondrial kynurenine aminotransferase with α-aminoadipate aminotransferase, *Biochim. Biophys. Acta,* 743, 323, 1983.
203. **Fellman, J. H., Roth, E. S., Avedovech, N. A., and McCarthy, K. D.,** Mammalian hypotaurine aminotransferase: isethionate is not a product, *Life Sci.,* 27, 1999, 1980.
204. **Fellman, J. H. and Roth, E. S.,** Hypotaurine aminotransferase, *Adv. Exp. Med. Biol.,* 139, 99, 1982.

Chapter 9

γ-GLUTAMYLTRANSFERASE

Nils-Erik Huseby

TABLE OF CONTENTS

I. INTRODUCTION

The major function of γ-glutamyltransferase (γ-glutamyltranspeptidase) is related to the interorgan metabolism of glutathione.[1-4] It initiates the degradation of both the reduced and the oxidized form of glutathione and acts also on several S-conjugates. γ-Glutamyltransferase catalyzes the hydrolysis of the γ-glutamyl-cysteine bond in glutathione, thereby releasing glutamate from the tripeptide. In the presence of various amino acids and peptides, the enzyme will also transfer the γ-glutamyl-group from glutathione to the amino acid or peptide, thereby producing γ-glutamyl-amino acid or γ-glutamyl-peptide. In addition, it may catalyze the glutaminase reaction in the presence of hippurate or maleate.

γ-Glutamyltransferase is a plasma membrane bound enzyme[5-7] exposed on the outside of cells primarily involved in secretion and absorption.[1,2] The enzyme is widely distributed in plants and animals, and has been characterized from several mammalian tissues; mostly from the kidney and liver.

The measurements of γ-glutamyltransferase in serum has been of considerable interest in diagnostic enzymology, as increased serum activity is a sensitive indication of liver disease.[8,9]

Several reviews have been published on γ-glutamyltransferase.[1,2,9,10] The purpose of this contribution has been to summarize recent findings on the catalytic properties, the structure and in vivo distribution, and the physiological functions of the enzyme.

II. CATALYTIC PROPERTIES: MEASUREMENT OF ACTIVITY

γ-Glutamyltransferase activity was first observed 70 years ago and termed antiglyoxalase due to its degradation of glutathione, the cofactor of glyoxalase.[11] Binkley and Nakamura[12] later named the enzyme glutathionase and showed that the enzyme catalyzes the initial step in the hydrolysis of glutathione, namely the breakdown of the γ-glutamyl bond in the tripeptide. Hanes and co-workers[13] demonstrated that the enzyme could catalyze both the hydrolysis reaction (Reaction 1) and the transfer or transpeptidation reaction (Reaction 2) which occurs in the presence of certain amino acids and peptides. The enzyme may also transfer the γ-glutamyl group to another molecule of the γ-glutamyl donor substrate (autotransfer, Reaction 3).

$$\gamma\text{-Glu-cys-gly} + H_2O \rightarrow \text{glutamate} + \text{cys-gly} \tag{1}$$

$$\gamma\text{-Glu-cys-gly} + \text{amino acid} \rightarrow \gamma\text{-glu-amino acid} + \text{cys-gly} \tag{2}$$

$$2\ \gamma\text{-Glu-cys-gly} \rightarrow \gamma\text{-glu-}\gamma\text{-glu-cys-gly} + \text{cys-gly} \tag{3}$$

The best acceptor substrates include the neutral amino acids glutamine, methionine, alanine, serine, and cystine, and some dipeptides such as glycylglycine. Branched-chain, acid, and basic amino acids are poor acceptors. D-Amino acids are inactive as acceptors but can act as γ-glutamyl donors. Both reduced and oxidized glutathione and various S-substituted derivatives can be utilized as γ-glutamyl donors.[14-17] Glutamine may also serve as a γ-glutamyl donor substrate, as γ-glutamyltransferase catalyzes the phosphate-independent glutaminase reaction.[18,19] This reaction is increased in the presence of maleate[19,20] or hippurate,[21] which will bind to the cysteinyl-glycine binding site and inhibit the transpeptidation and stimulate the hydrolytic reaction.

Several investigations on the kinetic properties of γ-glutamyltransferase have been published and reviewed.[2,10,22,23] The data from these studies are consistent with a ping-pong bi-bi mechanism in which the reaction proceeds through the formation of a γ-glutamyl-enzyme intermediate (Reaction 4). This activated intermediate can then react with the acceptor

Table 1
OPTIMIZED CONDITIONS FOR MEASUREMENTS OF γ-GLUTAMYLTRANSFERASE IN SERUM[23]

Temperature	30, 0°C
pH (30°C)	7, 90°C
L-γ-Glutamyl-3-carboxy-4-nitroanilide	6 mM
Glycylglycine	150 mM

Note: The concentrations apply to the complete reaction mixture. The volume fraction of serum is 1:11.

substrate; water, amino acids, or dipeptides (Reaction 5). The dipeptide acceptors bind to the region of the glutathione binding site vacated by cysteinyl-glycine, while amino acid acceptors bind to the cysteinyl binding site.

$$γ\text{-Glu-cys-gly} + \text{enzyme} \rightleftharpoons γ\text{-glu-enzyme} + \text{cys-gly} \tag{4}$$

$$γ\text{-Glu-enzyme} + \text{acceptor} \rightleftharpoons γ\text{-glu-acceptor} + \text{enzyme} \tag{5}$$

Separate determinations of the hydrolytic and transferase processes (Reactions 1 and 2) have shown that the optimal conditions for the two reactions are different.[24,25] Thus, the rate of the transferase reaction is higher than the hydrolysis reaction at a slightly alkaline pH (pH 8 to 9) and with acceptor substrate concentration at 50 mM or higher. With the optimized assay conditions[23] using the artificial substrate γ-glutamyl-3-carboxy-4-nitro-anilide (Table 1), the rate of the hydrolytic reaction is negligible and that of the autotransfer reaction (Reaction 3) is less than 1%.[26,27] On the other hand at physiological pH (pH 7.4) and in the presence of plasma concentrations of amino acids and glutathione, the hydrolytic reaction has been shown to account for 50 to 75% of the total activity of γ-glutamyltransferase.[24,25] Therefore, the hydrolytic process will dominate in the renal tubular lumen and in bile canaliculi, where significant amounts of γ-glutamyltransferase are concentrated.

Reversible inhibition of γ-glutamyltransferase activity can be achieved with a mixture of serine and borate.[28] Studies have indicated that these compounds interact with the γ-glutamyl binding site.[29] Rapid and irreversible inhibition occurs with the glutamine antagonists 6-diazo-5-oxo-L-norleucine (DON), O-diazoacetyl-L-serine (azaserine), and AT-125, L-(αS,5S)-α-amino-3-chloro-4,5-dihydro-5-isoxazolone-acetic acid (acivicin).[30-32] Of these, acivicin has the highest inactivation rate, being 20-fold greater than that with DON. These inhibitors have been used as highly effective affinity labels for the active site, and have also been of great value in studying the in vivo functions of γ-glutamyltransferase.

Prior to 1960 glutathione was the substrate used for measurements of γ-glutamyltransferase activity. Due to the low substrate specificity of the enzyme several artificial substrates have been introduced. Improved sensitivity and simplicity were gained with the kinetic method published by Szasz[33] in 1969, using γ-glutamyl-4-nitro-anilide in combination with glycylglycine as an acceptor. This method gained much attention and propagated a great interest for γ-glutamyltransferase as a clinical parameter.

Several papers describing modified conditions were subsequently published.[26,34,35] Recently, a reference method was proposed by the International Federation of Clinical Chemistry (IFCC)[23] which provides optimized reaction conditions (see Table 1). These assay conditions are most favorable for both the kinetic reactions and the technical aspects of the measurements. A method which gives a much higher sensitivity is based on the fluorogenic substrate γ-glutamyl-7-amino-4-methyl-coumarin.[36]

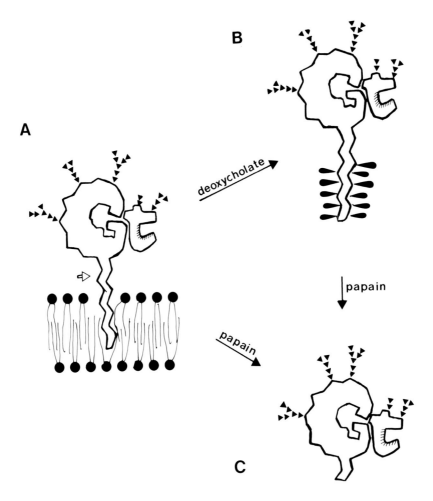

FIGURE 1.   Schematic representation of release of γ-glutamyl transferase from intact membranes by treatment with protease (papain) or detergent (deoxycholate). The enzyme is bound
to the membrane (A) via a hydrophobic domain of the large subunit. The active site is
indicated by the shaded ''pocket'' of the small subunit. Detergents will break up the membrane
and release the amphipathic enzyme as a detergent-enzyme complex (B). Proteases will
cleave the large subunit at a susceptible peptide bound (arrow) and release the enzyme in its
hydrophilic form (C). ▼: carbohydrate, and ➤: deoxycholate.

III. STRUCTURAL AND TOPOLOGICAL CHARACTERIZATION

The first attempts to purify γ-glutamyltransferase were hampered by its membrane-bound
state. Advances were made when detergents were introduced as solubilizing agents and also
when simpler chromogenic assays were employed for activity measurements. From 1974 to
1976 the enzyme from the rat kidney was extensively purified and obtained in a homogeneous
form.[18,19,37,38] The rat kidney enzyme has later been well characterized. Purifications to
apparent homogeneity have been obtained from human organs such as the kidney[39] and
liver.[40] The physical as well as the kinetic properties of γ-glutamyltransferase from these
sources are grossly the same as those of the rat kidney enzyme.

γ-Glutamyltransferase is an integral membrane glycoprotein.[1,2] The release of the enzyme
from membranes can occur with the use of either detergents or proteases, whereby two
different forms of the enzyme are produced (see Figure 1). Solubilization with detergents
releases γ-glutamyltransferase in an amphipathic form.[18,37,38] This form binds detergents in

a micellar complex when detergents are present in amounts above the critical micellar concentration. The molecular mass of this complex has been estimated to 169,000, half of which consists of detergent.[37] In lower concentrations, the amphipathic enzyme aggregates to a ''heavier'' form with molecular mass higher than 200,000, due to the hydrophobicity of the membrane-binding domain.[37,41] Proteases such as papain, trypsin, and bromelain will act upon a sensitive amino acid sequence close to this domain.[43] Proteolytic treatment of membranes will therefore result in the solubilization of a hydrophilic form of γ-glutamyl-transferase.[37,38] The enzyme seems protected against further proteolytic degradation,[42] probably due to the high amount of carbohydrate in the enzyme.

The enzyme is composed of two different subunits and both are heavily glycosylated.[37,38] The active site is located on the smaller subunit[30,31] while a domain of the large subunit is responsible for the membrane association.[43] This hydrophobic domain, which comprises 52 amino acids,[43] is a part of the NH_2-terminal segment and believed to span the membrane.[44] The molecular mass of the hydrophilic form of rat kidney γ-glutamyltransferase was estimated to 66,700 to 69,000 and the two different subunits being 45,000 to 46,000 and 22,000 to 23,000.[5,37,38]

Recent studies on the biosynthesis[45-47] of the rat kidney enzyme have demonstrated that γ-glutamyltransferase is synthesized as one single precursor (M_r 63,000), then transferred to the Golgi system and glycosylated (M_r 78,000). This form is integrated into the microsomal membranes and oriented analogously to that found on the brush-border membranes. The precursor is then cleaved into the two subunits of the active enzyme. Investigations on the turnover of the rat kidney enzyme indicated an apparent half-life of 3 to 4 days.[47,48]

Investigations on the amount and composition of the carbohydrate moiety have revealed that this part of the enzyme is very complex and heterogeneous.[46,49] The rat kidney enzyme possesses a large mixture of neutral and acidic oligosaccharides. This will explain the significant heterogeneity detected in isoelectric focusing of the kidney enzyme.[38] Variations in the content of both sialic acid and other carbohydrates have been described for γ-glutamyltransferase in human serum, liver, kidney, and other organs, but the polypeptide chains are apparently identical.[50-54] ''Novel forms'' of the enzyme have been described in neoplastic tissues, but these variants are not true isoenzymes, as they show identical antigenic properties to the enzymes in nonneoplastic tissue.[52,54,55]

IV. TISSUE DISTRIBUTION

The highest activity of γ-glutamyltransferase has been demonstrated in the kidney. Significant activities have also been detected in the pancreas, liver, and prostate.[2] The relative amounts of enzyme in various organs vary between different species. Thus, while the rat liver activity is very low, the human liver contains significantly higher activity.[27] Although the activity in homogenates of tissues may be low or negligible, significant enzyme activity can be demonstrated histochemically in certain regions and cellular membranes of such tissues.

The subcellular localization of γ-glutamyltransferase is of great importance in view of its in vivo function. The enzyme is bound to the plasma membranes and its active site is oriented on the outer surface of cells that primarily have a secretory or absorptive function.[5-7]

In the kidney, the highest concentration of γ-glutamyltransferase has been demonstrated in the brush border membranes of the proximal tubular cells.[1,56-58] Activity can also be demonstrated in the luminal membrane of distal tubules and collecting ducts. Renal γ-glutamyltransferase activity is also associated with basolateral cell membranes of proximal and distal tubular fragments.[57,58]

The cellular and subcellular localization in the liver differs in various animals. In the rat liver, high specific activity is found mainly in nonparenchymal cells[59,60] and especially in canalicular plasma membranes.[61] In the human and guinea pig liver, however, the major amount of γ-glutamyltransferase is located in the plasma membranes of hepatocytes.[7,59] Significant activity was demonstrated in both canalicular and sinusoidal plasma membranes in the guinea pig, whereas in the human liver the canalicular γ-glutamyltransferase activity was lower than the sinusoidal but increased in pathological conditions.

γ-Glutamyltransferase activity can also be demonstrated in several body fluids.[8,9] Very high activity has been reported in seminal plasma, and significant activity have been found in colostrum, bile, urine, and plasma.

V. PHYSIOLOGICAL FUNCTION

A. Glutathione Metabolism

It is generally accepted that γ-glutamyltransferase plays a crucial role in the regulation of glutathione and initiates the hydrolysis of both reduced and oxidized glutathione as well as several of its *S*-conjugates.[62,63] The turnover of glutathione is both an interorgan as well as an intraorgan process. The tripeptide is synthesized in most cells and organs, and maintained at millimolar concentrations in the cytosol. The initial step in glutathione turnover is its translocation out of the cells. Significant efflux has been demonstrated from rat hepatocytes[64] and specific carrier systems have been demonstrated.[65] Glutathione transported by plasma is largely extracted by the kidneys.[66] Renal extraction occurs by a glomerular filtration and a nonfiltrating peritubular mechanism.[67,68] The major amount is degraded by γ-glutamyltransferase and dipeptidase within the tubular lumen and at the basolateral plasma membranes, and the constituent amino acids are absorbed by sodium-dependent uptake. At the basolateral membranes a lesser but significant amount of γ-glutamyl-amino acids is formed by the γ-glutamyltransferase activity.[67-69] Whether these γ-glutamylpeptides are taken up by specific carriers is being discussed.

The intraorgan metabolism of glutathione is also initiated by the efflux of glutathione.[3] The kidney cells are excreting significant amounts of glutathione into the tubular lumen, which is then effectively degraded and reabsorbed as free amino acids.[3,65]

γ-Glutamyltransferase is involved in the metabolic conversion of glutathione conjugates of xenobiotics or their electrophilic metabolites.[16,70] The γ-glutamyl and glycine groups of these conjugates are removed by the action of γ-glutamyltransferase and dipeptidase and the resulting cysteine derivatives are acetylated to form mercapturic acids.[16] The presence of γ-glutamyltransferase and dipeptidase on the luminal surface of the proximal tubules in the kidney, bile ducts in the liver, acinar cells of the pancreas, seminal vesicles, and epithelium of the small intestine, allows the reabsorption of the amino acids of reduced and oxidized glutathione or its derivatives from fluids being excreted.[1,71] The recent interest in the role of γ-glutamyltransferase in inflammation and allergy is connected to the metabolism of the leukotrienes C and D which are constituents of the slow-reacting substance of anaphylaxis.[72] Leukotriene C is a glutathione-*S*-derivative, and γ-glutamyltransferase catalyzes its transformation into leukotriene D.[17]

B. γ-Glutamyl Cycle

The low specificity for amino acids as acceptor substrates in the transpeptidation reaction, and the widespread distribution of γ-glutamyltransferase in cells involved in secretory and absorptive functions, lead to the suggestion that γ-glutamyltransferase was involved in amino acid transport. Meister proposed the γ-glutamyl-cycle which consists of six enzymatic reactions for the synthesis and degradation of glutathione.[73] The transport of amino acids into cells should be coupled to the cycle by the transpeptidation reaction (Reaction 2). The products, γ-glutamyl-amino acids, should be carried through the cellular membranes and transformed to free amino acid and 5-oxoproline by intracellular γ-glutamylcyclotransferase. Data in support of this cycle have been reviewed.[4]

However, the significance of the cycle has been debated. Cellular uptake of amino acid does not appear to be dependent upon γ-glutamyltransferase.[74,75] Patients lacking γ-glutamyltransferase have been described and their amino acid patterns in serum and urine were normal.[76] These patients, as well as animals given γ-glutamyltransferase inhibitors, showed significant glutathionemia and severe glutathionuria.[76-78] Further, the kinetic properties of γ-glutamyltransferase favor the hydrolysis reaction.[1,22,27,65] The major function of γ-glutamyltransferase is apparently to act as a glutathionase.

C. Glutaminase

γ-Glutamyltransferase may utilize glutamine as the substrate. The rate will be 1 to 2% of the rate at which it will utilize glutathione.[18] In the presence of 10 to 50 mM maleate[19] or hippurate,[21] the glutaminase reaction is increased seven to ten times. This reaction is independent of phosphate and has been termed the phosphate-independent glutaminase (PIG) or maleate activated glutaminase (MAG) reaction. Although Katunuma[79] described the presence of this PIG reaction in the rat kidney, liver, and brain, several later studies have failed to establish the presence of PIG activity in the brain.[80] The activity of γ-glutamyltransferase, however, has been located in several brain structures.

Suggestions have been made that the glutaminase reaction would contribute significantly to the catalysis by γ-glutamyltransferase in vivo.[21,81] In a recent publication using cultured rat kidney cells, Dass and Wu[82] claimed that γ-glutamyltransferase utilizes glutamine and forms glutamate and γ-glutamylpeptides. However, Curthoys et al.[83] argue against such a glutaminase function of the enzyme. The approximate K_m value estimated for glutamine is greater than the plasma concentration of glutamine. On the other hand, the K_m value for glutathione is less than the plasma concentration of glutathione. Thus, kinetically, glutathione will be the preferred substrate. Further, it has been considered unlikely that the rather high hippurate concentration necessary for this reaction will be reached in vivo,[83] although increases in hippurate concentrations have been noted in metabolic acidosis.[81] The use of the γ-glutamyltransferase inhibitor acivicin (or AT-125) did not alter the ammonia excretion from rats that were made acute or chronic acidotic.[84] In addition, the acivicin treatment did not affect the plasma glutamine concentration and the acidification of urine in acute acidosis. However, large amounts of glutathione were detected in the urine of these rats.

VI. ROLE IN CARCINOGENESIS

Rat hepatomas contain very high level of γ-glutamyltransferase activity when compared to the low level in the normal liver. High activity has also been indicated in preneoplastic foci that have been isolated from livers of rats during hepatocarcinogenesis.[71] Therefore, the enzyme has been widely used as a marker in preneoplastic lesions in the liver during chemical carcinogenesis.[85-87] A model for the role of γ-glutamyltransferase in carcinogenesis has been suggested.[71] In the promotion phase the liver is subjected to stress which could include a depletion of cellular glutathione. Hepatocytes with high levels of γ-glutamyltransferase on their cellular surface will be able to degrade and take up higher amounts of amino acids needed for glutathione synthesis. This will give these cells a selective advantage during the promotion. γ-Glutamyltransferase may thus not be a marker of fetal phenotype in preneoplastic cells, but the enzyme provides the cell a selective advantage during stress and intracellular depletion of glutathione. This model may also have implications for cellular toxicity.

VII. ROLE IN CLINICAL ENZYMOLOGY

The measurement of γ-glutamyltransferase activity in serum has been a sensitive test for liver pathology. Rosalki[8] stated in his review in 1975 that γ-glutamyltransferase is the best screening parameter for liver obstructive diseases. γ-Glutamyltransferase has also been suggested as a parameter of alcohol abuse as it frequently is increased in alcoholic liver injury. However, as γ-glutamyltransferase activity is also increased in other diseases such as diabetes and cardiac and neurological diseases, the specificity of γ-glutamyltransferase as a liver test is limited. Goldberg concluded in his critical review[9] that the measurement of γ-glutamyltransferase "has yet to find a genuinely useful diagnostic role substantiated by a convincing body of scientific data."

In serum γ-glutamyltransferase is present in several multiple forms. These have been demonstrated to be complexes of the enzyme with serum lipoproteins and lipid aggregates.[88,89] There are some indications that such multiple forms might increase the specificity of γ-glutamyltransferase as a cholestatic marker.

REFERENCES

1. **Curthoys, N. P. and Hughey, R. P.**, Characterization and physiological function of rat renal γ-glutamyltranspeptidase, *Enzyme*, 24, 383, 1979.
2. **Tate, S. S. and Meister, A.**, γ-Glutamyl transpeptidase: catalytic, structural and functional aspects, *Mol. Cell. Biochem.*, 39, 357, 1981.
3. **Curthoys, N. P., Frielle, T., Tsao, B., McIntyre, T. M., and Hughey, R. P.**, The amphipathic structure and membrane topology of enzymes involved in the renal catabolism of glutathione, in *Glutathione: Storage, Transport and Turnover in Mammals*, Sakamoto, Y., Higashi, T., and Tateishi, N., Eds., VNU Science Press BV, Utrecht, 1983, 147.
4. **Meister, A.**, New aspects of glutathione biochemistry and transport: selective alteration of glutathione metabolism, *Fed. Proc., Fed. Am. Soc. Exp. Biol.*, 43, 3031, 1984.
5. **Horiuchi, S., Inoue, M., and Morino, Y.**, γ-Glutamyl transpeptidase: sidedness of its active site on renal brush border membrane, *Eur. J. Biochem.*, 87, 429, 1978.
6. **Hughey, R. P., Coyle, P. J., and Curthoys, N. P.**, Comparison of the association and orientation of γ-glutamyltranspeptidase in lecithin vesicles and in native membranes, *J. Biol. Chem.*, 254, 1124, 1979.
7. **Huseby, N. E.**, Subcellular localization of γ-glutamyltransferase activity in guinea pig liver. Effect of phenobarbital on the enzyme activity level, *Clin. Chim. Acta*, 94, 163, 1979.
8. **Rosalki, S. B.**, Gamma-glutamyl transpeptidase, in *Advances in Clinical Chemistry*, Vol. 17, Bodansky, O. and Latner, A. L., Eds., Academic Press, New York, 1975, 53.
9. **Goldberg, D. M.**, Structural, functional and clinical aspects of γ-glutamyltransferase, *Crit. Rev. Clin. Lab. Sci.*, 12, 1, 1980.
10. **Meister, A., Tate, S. S., and Ross, L. L.**, Membrane bound γ-glutamyl transpeptidase, in *The Enzymes of Biological Membranes: Enzymes, Transport Systems and Receptors*, Vol. 3, Martonosi, A., Ed., Plenum Press, New York, 1976, 315.
11. **Dakin, H. D. and Dudley, H. W.**, Glyoxalase III. The distribution of the enzyme and its relation to the pancreas, *J. Biol. Chem.*, 15, 463, 1913.
12. **Binkley, F. and Nakamura, K.**, Metabolism of glutathione hydrolysis by tissues of the rat, *J. Biol. Chem.*, 173, 411, 1948.
13. **Hanes, C. S., Hird, F. J. R., and Isherwood, F. A.**, Enzymic transpeptidation reactions involving γ-glutamyl peptides and α-amino-acyl peptides, *Biochem. J.*, 51, 25, 1952.
14. **Tate, S. S. and Meister, A.**, Interactions of γ-glutamyl transpeptidase with amino acids, dipeptides, and derivatives and analogs of glutathione, *J. Biol. Chem.*, 249, 7593, 1974.
15. **Thompson, G. A. and Meister, A.**, Interrelationships between the binding site for amino acids, dipeptides and γ-glutamyl donors in γ-glutamyl transpeptidase, *J. Biol. Chem.*, 252, 6792, 1977.
16. **Tate, S. S.**, Enzymes of mercapturic acid formation, in *Enzymatic Basis of Detoxification*, Jacoby, W., Ed., Academic Press, New York, 1980, 95.
17. **Örning, L. and Hammarström, S.**, Leukotriene D: a slow reacting substance from rat basophilic leukemic cells, *Proc. Natl. Acad. Sci. U.S.A.*, 77, 2014, 1980.
18. **Tate, S. S. and Meister, A.**, Identity of maleate-stimulated glutaminase activity with γ-glutamyl transpeptidase in rat kidney, *J. Biol. Chem.*, 250, 4619, 1975.
19. **Curthoys, N. P. and Kuhlenschmidt, T.**, Phosphate-independent glutaminase from rat kidney. Partial purification and identity with γ-glutamyltranspeptidase, *J. Biol. Chem.*, 250, 2099, 1975.

20. **Thompson, G. A. and Meister, A.,** Modulation of the hydrolysis, transfer and glutaminase activities of γ-glutamyl transpeptidase by maleate bound at the cysteinylglycine binding site of the enzyme, *J. Biol. Chem.,* 254, 2956, 1979.

21. **Thompson, G. A. and Meister, A.,** Modulation of γ-glutamyl-transpeptidase activities by hippurate and related compounds, *J. Biol. Chem.,* 255, 2109, 1980.

22. **Elce, J. C.,** Kinetics and mechanism of rat kidney γ-glutamyltransferase, in *Gamma-Glutamyltransferases,* (Adv. Biochem. Pharmacol., 3rd ser.), Siest, G. and Heusghem, C., Eds., Masson, Paris, 1982, 15.

23. **International Federation of Clinical Chemistry,** IFCC methods for the measurement of catalytic concentration of enzymes. IV. IFCC method for γ-glutamyltransferase, *J. Clin. Chem. Clin. Biochem.,* 21, 633, 1983.

24. **McIntyre, T. M. and Curthoys, N. P.,** Comparison of the hydrolytic and transfer activities of rat renal γ-glutamyl transpeptidase, *J. Biol. Chem.,* 254, 6499, 1979.

25. **Allison, R. D. and Meister, A.,** Evidence that transpeptidation is a significant function of γ-glutamyl transpeptidase. *J. Biol. Chem.,* 256, 2988, 1981.

26. **Shaw, L. M., London, J. W., Fetterolf, D., and Garfinkel, D.,** γ-Glutamyltransferase: kinetic properties and assay conditions when γ-glutamyl-4-nitroanilide and its 3-carboxy derivative are used as donor substrates, *Clin. Chem.,* 23, 79, 1977.

27. **Shaw, L. M. and Newman, D. A.,** Hydrolysis of glutathione by human liver γ-glutamyltransferase, *Clin. Chem.,* 25, 75, 1979.

28. **Revel, J. P. and Ball, E. G.,** The reaction of glutathione with amino acids and related compounds as catalyzed by γ-glutamyl transpeptidase, *J. Biol. Chem.,* 234, 577, 1959.

29. **Tate, S. S. and Meister, A.,** Serine-borate complex as a transition state inhibitor of γ-glutamyl transpeptidase, *Proc. Natl. Acad. Sci. U.S.A.,* 75, 4806, 1978.

30. **Tate, S. S. and Meister, A.,** Affinity labeling of γ-glutamyl transpeptidase and location of the γ-glutamyl binding site on the light subunit, *Proc. Natl. Acad. Sci. U.S.A.,* 74, 931, 1977.

31. **Inoue, M., Horiuchi, S., and Morino, Y.,** Affinity labeling of rat kidney γ-glutamyl transpeptidase, *Eur. J. Biochem.,* 73, 335, 1977.

32. **Gardell, S. J. and Tate, S. S.,** Affinity labeling of γ-glutamyl transpeptidase by glutamine antagonists. Effects on the γ-glutamyl transfer and proteinase activities, *FEBS Lett.,* 122, 171, 1980.

33. **Szasz, G.,** A kinetic photometric method for serum γ-glutamyl transpeptidase, *Clin. Chem.,* 15, 124, 1969.

34. **Huseby, N. E. and Strömme, J. H.,** Practical points regarding routine determination of γ-glutamyltransferase (γ-GT) in serum with a kinetic method at 37°C, *Scand. J. Clin. Lab. Invest.,* 34, 357, 1974.

35. **Committee on Enzymes,** the Scandinavian Society for Clinical Chemistry and Clinical Physiology, Recommended method for the determination of γ-glutamyltransferase in blood, *Scand. J. Clin. Lab. Invest.,* 36, 119, 1976.

36. **Smith, G. D., Ding, J. L., and Peters, T. J.,** A sensitive fluorometric assay for γ-glutamyl transferase, *Anal. Biochem.,* 100, 136, 1979.

37. **Hughey, R. P. and Curthoys, N. P.,** Comparison of the size and physical properties of γ-glutamyltranspeptidase purified from rat kidney following solubilization with papain or with Triton X-100, *J. Biol. Chem.,* 251, 7863, 1976.

38. **Tate, S. S. and Meister, A.,** Subunit structure and isozymic forms of γ-glutamyl transpeptidase, *Proc. Natl. Acad. Sci. U.S.A.,* 73, 2599, 1976.

39. **Tate, S. S. and Ross, M. E.,** Human kidney γ-glutamyl transpeptidase. Catalytic properties, subunit structure and localization of γ-glutamyl binding site on the light subunit, *J. Biol. Chem.,* 252, 6042, 1977.

40. **Huseby, N. E.,** Purification and some properties of γ-glutamyltransferase from human liver, *Biochim. Biophys. Acta,* 483, 46, 1977.

41. **Huseby, N. E.,** Multiple forms of γ-glutamyltransferase in normal human liver, bile and serum, *Biochim. Biophys. Acta,* 522, 354, 1978.

42. **Huseby, N. E.,** Hydrophilic form of γ-glutamyltransferase: proteolytic formation in liver homogenates and its estimation in serum, *Clin. Chim. Acta,* 124, 113, 1982.

43. **Matsuda, Y., Tsuji, A., and Katunuma, N.,** Studies on the structure of γ-glutamyltranspeptidase. III. Evidence that the aminoterminus of the heavy subunit is the membrane binding segment, *J. Biochem.,* 93, 1427, 1983.

44. **Tsao, B. and Curthoys, N. P.,** Evidence that the hydrophobic domain of rat renal γ-glutamyltranspeptidase spans the brush border membrane, *Biochim. Biophys. Acta,* 690, 199, 1982.

45. **Nash, B. and Tate, S. S.,** Biosynthesis of rat renal γ-glutamyl transpeptidase. Evidence for a common precursor of the two subunits, *J. Biol. Chem.,* 257, 585, 1982.

46. **Capraro, M. A. and Hughey, R. P.,** Processing of the propeptide form of rat renal γ-glutamyltranspeptidase, *FEBS Lett.,* 157, 139, 1983.

47. **Matsuda, Y., Tsuji, A., Kuno, T., and Katunuma, N.,** Biosynthesis and degradation of γ-glutamyltranspeptidase of rat kidney, *J. Biochem.,* 94, 755, 1983.

48. **Capraro, M. A. and Curthoys, N. P.,** Use of acivicin in the determination of rate constants for turnover of rat renal γ-glutamyltranspeptidase, *J. Biol. Chem.,* 260, 3408, 1985.

49. **Yamashita, K., Hitoi, A., Matsuda, Y., Tsuji, A., Katumuna, N., and Kobata, A.,** Structural studies of the carbohydrate moieties of rat kidney γ-glutamyltranspeptidase. An extremely heterogeneous pattern enriched with nonreducing terminal N-acetylglucosamine residues, *J. Biol. Chem.,* 258, 1098, 1983.

50. **Huseby, N. E.,** Separation and characterization of human γ-glutamyltransferases, *Clin. Chim. Acta,* 111, 39, 1981.

51. **Lilja, H., Jeppsson, J. O., and Kristensson, H.,** Evaluation of serum γ-glutamyltransferase by electrofocusing, and variations in isoform patterns, *Clin. Chem.,* 29, 1034, 1983.

52. **Tsuchida, S., Yamazaki, T., Camba, E. M., Morita, T., Matsue, H., Yoshida, Y., and Sato, K.,** Comparison of the peptide and saccharide moieties of γ-glutamyltransferase isolated from neoplastic and non-neoplastic human liver tissue, *Clin. Chim. Acta,* 152, 17, 1985.

53. **Shaw, L. M., Petersen-Archer, L., London, J. W., and Marsh, E.,** Electrophoretic, kinetic, and immunoinhibition properties of γ-glutamyltransferase from various tissues compared, *Clin. Chem.,* 26, 1523, 1980.

54. **Huseby, N. E. and Eide, T. J.,** Variant γ-glutamyltransferases in colorectal carcinomas, *Clin. Chim. Acta,* 135, 301, 1983.

55. **Hada, T., Higashino, K., Yamamoto, H., Okochi, T., Sumikawa, K., and Yumamura, Y.,** Further investigations on a novel γ-glutamyltranspeptidase in human renal carcinoma, *Clin. Chim. Acta,* 112, 135, 1981.

56. **Spater, H. W., Poruchynski, M. S., Quintana, N., Inoue, M., and Novikoff, A. B.,** Immunocytochemical localization of γ-glutamyltransferase in rat kidney with protein A-horseradish peroxidase, *Proc. Natl. Acad. Sci. U.S.A.,* 79, 3547, 1982.

57. **Pfaller, W., Gstrunthaler, G., Kotanko, P., Wolf, H., and Curthoys, N. P.,** Immunocytochemical localization of γ-glutamyl transferase on isolated renal cortical tubular fragments, *Histochemie,* 80, 289, 1984.

58. **Dass, P. D., Misra, R. P., and Welbourne, T. C.,** Renal γ-glutamyl-transpeptidase in situ antiluminal localization, *J. Histochem. Cytochem.,* 30, 148, 1982.

59. **Desmet, V.,** Histochemical variations of GGT in normal and pathological liver, in *Gammaglutamyltransferases,* (Adv. Biochem. Pharmacol., 3rd series), Siest, G. and Heusgheur, C., Eds., Massou, Paris, 1982, 175.

60. **Galteau, M. M., Siest, G., and Ratanasavahn, D.,** Effect of phenobarbital on the distribution of gamma-glutamyltransferase between hepatocytes and nonparenchymal cells in the rat, *Cell. Mol. Biol.,* 26, 267, 1980.

61. **Inoue, M., Akerboom, T. P. M., Sies, H., Kinne, R., Thao, T., and Arias, I. M.,** Biliary transport of glutathione S-conjugate by rat liver canalicular membrane vesicles, *J. Biol. Chem.,* 259, 4998, 1984.

62. **Higashi, T. and Yamaguchi, K.,** Retrospects and prospects, in *Glutathione: Storage, Transport and Turnover in Mammals,* Sakamoto, Y., Higashi, T., and Tateishi, N., Eds., VNU Science Press BV, Utrecht, 1983, 3.

63. **Meister, A. and Anderson, M. E.,** Glutathione, *Ann. Rev. Biochem.,* 52, 711, 1983.

64. **Sies, H.,** Reduced and oxidized glutathione efflux from liver, in *Glutathione: Storage, Transport and Turnover in Mammals,* Sakamoto, Y., Higashi, T., and Tateishi, N., Eds., VNU Science Press BV, Utrecht, 1983, 63.

65. **Inoue, M. and Morino, Y.,** Direct evidence for the role of the membrane potential in glutathione transport by renal brush-border membrane, *J. Biol. Chem.,* 260, 326, 1985.

66. **Haberle, D. A., Wahlander, A., and Sies, H.,** Assessment of the kidney function in maintenance of plasma glutathione concentration and redox state in anaesthetized rats, *FEBS Lett.,* 108, 335, 1979.

67. **Abbott, W. A., Bridges, R. J., and Meister, A.,** Extracellular metabolism of glutathione accounts for its disappearance from the basolateral circulation of the kidney, *J. Biol. Chem.,* 259, 15393, 1984.

68. **Rankin, B. B., Wells, W., and Curthoys, N. P.,** Rat renal peritubular transport and metabolism of plasma ^{35}S-glutathione, *Am. J. Physiol.,* 249, F198, 1985.

69. **Bridges, R. J. and Meister, A.,** γ-Glutamyl amino acids. Transport and conversion to 5-oxoproline in the kidney, *J. Biol. Chem.,* 260, 7304, 1985.

70. **Okajima, K., Inoue, M., Itoh, K., Horiuchi, S., and Morino, Y.,** Interorgan cooperation in enzymic processing and membrane transport of glutathione S-conjugates, in *Glutathione: Storage, Transport and Turnover in Mammals,* Sakamoto, Y., Higashi, T., and Tateishi, N., Eds., VNU Science Press BV, Utrecht, 1983, 129.

71. **Hanigan, M. H. and Pitot, H. C.,** Gamma-glutamyl transpeptidase — its role in hepatocarcinogenesis, *Carcinogenesis,* 6, 165, 1985.

72. **Örning, L. and Hammarström, S.,** Kinetics of the conversion of leukotriene C by γ-glutamyltranspeptidase, *Biochem. Biophys. Res. Commun.,* 106, 1304, 1982.

73. **Orlowski, M. and Meister, A.,** The γ-glutamyl cycle: a possible transport system for amino acids, *Proc. Natl. Acad. Sci. U.S.A.,* 67, 1248, 1970.

74. **Ormstad, K., Tanaka, M., and Orrenius, S.,** Functions of γ-glutamyltransferase in kidney, in *Gamma-glutamyltransferases,* (Adv. Biochem. Pharmacol., 3rd ser.), Siest, G. and Heusghem, C., Eds., Masson, Paris, 1982, 7.

75. **Pellefigue, F., Butler, J. D., Spielberg, S. P., Hollenberg, M. D., Goodman, S. I., and Schulman, J. D.,** Normal amino acid uptake by cultured human fibroblasts does not require gamma-glutamyl transpeptidase, *Biochem. Biophys. Res. Commun.,* 73, 997, 1976.

76. **Schulman, J. D., Goodman, S. I., Mace, J. W., Patrick, A. D., Tietze, E., and Butler, E. J.,** Glutathionuria: inborn errors of metabolism due to tissue deficiency of gamma-glutamyl transpeptidase, *Biochem. Biophys. Res. Commun.,* 65, 68, 1975.

77. **Griffith, O. W. and Meister, A.,** Translocation of intracellular glutathione to membrane-bound γ-glutamyl transpeptidase as a discrete step in γ-glutamyl cycle: glutathionuria after inhibition of transpeptidase, *Proc. Natl. Acad. Sci. U.S.A.,* 76, 268, 1979.

78. **Anderson, M. E., Bridges, R. J., and Meister, A.,** Direct evidence for inter-organ transport of glutathione and that the non-filtration renal mechanism for glutathione utilization involves γ-glutamyl transpeptidase, *Biochem. Biophys. Res. Commun.,* 96, 848, 1980.

79. **Katunuma, N., Tomino, L., and Nishino, H.,** Glutaminase isoenzymes in rat kidney, *Biochem. Biophys. Res. Commun.,* 22, 321, 1966.

80. **Kvamme, E.,** Enzymes of cerebral glutaminase metabolism, in *Glutamine Metabolism in Mammalian Tissues,* Häussinger, D. and Sies, H., Eds., Springer-Verlag, Berlin, 1984, 32.

81. **Welbourne, T. C. and Dass, P. D.,** Role of hippurate in acidosis in the renal γ-glutamyltranspeptidase, *Life Sci.,* 29, 253, 1981.

82. **Dass, P. D. and Wu, M.,** Uptake and metabolism of glutamine in cultured kidney cells, *Biochim. Biophys. Acta,* 845, 94, 1985.

83. **Curthoys, N. P., Shapiro, R. A., and Haser, W. G.,** Enzymes of renal glutaminase metabolism, in *Glutamine Metabolism in Mammalian Tissues,* Häussinger, D. and Sies, H., Eds., Springer-Verlag, Berlin, 1984, 16.

84. **Shapiro, R. A. and Curthoys, N. P.,** Differential effects of AT-125 on rat renal glutaminase activities, *FEBS Lett.,* 133, 131, 1981.

85. **Peraino, C., Richards, W. L., and Stevens, F. J.,** Multistage-hepatocarcinogenesis, *Environ. Health Perspect.,* 50, 1, 1983.

86. **Fiala, S., Fiala, A. E., and Dixon, B.,** Gamma-glutamyl transpeptidase in transplantable, chemically induced rat hepatomas and 'spontaneous' mouse hepatomas, *J. Natl. Cancer Inst.,* 48, 1393, 1972.

87. **Kalengayi, M. M., Ronchi, G., and Desmet, V. J.,** Histochemistry of gamma-glutamyltranspeptidase in rat liver during aflatoxin B_1 induced carcinogenesis, *J. Natl. Cancer Inst.,* 55, 579, 1975.

88. **Huseby, N. E.,** Multiple forms of serum γ-glutamyltransferase. Association of the enzyme with lipoproteins, *Clin. Chim. Acta,* 124, 103, 1982.

89. **Wenham, P. R., Horn, D. B., and Smith, A. F.,** Multiple forms of γ-glutamyltransferase: a clinical study, *Clin. Chem.,* 31, 569, 1985.

Extranervous Metabolism of Glutamine and Glutamate

Chapter 10

GLUTAMINE: AN ENERGY SOURCE FOR MAMMALIAN TISSUES

J. Tyson Tildon and H. Ronald Zielke

TABLE OF CONTENTS

I. INTRODUCTION

Glutamine and alanine are the major amino acids released from the muscle[1-4] and subsequent utilization of alanine has been proposed to occur via an alanine-glucose cycle[5,6] very similar to the recycling of lactate in the Cori cycle.[7] The major metabolic fate of glutamine has not been well defined; however, this has been the object of intense investigation in several laboratories.

A review of the literature provides evidence that glutamine is an oxidative fuel for multiple tissues and that lactate and alanine, by-products of its metabolism, may be gluconeogenic precursors via a glutamine-glucose cycle. These functions of glutamine are in addition to its role in protein,[8] purine,[9] and neurotransmitter[10-14] synthesis, and acid-base balance.[15] The conclusion that glutamine is a major respiratory substrate for mammalian organisms is based on its availability following release by the muscle, its elevated concentration in tissue and body fluids, its uptake by tissues such as the intestine, its oxidation by these tissues and by cultured cells, and its ability to support growth in vitro in the absence of other energy sources. A comparison of the rates of utilization of various potential energy sources indicates that the intestine, fibroblasts, tumor cells, lymphocytes, brain, heart, chondrocytes, reticulocytes, eye lens, and oocytes are among tissues that are likely candidates for the utilization of glutamine as a respiratory substrate.

A major consideration in a review of the utilization of glutamine as an energy source is the methodology and systems being employed for the various studies. Some studies have measured ATP production[16,17] while others have used cell growth in culture.[18-20] Other investigators have measured uptake or transport into isolated cells[21-23] or subcellular components such as mitochondria or synaptosomes.[24,25] Similar types of uptake studies have been performed with isolated perfused organs and measuring changes in arteriovenous concentrations[26,27] using several different animal species. In our studies we have focused mainly on CO_2 production from labeled precursors. Several of our studies compared the utilization of substrates by whole homogenates and by dissociated cells from brain tissue. The use of these two systems revealed striking differences in the rates of oxidation of several substrates especially when comparisons are made at various times during development.[28,29] This approach has also allowed for extensive examination of the kinetics of oxidation as well as the transport. All experimental approaches have their limitations, but by using several different systems it has become reasonable to draw the conclusion that glutamine metabolism plays a central role in the energetic homeostasis of the mammalian organism.

II. GLUTAMINE AS AN ENERGY SOURCE FOR CULTURED FIBROBLASTS

During early studies of factors required for maintenance of tissue cells in vitro Ehrensvärd et al.[30] identified glutamine as an obligate factor of tissue culture nutrition. Although glutamine is not an essential amino acid for humans, the cell culture requirement was due in part to the low activity of glutamine synthetase activity in cultured cells. Some cell lines were able to grow in a medium with 20 m*M* glutamate, but lacking glutamine, because of the induction of glutamine synthetase.[31,32] When Eagle[33] empirically determined the in vitro cellular requirement for amino acids, he noted that glutamine was required at a concentration 10- to 100-fold greater than other amino acids and that it was extensively metabolized. The rate of disappearance of glutamine from the medium was greater than for other amino acids;[20,34-36] this disappearance primarily reflected utilization rather than chemical decomposition.[20,37] In early studies with radioactively labeled glutamine, Stoner and Merchant[20] reported that 56% of the utilized glutamine could be accounted for in $^{14}CO_2$, 15% in other amino acids, and 17% in cellular material. In spite of these reports it was generally maintained that glucose was the primary, if not sole, energy source for cultured cells.[38]

Table 1
RECIPROCAL INHIBITION OF GLUCOSE
AND GLUTAMINE OXIDATION BY
HUMAN FIBROBLASTS

[14]C-Substrate	Addition	[14]CO$_2$ Released (nmol/ mg protein/hr)
Glutamine-1-[14]C	—	310
	Glucose	54
Glutamine-5-[14]C	—	80
	Glucose	13
Glucose-1-[14]C	—	30
	Glutamine	53
Glucose-6-[14]C	—	7.5
	Glutamine	0.9

Note: The oxidative rates are the mean of four samples using cells obtained during logarithmic growth phase. Labeled substrates were added in 2 mℓ of MEM (minimal essential medium) plus 10% dialyzed fetal calf serum. The concentration of radioactive or nonradioactive glucose and glutamine, when present in these experiments, was 5.5 or 2.0 m*M*, respectively.[40]

This conclusion was questioned by a series of papers on glucose and glutamine metabolism in human diploid fibroblasts. Tildon[16] observed that fibroblasts from a patient with succinyl-CoA:3-ketoacid-CoA transferase deficiency exhibited normal growth but utilized only 20% as much glucose as control cells, suggesting that an alternative energy source, perhaps glutamine, was used by the enzyme-deficient cells. Zielke et al.[37] reported that fibroblasts were not dependent on glucose for their energy if low levels of nucleosides were included in the medium to allow cellular replication. Under these conditions the rate of glutamine utilization increased twofold. Other experiments demonstrated that there was reciprocal regulation of glucose and glutamine oxidation (Table 1). The rate of L[1- or 5-^{14}C] glutamine oxidation was sixfold greater in the absence of glucose than in its presence (Crabtree effect). In an analogous manner D[6-^{14}C]glucose oxidation was eightfold greater in the absence of glutamine than in its presence. Furthermore, the oxidation of D[1-^{14}C]glucose, which proceeds via the hexose-monophosphate shunt and provides a precursor for nucleic acid biosynthesis, was stimulated by glutamine, itself a nucleic acid precursor. These experiments demonstrate the importance of measuring metabolic rates under conditions which allow for the interactive metabolism of several potential energy sources. Other potential energy sources such as fatty acids and ketone bodies were not oxidized by fibroblasts and lacked an effect on glutamine oxidation.[39] Based on these studies Zielke et al.[18,40] calculated that glutamine was utilized as the primary energy source in the absence of glucose, and that even in the presence of physiological concentrations of glucose, glutamine was the primary respiratory substrate and provided at least one third of the energy of growing fibroblasts.

Similar conclusions were reached by other investigators through studies with mutant fibroblast cultures. DeFrancesco et al.[42] described a Chinese hamster cell mutant with a defect in tricarboxylic acid (TCA) cycle activity. These cells had a 90% decrease in their oxygen uptake, a decreased rate of glucose oxidation, and an increased metabolism of glucose to lactate.[43] Based on the increased rate of glycolysis in the absence of respiration, Donnelly and Scheffler[43] estimated that the hamster cells obtained 40% of their energy from respiration, primarily glutamine, and 60% from glycolysis. These results correlate well with our findings and indicate that fibroblasts increase their utilization of alternative substrates when the

Table 2

GLUCOSE AND GLUTAMINE OXIDATION BY MUTANT CHINESE HAMSTER LUNG FIBROBLASTS

	$^{14}CO_2$ Released (nmol/mg protein/hr)					
	Glutamine-1-^{14}C		Glutamine-5-^{14}C		Glucose-6-^{14}C	
Cell line	− Glc	+ Glc	− Glc	+ Glc	− Gln	+ Gln
O_{23} (Normal)	5.7 ± 1.0	1.3 ± 0.5	2.0 ± 0.4	0.5 ± 0.1	1.3 ± 0.7	2.0 ± 1.0
DS_7 (PGI def)	14.9 ± 2.0	15.8 ± 2.9	10.2 ± 2.6	9.1 ± 0.8	0	0.1 ± 0.2
GSK_3 (RESP def)	0.5 ± 0.4	1.4 ± 1.0	0.2 ± 0.2	0.1 ± 0.1	0.6 ± 0.3	1.4 ± 1.0

Note: The concentrations of radioactive glutamine were 0.5 mM and of radioactive glucose were 1.0 mM. The concentration of nonradioactive glutamine, when present, was 2.0 mM and nonradioactive glucose, when present, was 5.5 mM. n = 4. PGI def = Phosphoglucose isomerase deficient and RESP def = respiratory chain deficient. The Chinese hamster lung fibroblast cells for this study were obtained from Dr. J. Pouysségur.

availability of one substrate is decreased either by exclusion or due to an enzyme defect. A subsequent study demonstrated that the high-energy phosphate state of the two cell types was similar but that the adenylate pool was smaller in the respiratory mutants than in control fibroblasts.[44] Pouysségur et al.[45] and Franchi et al.[46] described two mutants of Chinese hamster lung fibroblasts, one of which was dependent on respiration because of a lack of phosphoglucose isomerase activity (DS_7) and a second mutant that was dependent on glycolysis because of a defect in respiration (GSK_3). The existence of these two mutants demonstrates that these cells can alternatively use either respiration or glycolysis for energy when one of these pathways is missing. As anticipated, the GSK_3 cells have a very low rate of glutamine oxidation while DS_7 cells have a rate nearly triple that of the wild-type parental cell (O_{23}) (Table 2). The rate of glucose oxidation is low compared to glutamine oxidation, especially for the DS_7 cells. Glutamine oxidation by the normal parental cells was inhibited about 75% by glucose, similar to the inhibition observed with human fibroblasts. However, glutamine oxidation by DS_7 cells was not inhibited by glucose suggesting that either a metabolite of glucose or the energy state of the cell regulates glutamine oxidation in normal cells. It is surprising that the rate of glutamine oxidation by hamster fibroblasts is much lower than for human fibroblasts (compare Tables 1 and 2). However, the rates for glucose oxidation reported here for the hamster cells are similar to those reported by Franchi et al.[46] From these types of studies with fibroblasts, one can conclude that normal cells use two energy sources: glucose via glycolysis and glutamine for respiration. Under conditions where one pathway is impaired, the second compensates with increases in rates. Likewise, under experimental conditions in which glucose is supplied at a low level, cell growth is maintained through increased glutamine oxidation[40] and a greater proportion of the limited glucose is metabolized to the ribose moiety of nucleosides.[47]

Stoner and Merchant[20] reported that CO_2 was the major metabolite of glutamine metabolism. Table 3 summarizes the products of glutamine metabolism by cultured cells. Surprisingly, over 10% of the glutamine is converted to lactate. It has been proposed that the malic enzyme converts malate, formed from glutamine, to pyruvate which is then reduced to lactate.[17,48] Glutamine can also be a good precursor for lipid biosynthesis in fibroblasts[49] which is consistent with the rapid rate of glutamine oxidation observed in the absence of glucose (Table 1). Under these conditions glutamine supplies both the oxalacetate and the acetyl-CoA unit to maintain a functioning TCA cycle.

Table 3
PRODUCTS OF GLUTAMINE
METABOLISM BY CULTURED
MAMMALIAN CELLS

Product	Percent of metabolized glutamine	Ref.
CO_2	35—56	17,20
Glutamate	17	48
Lactate	13	17,48
Pyruvate	2	17
Citrate	3	17
Malate	1	17
Aspartate	<1	17
Cellular material	2	17,48

From Zielke, H. R., Sumbilla, C. M., Zielke, C. L., Tildon, J. T., and Ozand, P. T., *Glutamine Metabolism in Mammalian Tissues*, Häussinger, D. and Sies, H., Eds., Springer-Verlag, New York, 1984, 247. With permission.

III. GLUTAMINE AS AN ENERGY SOURCE FOR CANCER CELL LINES

The bioenergetics of cancer cells have been extensively studied since Warburg[50] proposed that cancer cells may have an impaired respiratory capacity which is compensated by increased rate of glycolysis. Subsequent studies have shown variation in the bioenergetic mechanisms used by different cancer cells.[51] Even with an elevated rate of glycolysis, 50 to 85% of the energy produced in tumor cells is derived from mitochondrial oxidative phosphorylation.[52] In addition to glucose, tumor cells can utilize fatty acids,[53,54] amino acids, especially glutamine,[17,33,55,56] and ketone bodies.[57] The rate and the identity of preferential substrates varies with the origin, degree of differentiation, and rate of growth of the tumor.[51]

Kvamme and Svenneby[58,59] observed that Ehrlich ascites cells rapidly metabolized glutamine, consistent with a role in energy production. This was supported by additional studies using these cells.[60] Kovačević and Morris[55] measured rates of glutamine oxidation in Morris hepatomas which correlated with growth rate. It has been demonstrated that glutaminase activity in extracts is proportional to growth rate;[61,62] however, the interpretation of these results is uncertain because of the difference between glutaminase activity in extracts and whole cells (see Section VI). Glutamine is also the primary respiratory substrate for lymphoma cells[63] and hematopoietic tumors.[64] Detailed studies on the energy production by HeLa cells in the presence of various hexoses revealed that in the presence of fructose or galactose essentially all of the cellular energy was obtained from glutamine oxidation, and that in the presence of glucose over one half of the cellular energy was obtained from glutamine.[17] Under aerobic conditions HeLa cells were able to maintain their intracellular ATP levels in the absence of hexoses if glutamine was available. However, not all tumor lines have a strict requirement for glutamine and the proportion of energy derived from glutamine may also vary[65,66] reflecting the variability and adaptivity of tumor cells.

A role for glutamine as a respiratory fuel for tumors is also supported by studies in vivo. Roberts and Simonsen[67] demonstrated a lower glutamine content in malignant tumors than in normal tissue. Sebolt and Weber[68] reported a negative correlation of glutamine content with proliferation rate of implanted rat hepatomas. The data suggest that the more rapidly growing tumors utilize glutamine at a rapid rate, therefore, resulting in a lower glutamine content in the tumor. The rapid utilization of glutamine by tumor cells has been proposed as a point of attack in the treatment of malignancies.[69-71] The utilization of glutamine as an

Table 4

**COMPARISON OF THE RATES OF GLUCOSE AND
GLUTAMINE OXIDATION BY WHOLE
HOMOGENATES OF BRAIN AND DISSOCIATED
BRAIN CELLS**

Substrate conc (mM)	Dissociated brain cells		Brain whole homogenates	
	Glucose	**Glutamine**	**Glucose**	**Glutamine**
0.5	4.02 ± 0.43	12.5 ± 1.6	2.7 ± 0.36	15.5 ± 1.33
1.0	4.35 ± 0.56	14.5 ± 1.5	4.09 ± 0.37	22.5 ± 1.06
2.0	4.36 ± 0.31	16.7 ± 1.0	6.07 ± 0.46	27.5 ± 1.12
5.0	4.45 ± 0.45	19.3 ± 1.2	5.18 ± 0.42	30.6 ± 1.35

Note: Rates of oxidation (mean ± SEM) are expressed as nmol/hr/mg protein of substrates converted to $^{14}CO_2$ at 37°C. U-^{14}C-Glutamine and 6-^{14}C-glucose were used in these experiments. For glucose, n = 4; for glutamine, n = 3.[74]

energy source may be a general phenomenon for normal tissue which is rapidly growing or regenerating. Tissue such as testis, intestinal mucosa, spleen, and thymus contained 18 to 46% as much glutamine as normal liver. These results are consistent with the rapid utilization of glutamine by the small intestines.[26] It also suggests that tissues rapidly regenerating following damage due to trauma may utilize increased amounts of glutamine during the healing process.

The question of why tumor cells, as well as fibroblasts, primarily metabolize glucose to lactate rather than oxidize pyruvate totally to CO_2 via the TCA cycle is still unresolved. This topic has been extensively reviewed by Pederson.[51] However, his suggestion that cultured cells may have reduced capacity to oxidize pyruvate is questionable. The oxidation rate of 100 μM[1-^{14}C] pyruvate by human fibroblasts was 4.9 compared to 36.0 nmol/hr/ mg protein for 500 μM pyruvate.[71a] Glutamine had no effect on the rate of pyruvate oxidation, nor did pyruvate affect the rate of glutamine oxidation.[18] The oxidation rate of pyruvate is greater than that of glucose (see Table 1). The greater oxidation rate with 500 μM pyruvate compared to 100 μM pyruvate may indicate that pyruvate inactivates the pyruvate dehydrogenase kinase, an inhibitor of pyruvate dehydrogenase.[72] The concentration effect of pyruvate is probably not related to the K_m (pyruvate) of pyruvate dehydrogenase which is 42 μM.[73]

IV. GLUTAMINE AS AN ENERGY SOURCE FOR THE BRAIN

One of the strongest arguments for the utilization of glutamine as an energy source are studies showing the production of $^{14}CO_2$ from labeled glutamine. Results from our laboratory[29,74] as well as those by Hertz and colleagues[23,75] have demonstrated a metabolic flux of glutamine via α-ketoglutarate (2-oxoglutarate) to CO_2. Perhaps most revealing were the results showing the rate of glutamine oxidation to be greater than the rate of glucose oxidation (Table 4). The oxidation rates of [U-^{14}C]glutamine by two preparations (dissociated brain cells and brain whole homogenates) were determined at several different substrate concentrations. The results reveal that the rate of oxidation of [U-^{14}C] glutamine by dissociated brain cells is three- to fourfold greater than the rate of oxidation of [6-^{14}C] glucose. Using brain whole homogenates the difference was even greater. It should be noted that using homogenates, the rates for glutamine and glucose oxidation doubled when the initial substrate concentration was increased tenfold over the range of 0.5 to 5.0 mM. In our studies with both freshly prepared dissociated brain cells as well as whole brain homogenates, glutamine oxidation was inhibited by about 80% with either rotenone or antimycin A, suggesting a role for the electron transport chain in the oxidation of glutamine. Furthermore, only 40% of the glutamine oxidation was inhibited by aminooxyacetate, an inhibitor of glutamine decarboxylase and glutamine oxaloacetate transferase. Yu et al.[23] using primary astrocytes observed that there was essentially no inhibition of glutamine oxidation by aminooxyacetate. These results indicate that significant amounts of glutamine are metabolized by these tissues via a reaction sequence that includes the formation of α-ketoglutarate as catalyzed by glutamate dehydrogenase with subsequent metabolism via the TCA cycle.

In a companion series of studies employing either brain whole homogenates or dissociated brain cells we compared the rates of oxidation using specifically labeled substrates.[74] The rate of [1-^{14}C]glutamine oxidation was consistently threefold greater than that of either uniformly labeled glutamine or [5-^{14}C]glutamine. This higher rate was more susceptible to inhibition by aminooxyacetate suggesting that it reflected a more rapid decarboxylation of the C-1 unit for the production of the neurotransmitter GABA. Furthermore, the rates of $^{14}CO_2$ production from [5-^{14}C] and [U-^{14}C] glutamine were essentially the same. The addition of GABA also showed little or no effect on the rate of $^{14}CO_2$ production from [U-^{14}C] glutamine, providing additional evidence that the major portion of glutamine oxidation by these preparations of the brain does not proceed via its conversion to GABA. Ammonia is also a product of glutamine metabolism but it also had essentially no effect on the rate of glutamine oxidation.

A unique aspect of glutamine oxidation by the two experimental systems (i.e., whole homogenates and dissociated brain cells) was revealed in the kinetic analysis of the data. The rates of glutamine oxidation by dissociated cells showed saturation kinetics with an apparent K_m of 0.30 mM.[29] In that same report, Lineweaver-Burk plots of glutamine oxidation by homogenates revealed two linear segments with two apparent K_m values (0.58 and 3.0 mM). However, in the presence of aminooxyacetate there was only one linear segment with a single K_m of 0.47 mM. It was concluded that these results reflect the heterogeneity of the in vitro preparations with differences depending upon the activity of a given enzyme pathway. The kinetic differences between the dissociated cells and the whole homogenates also suggested a role for the cell membrane in the regulation of glutamine utilization since the rate of glutamine oxidation was much higher using whole homogenates than using intact cells. Another explanation for the different profiles of glutamine oxidation by homogenates and dissociated cells may be a differential selection of specific cellular and subcellular populations in these two preparations. Supportive of this latter position is the fact that homogenates would contain synaptosomes while the preparations of intact cells contain relatively few of these subcellular components.

Although these in vitro results provide strong support for the proposal that glutamine may be an energy source for the brain, this conclusion is also supported by other lines of evidence. First, the brain contains abundant enzymatic activity required for glutamine oxidation. Second, the brain contains large amounts of glutamine (4.4 μmol/g wet weight). A major consideration of the use of glutamine by the brain is the question of whether there is a net uptake of this amino acid. Several workers[27,76-78] have reported a net uptake of glutamine. However, other workers have reported a net release of glutamine by the brain.[79] These discrepancies are unresolved but species differences and differences in dietary status and/or hormonal factors may contribute to the variable results.

The brain is heterogeneous and this complexity gives rise to metabolic compartmentation.[74,80,81] Therefore, it is not unreasonable to conclude that one or more of these compartments may use glutamine as an energy source. Yu et al.[23] determined the metabolic fate of glutamate in primary astrocytes and concluded that this amino acid can substitute for glucose as a metabolic substrate for astrocytes. Since glutaminase is present in these cells,[21,82] it seems reasonable that after its conversion to glutamate, glutamine could be oxidized via the TCA cycle in astrocytes. Similar results were obtained using GABAergic preparations of cerebral cortical neurons in primary culture even though a small portion of the glutamine was converted to GABA.[75] Bradford et al.[10] have also shown that glutamine can be the major substrate for isolated synaptosomes. Other workers[22,25] provide additional evidence that glutamine can be metabolized via a variety of routes. The results have implications which must be considered in the overall homeostasis of the brain. In addition to its role as a major precursor for neurotransmitters such as glutamate and GABA,[83] glutamine has the potential to be utilized as an energy source in this tissue. Although absolute proof is still required, the evidence strongly supports this conclusion.

V. GLUTAMINE UTILIZATION BY OTHER CELLS AND TISSUES

The fact that glutamine is oxidized by numerous tissues identifies this amino acid as a respiratory fuel for a variety of tissues. The classical studies of Windmueller and Spaeth[26] demonstrated a net uptake of glutamine by the small intestines. These workers also demonstrated that labeled glutamine rapidly appeared as $^{14}CO_2$ in the venous blood. They concluded that glutamine along with ketone bodies were the major respiratory fuels for the intestines. Lymphocytes and thymocytes of the rat have been shown to generate a significant portion of their respiratory energy from glutamine.[84-86] The suggestion that glutamine may be an energy source for lymphocytes could have important implications for the immune system. Studies have revealed that lymphocytes have an absolute requirement for glutamine in order to respond to mitogen stimulation.[84,87] In addition, the review by Kafkewitz and Bendich[88] supports the proposal that glutamine deficiency induced by administration of asparaginase, a glutamine-catabolizing enzyme, may be immunosuppressive. Glutamine is also the substrate for up to 50% of the CO_2 formed by reticulocytes,[89,90] and rapid utilization of glutamine has been reported for chicken epiphyseal chondrocytes[91] and the bovine lens.[92]

Freshly isolated kidney tubules from rats with metabolic alkalosis oxidize about 15% of the utilized glutamine to CO_2 while converting the majority of metabolized glutamine to glucose.[93] Tubules from fed rats oxidized 7% of the utilized glutamine to CO_2 while tubules isolated from fasted or acidic rats showed little CO_2 production until after 30 min of incubation. Although Vinay et al.[93] dismissed this as a quantitatively unimportant metabolic pathway, total oxidation of 15% of the most abundant amino acid present in the blood could be significant. Furthermore, cultured kidney cells also oxidize 13 to 15% of the utilized glutamine to CO_2.[94]

In a comparison of potential energy sources for the cultured heart muscle and HeLa cells Stanisz et al.[95] noted that although cultured heart cells retained the property of oxidizing fatty acids, a surprising 50% of the energy of both cell types was derived from glutamine oxidation. Some alteration of metabolic pathways due to in vitro growth may have contributed to this observation; however, the retention of heart-specific characteristics suggests that glutamine oxidation by heart tissue needs further exploration.

Maturation of rabbit follicular oocytes requires glutamine, but not glucose, for energy and biosynthesis of cellular material.[20,96] Likewise, glutamine may have a critical role in differentiation of HL-60 cells.[97] It has not been established whether these effects of glutamine are related to its role as an energy source or some other function.

Although this list is not exhaustive, it demonstrates that numerous cells and tissues can oxidize glutamine in varying degrees. The contribution of glutamine to the overall energy production in these cells usually ranges between 30 to 50%, a very significant proportion of their total energy needs.

VI. REGULATION AND INTERACTIONS

The regulation of glutamine metabolism occurs at several levels. In the whole animal circulating levels of glutamine are modulated by the diet as well as by hormones. The utilization of glutamine is regulated at the tissue levels by enzyme activities and transport properties of the individual cells. This latter property is regulated by Na^+/K^+ concentrations. Another major regulatory component is the interaction among substrates.

The enzymes of glutamine metabolism adapt to a variety of conditions in vivo and in vitro. In the kidney, glutaminase activity increases threefold in response to acute acidosis.[98] This enzyme is also subject to allosteric regulation by phosphate and an extensive review of these properties has been described by Curthoys et al.[99] Glutamine synthetase is present in most tissues and appears to be regulated by glucocorticoids[100-102] as well as by triiodo-thyronine.[101,103] Other workers[104] have proposed a role for fatty acids in the simultaneous regulation of both glutaminase and glutamine synthetase.

The enzymatic activities of glutamine metabolism change dramatically during early ontogeny and these changes probably reflect the varying dynamic requirements of the individual cells or level of differentiation. Glutamine synthetase increases from a low level in the fetal liver and gradually reaches adult levels in 2 to 3 weeks postpartum.[101,105] A striking change in this enzyme also occurs in the brain where the change is more than eightfold during the first 20 days of life.[106] Although glutaminase also follows a similar developmental pattern in the brain, glutamate dehydrogenase has a unique ontological profile increasing early in postnatal development then decreasing to the same levels found in the newborn rat brain.[106] None of these enzyme activities appear to be the sole regulator of glutamine utilization in brain tissue. Hotta and Levinson[107] proposed a role for glutamate dehydrogenase in the regulation of glutamate. The activity of glutaminase is more than ten times that of other enzymes suggesting that it is not the rate-limiting step in glutamine utilization. However, the possible role of glutaminase as a regulator is supported by the report that the amount of glutamine utilization is correlated with glutaminase activity.[108]

As stated above and also demonstrated by studies in our laboratory,[106,108] the enzymes of glutamine metabolism are subject to dietary manipulations. Long-term exposure to elevated levels of 3-hydroxybutyrate and acetoacetate caused dramatic alterations in the developmental profile of both glutaminase and glutamate dehydrogenase, but this treatment had no effect on glutamine synthetase. These findings suggest that enzyme activities can be altered by the interactions among various substrates. Studies by Roeder et al.[109,110] have shown that the presence of 3-hydroxybutyrate or acetoacetate can have dramatic effects on the in vitro rates of glutamine oxidation by homogenates of young rat brains. In their in vitro studies, they demonstrated a striking inhibition of glucose and ketone body oxidation by glutamine suggesting a series of interactions that represented more than substrate dilution.

The enzymes of glutamine metabolism are discussed in detail in other chapters; however, one observation regarding the expression of glutaminase activity needs special emphasis. Based on the concentration of glutamine and phosphate in the brain, and the maximal rates of glutaminase activity observed under optimal conditions in vitro, Kvamme[111] estimated that 5 to 10% of the maximal activity was expressed in vivo. Zielke et al.[112] developed a flow-through assay in which ^3H_2O was released from L[2-^{3}H] glutamine metabolism to L[2-^{3}H]glutamate and subsequently to α-ketoglutarate and ^3H_2O. This assay allows the direct measurement of glutamine metabolism in whole cells by determining the quantity of ^3H_2O released into the medium. The application of this assay to intact mammalian cells is shown in Table 5. The percentage of intracellular glutaminase activity in human fibroblasts (HDF) was less than 1% of the activity measured in extracts. However, the intracellular rate of glutaminase activity in fibroblasts was equal or greater than the rate of CO_2 release from L[1-^{14}C]glutamine (data not shown). ^3H_2O release was also measured in growing Chinese

Table 5
COMPARISON OF GLUTAMINASE ACTIVITY MEASURED WITH THE ³H₂O ASSAY IN GROWING CELLS AND IN CELL EXTRACTS

Cell line	Phenotype (nmol/mg protein/hr)	Extracts (nmol/ mg protein/hr)	Growing cells (nmol/mg protein/hr)	Activity in extracts (%)
F-134	HDF	9312 ± 656	56 ± 6[a]	0.6
O₂₃	CHF	4650 ± 75	61 ± 4	1.3
DS₇	PGI def	9288 ± 250	142 ± 27	1.5
GSK₃	RESP def	5675 ± 150	59 ± 4	1.0

[a] nmol/mg protein/hr ± SD; n = 4. The Chinese hamster cells for this study were obtained from Dr. J. Pouysségur.

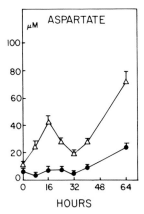 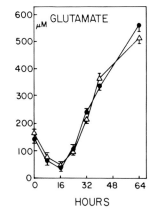

FIGURE 1. Accumulation of aspartate and glutamate in medium at different glucose concentrations. The human fibroblasts were grown in minimal essential medium with 5.5 mM glucose in 60-mm diameter petri dishes for 5 days to achieve near confluency and then refed with 10.0 mℓ of medium containing 1.5 mM glucose ($\bullet$) or 55 μM glucose plus 100 μM inosine, 40 μM thymidine, and 100 μM uridine ($\triangle$). Both media contained 10% dialyzed fetal calf serum, 100 μM pyruvate, and 1 mM glutamine. Each point is the average of 12 dishes.[115]

hamster fibroblasts (CHF) and their extracts. The elevated rate of ³H₂O release by glycolysis-deficient DS₇ cells relative to the normal parental cells (O₂₃) is consistent with a total dependence of DS₇ cells on respiratory energy generation. The release of ³H₂O by the respiratory-deficient GSK₃ cells was identical to the O₂₃ cells. This suggests that the regulation of glutamine oxidation by glucose does not appear to occur at the glutaminase step. Further information about the exact flux of these metabolites should be obtained by determining the products of glutamine metabolism by the GSK₃ cells.

The role of glutamine as a precursor as well as its interactions with other substrates have been evaluated by Zielke et al.[18,41,113] in their studies of glutamine utilization by fibroblasts. Aspartate production from glutamine is very sensitively regulated in this system and it appears to depend on the level of glucose present. Figure 1 shows that aspartate accumulated when glucose levels were low and not when glucose was high. In contrast, the level of glutamate did not differ between these two conditions, suggesting that these regulatory events occur at a site distal to glutaminase activity. However, glutamine does appear to be the precursor

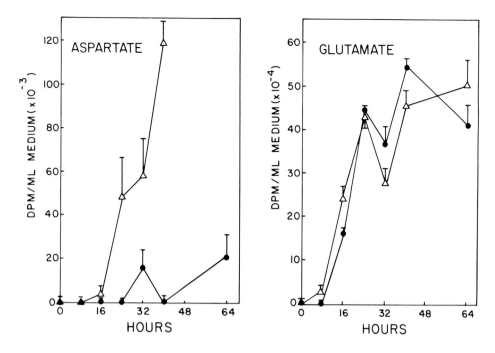

FIGURE 2. Label accumulation in aspartate and glutamate from U-^{14}C glutamine. Triplicate dishes were grown and refed as in Figure 1. Each dish contained 5 μ Ci U-^{14}C glutamine (1 m*M*, 0.5 Ci/mol) and either 1.5 m*M* glucose (●) or 55 μ*M* glucose (△).[115]

for this aspartate since the accumulation of label (from [U-^{14}C] glutamine) in aspartate decreased dramatically when glucose was present (Figure 2).

Earlier studies by Zielke et al.[48] have also shown that lactate is a major product of glutamine metabolism by fibroblasts accounting for more than 13% of the glutamine metabolized, and confirmed the active conversion of 4-carbon TCA intermediates to three carbon components. These studies are consistent with the broader proposal that glutamine, a major product of the skeletal muscle, is used directly as an energy source by several tissues under some physiological conditions and under other conditions it may be converted into glycolytic precursors. When these results are combined with the other studies, particularly those of Windmueller et al.,[26] the selective conversion of amino acid components of skeletal muscle protein into glutamine provides the body with a special system for maintaining its energy requirements via a multipurpose substance.

VII. CONCLUSIONS

The circulating level of glutamine is about 0.8 m*M* and represents about 50% of the total amino acids that are released from the muscle. However, the exact metabolic fate of this amino acid has not been characterized. Based on the information described above, and as diagrammed in Figure 3, we propose that a large portion of the glutamine released by the muscle is taken up by fibroblasts, lymphocytes, intestines, the brain, and other tissues. In these tissues it is converted to glutamate, and then to α-ketoglutarate which enters the TCA cycle and is converted to malate or oxaloacetate. In this partial turn through the cycle one carbon unit is converted to CO_2 with the production of energy (ATP units) equivalent to 75% of that obtained from acetyl-CoA. The ammonia released by this series of reactions is carried to the liver where it is used to form urea.

We postulate that, in these tissues, there is an active conversion of 4-carbon units (malate or oxaloacetate) to 3-carbon components (indicated in the scheme as pyruvate). This pyruvate

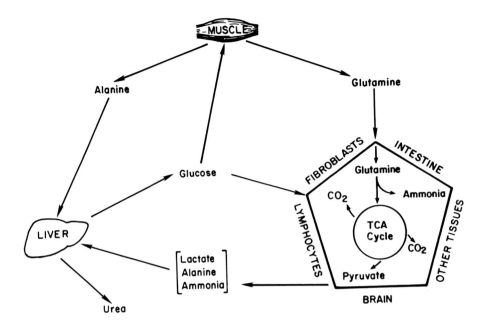

FIGURE 3.   The metabolic fate of glutamine and alanine in mammalian tissues.

may be transaminated to alanine or reduced to lactate, both of which would then be transported to the liver to be converted via gluconeogenesis to glucose. This glucose then returns to the muscle and to other tissues to be further utilized.

The obvious advantage of the proposed scheme is that it helps explain the overall fate of the largest quantity of amino acids released from the muscle. It also incorporates the results from many laboratories. The physiological importance of these series of metabolic events is apparent from the total CO_2 produced by the various tissues. In addition, however, it is obvious that by having two amino acid products follow different initial pathways this allows for greater flexibility as well as increased regulation.

The metabolic scheme outlined in Figure 3 augments the accepted glucose-alanine cycle. It is not proposed that these series of reactions occur equally in all the tissues indicated. Indeed, the exact nature of the events will be dependent upon a variety of circumstances including dietary status and the level of many hormones and effectors. The overriding value of the proposed model is that it can be evaluated by a variety of experimental approaches and it is presented here for that purpose.

ACKNOWLEDGMENT

Supported in part by NIH grant HD16596 and a grant from the Bressler Fund.

REFERENCES

1. **Ruderman, N. B. and Lund, P.,** Amino acid metabolism in skeletal muscle: regulation of glutamine and alanine release in the perfused rat hindquarters, *Isr. J. Med. Sci.,* 8, 295, 1972.
2. **Garber, A. J., Karl, I. E., and Kipnis, D. M.,** Alanine and glutamine synthesis and release from skeletal muscle. I. Glycolysis and amino acid release from skeletal muscle, *J. Biol. Chem.,* 251, 826, 1976.

3. **Garber, A. J., Karl, I. E., and Kipnis, D. M.,** Alanine and glutamine synthesis and release from skeletal muscle. II. The precursor role of amino acids in alanine and glutamine synthesis, *J. Biol. Chem.,* 251, 836, 1976.

4. **Goldstein, L. and Newsholme, E. A.,** The formation of alanine from amino acids in diaphragm muscle of the rat, *Biochem. J.,* 154, 555, 1976.

5. **Mallette, L. E., Exton, J. H., and Park, C. R.,** Control of gluconeogenesis from amino acids in the perfused rat liver, *J. Biol. Chem.,* 244, 5713, 1969.

6. **Felig, P., Pozefsky, T., Marliss, E., and Cahill, G. F., Jr.,** Alanine: key role in gluconeogenesis, *Science,* 167, 1003, 1970.

7. **Cahill, G. F., Jr., Herrera, M. G., Morgan, A. P., Soeldner, J. S., Steinke, J., Levy, P. L., Reichard, G. A., Jr., and Kipnis, D. M.,** Hormone-fuel interrelationships during fasting, *J. Clin. Invest.,* 45, 1751, 1966.

8. **Levintow, L., Eagle, H., and Piez, K. A.,** The role of glutamine in protein biosynthesis in tissue culture, *J. Biol. Chem.,* 227, 929, 1957.

9. **Salzman, N. P., Eagle, H., and Sebring, E. D.,** The utilization of glutamine, glutamic acid, and ammonia for the biosynthesis of nucleic acid bases in mammalian cell cultures, *J. Biol. Chem.,* 230, 1001, 1958.

10. **Bradford, H. F., Ward, H. K., and Thomas, A. J.,** Glutamine, a major substrate for nerve endings, *J. Neurochem.,* 30, 1453, 1978.

11. **Hamberger, A. C., Chiang, G. H., Nylen, E. S., Scheff, S. W., and Cotman, C. W.,** Glutamate as a CNS transmitter: evaluation of glucose and glutamine as precursors for the synthesis of preferentially released glutamate, *Brain Res.,* 168, 513, 1979.

12. **Hamberger, A. C., Chiang, G. H., Sandoval, E., and Cotman, C. W.,** Glutamate as a CNS transmitter: regulation of synthesis in the releasable pool, *Brain Res.,* 168, 531, 1979.

13. **Shank, R. P. and Aprison, H. M.,** Biochemical aspects of the neurotransmitter function of glutamate, in *Glutamic Acid: Advances in Biochemistry and Physiology,* Filer, L. J., Garattini, S., Kare, M. R., Reynolds, W. A., and Wurtman, R. J., Eds., Raven Press, New York, 1979, 139.

14. **Reubi, J. C.,** Comparative study of the release of glutamate and GABA, newly synthesized from glutamine in various regions of the central nervous system, *Neuroscience,* 5, 2140, 1980.

15. **Welbourne, T. C. and Phromphetcharat, V.,** Renal glutamine metabolism and hydrogen ion homeostasis, in *Glutamine Metabolism in Mammalian Tissues,* Häussinger, D. and Sies, H., Eds., Springer-Verlag, New York, 1984, 16.

16. **Tildon, J. T.,** An alteration in glucose metabolism associated with a defect in ketone body metabolism, *Proc. Natl. Acad. Sci. U.S.A.,* 70, 210, 1973.

17. **Reitzer, L. J., Wice, B. M., and Kennell, D.,** Evidence that glutamine, not sugar, is the major energy source for cultured HeLa cells, *J. Biol. Chem.,* 254, 2667, 1979.

18. **Zielke, H. R., Zielke, C. L., and Ozand, P. T.,** Glutamine: a major energy source for cultured mammalian cells, *Fed. Proc., Fed. Am. Soc. Exp. Biol.,* 43, 121, 1984.

19. **Cristofalo, V. J. and Kritchevsky, D.,** Growth and glycolysis in the human diploid cell strain WI-38, *Proc. Soc. Exp. Biol. Med.,* 118, 1109, 1965.

20. **Stoner, G. D. and Merchant, D. J.,** Amino acid utilization by L-M strain mouse cells in a chemically defined medium, *In Vitro,* 7, 330, 1972.

21. **Schousboe, A., Hertz, L., Svenneby, G., and Kvamme, E.,** Phosphate activated glutaminase activity and glutamine uptake in astrocytes in primary cultures, *J. Neurochem.,* 32, 943, 1979.

22. **Ramaharobandro, N., Borg, J., Mandel, P., and Mark, J.,** Glutamine and glutamate transport in cultured neuronal and glial cells, *Brain Res.,* 244, 113, 1982.

23. **Yu, A. C., Schousboe, A., and Hertz, L.,** Metabolic fate of ^{14}C-labeled glutamate in astrocytes in primary cultures, *J. Neurochem.,* 39, 954, 1982.

24. **Weiler, C. T., Nystrom, B., and Hamberger, A.,** Characteristics of glutamine vs. glutamate transport in isolated glia and synaptosomes, *J. Neurochem.,* 32, 559, 1979.

25. **Minn, A.,** Glutamine uptake by isolated rat brain mitochondria, *Neuroscience,* 7, 2859, 1982.

26. **Windmueller, H. G. and Spaeth, A. E.,** Uptake and metabolism of plasma glutamine by the small intestine, *J. Biol. Chem.,* 249, 5070, 1974.

27. **Eriksson, L. S., Law, D. H., Hagenfeldt, L., and Wahren, J.,** Nitrogen metabolism of the human brain, *J. Neurochem.,* 41, 1324, 1983.

28. **Tildon, J. T., Merrill, S., and Roeder, L. M.,** Differential substrate oxidation by dissociated brain cells and homogenates during development, *Biochem. J.,* 216, 21, 1983.

29. **Tildon, J. T. and Roeder, L. M.,** Glutamine oxidation by dissociated cells and homogenates of rat brain: kinetics and inhibitor studies, *J. Neurochem.,* 42, 1069, 1984.

30. **Ehrensvärd, G., Fisher, A., and Stjernholm, R.,** Protein metabolism of tissue cells in vitro. VII. The chemical nature of some obligate factors of tissue cell nutrition, *Acta Physiol. Scand.,* 18, 218, 1949.

31. **DeMars, R.,** The inhibition by glutamine of glutamyl transferase formation in cultures of human cells, *Biochim. Biophys. Acta,* 27, 435, 1958.

32. **Viceps, D. and Cristofalo, V. J.**, Glutamine synthetase activity in WI-38 cells, *J. Cell. Physiol.*, 86, 9, 1975.
33. **Eagle, H.**, Amino acid metabolism in mammalian cell cultures, *Science*, 130, 432, 1959.
34. **McCarty, L.**, Selective utilization of amino acids by mammalian cells cultures, *Exp. Cell Res.*, 27, 230, 1962.
35. **Griffiths, J. B. and Pirt, S. J.**, The uptake of amino acids by mouse cells (strain LS) during growth in batch culture and chemostat culture: the influences of cell growth rate, *Proc. R. Soc. London, Ser. B.*, 168, 421, 1967.
36. **Griffiths, J. B.**, The quantitative utilization of amino acids and glucose and contact inhibition of growth in cultures of the human diploid cell, WI-38, *J. Cell Sci.*, 6, 739, 1970.
37. **Zielke, H. R., Ozand, P. T., Tildon, J. T., Sevdalian, D. A., and Cornblath, M.**, Growth of human fibroblasts in the absence of glucose utilization, *Proc. Natl. Acad. Sci. U.S.A.*, 73, 4110, 1976.
38. **Paul, J.**, Carbohydrate and energy metabolism, in *Cells and Tissues in Culture*, Willmer, E. N., Ed., Academic Press, New York, 1965, 239.
39. **Sumbilla, C. M., Zielke, C. L., Reed, W. D., Ozand, P. T., and Zielke, H. R.**, Comparison of the oxidation of glutamine, glucose, ketone bodies and fatty acids by human diploid fibroblasts, *Biochim. Biophys. Acta*, 657, 301, 1981.
40. **Zielke, H. R., Ozand, P. T., Tildon, J. T., Sevdalian, D. A., and Cornblath, M.**, Reciprocal regulation of glucose and glutamine utilization by cultured human diploid fibroblasts, *J. Cell Physiol.*, 95, 41, 1978.
41. **Zielke, H. R., Sumbilla, C. M., Zielke, C. L., Tildon, J. T., and Ozand, P. T.**, Glutamine metabolism by cultured mammalian cells, in *Glutamine Metabolism in Mammalian Tissues*, Häussinger, D. and Sies, H., Eds., Springer-Verlag, New York, 1984, 247.
42. **De Francesco, L., Werntz, D., and Scheffler, I. E.**, Conditionally lethal mutations in Chinese hamster cells. Characterization of a cell line with a possible defect in the Krebs cycle, *J. Cell. Physiol.*, 85, 293, 1975.
43. **Donnelly, M. and Scheffler, I. E.**, Energy metabolism in respiration-deficient and wild type Chinese hamster fibroblasts in culture, *J. Cell. Physiol.*, 89, 39, 1976.
44. **Soderberg, K., Nissinen, E., Bakay, B., and Scheffler, I. E.**, The energy charge in wild-type and respiration-deficient Chinese hamster cell mutants, *J. Cell. Physiol.*, 103, 169, 1980.
45. **Pouysségur, J., Franchi, A., Salomon, J.-C., and Silvestre, P.**, Isolation of a Chinese hamster fibroblast mutant defective in hexose transport and aerobic glycolysis: its use to dissect the malignant phenotype, *Proc. Natl. Acad. Sci. U.S.A.*, 77, 2698, 1980.
46. **Franchi, A., Silvestre, P., and Pouysségur, J.**, A genetic approach to the role of energy metabolism in the growth of tumor cells: tumorigenicity of fibroblast mutants deficient either in glycolysis or in respiration, *Int. J. Cancer*, 27, 819, 1981.
47. **Renner, E. D., Plagemann, P. G. W., and Bernlohr, R. W.**, Permeation of glucose by simple and facilitated diffusion by Novikoff rat hepatoma cells in suspension culture and its relationship to glucose metabolism, *J. Biol. Chem.*, 247, 5765, 1972.
48. **Zielke, H. R., Sumbilla, C. M., Sevdalian, D. A., Hawkins, R. L., and Ozand, P. T.**, Lactate: a major product of glutamine metabolism by human diploid fibroblasts. *J. Cell. Physiol.*, 104, 433, 1980.
49. **Reed, W. R., Zielke, H. R., Baab, P. J., and Ozand, P. T.**, Ketone bodies, glucose, and glutamine as lipogenic precursors in human diploid fibroblasts, *Lipids*, 9, 677, 1981.
50. **Warburg, O.**, *Metabolism of Tumors*, Arnold Constable, London, 1930.
51. **Pedersen, P. L.**, Tumor mitochondria and the bioenergetics of cancer cells, *Prog. Exp. Tumor Res.*, 22, 190, 1978.
52. **Aisenberg, A. C. and Morris, H. P.**, Energy pathways of hepatoma, *Nature*, 191, 1314, 1961.
53. **Block-Frankenthal, L., Langan, J., Morris, H. P., and Weinhouse, S.**, Fatty acid oxidation and ketogenesis in transplantable liver tumors, *Cancer Res.*, 25, 732, 1965.
54. **Weinhouse, S.**, Glycolysis, respiration, and anomalous gene expression in experimental hepatomas, *Cancer Res.*, 32, 2007, 1972.
55. **Kovačević, A. and Morris, H. P.**, The role of glutamine in the oxidative metabolism of malignant cells, *Cancer Res.*, 32, 326, 1972.
56. **Moreadith, R. W. and Lehninger, A. L.**, The pathways of glutamate and glutamine oxidation by tumor cell mitochondria, *J. Biol. Chem.*, 259, 6215, 1984.
57. **Fenselau, A. and Wallis, K.**, Ketone body oxidation by mouse hepatoma BW 7756, *Life Sci.*, 12, 185, 1973.
58. **Kvamme, E. and Svenneby, G.**, Effect of anaerobiosis and addition of keto acids on glutamine utilization by Ehrlich ascites-tumor cells, *Biochim. Biophys. Acta*, 42, 187, 1960.
59. **Kvamme, E. and Svenneby, G.**, The effect of glucose on glutamine utilization by Ehrlich ascites tumor cells, *Cancer Res.*, 21, 92, 1961.
60. **Coles, N. W. and Johnstone, R. N.**, Glutamine metabolism in Ehrlich ascites carcinoma cells, *Biochem. J.*, 83, 284, 1961.

61. **Knox, W. E., Horowitz, M. L., and Friedell, G. H.,** The proportionality of glutaminase content to growth rate and morphology of rat neoplasms, *Cancer Res.*, 29, 669, 1969.
62. **Linder-Horowitz, M., Knox, W. E., and Morris, H. P.,** Glutaminase activities and growth rates of rat hepatomas, *Cancer Res.*, 29, 1195, 1969.
63. **Lavietes, B. B., Regan, D. H., and Demopoulos, H. B.,** Glutamate oxidation in 6C3HED lymphoma: effects of L-asparaginase on sensitive and resistant lines, *Proc. Natl. Acad. Sci. U.S.A.*, 71, 3993, 1974.
64. **Abou-Khalil, W. H., Yunis, A. A., and Abou-Khalil, S.,** Prominent glutamine oxidation activity in mitochondria of hematopoietic tumors, *Cancer Res.*, 43, 1990, 1983.
65. **Nakashima, R. A., Paggi, M. G., and Pedersen, P. L.,** Contributions of glycolysis and oxidative phosphorylation to adenosine-5'-triphosphate productions in AS-30D hepatoma cells, *Cancer Res.*, 44, 5702, 1984.
66. **Dranoff, G., Elion, G. B., Freidman, H. S., Campbell, G. LeM., and Bigner, D. D.,** Influence of glutamine on the growth of human glioma and medulloblastoma in culture, *Cancer Res.*, 45, 4077, 1985.
67. **Roberts, E. and Simonsen, D. G.,** Free amino acids and similar substances in normal and neoplastic tissue, in *Amino Acids, Proteins and Cancer Biochemistry*, Edsall, J. T., Ed., Academic Press, New York, 1960, 127.
68. **Sebolt, J. S. and Weber, G.,** Negative correlation of L-glutamine concentration with proliferation rate in rat hepatomas, *Life Sci.*, 34, 306, 1984.
69. **Dranoff, G., Elion, G. B., Friedman, H. S., and Bigner, D. D.,** Combination chemotherapy in vitro exploiting glutamine metabolism of human glioma and medulloblastoma, *Cancer Res.*, 45, 4082, 1985.
70. **Neil, G. L., Berger, A. E., Bhuyan, B. K., Blowers, C. L., and Kuentzel, S. L.,** Studies of the biochemical pharmacology of the fermentation-derived antitumor agent, (alpha S, 5S)-alpha-amino-3-chloro-4,5-dihydro-5-isoxazoleactic acid (AT-125), *Adv. Enzyme Regul.*, 17, 375, 1978.
71. **Weber, G., Lui, M. S., Seboldt, J., and Faderan, M. A.,** Molecular targets of antiglutamine therapy with acivicin in cancer cells, in *Glutamine Metabolism in Mammalian Tissues*, Häussinger, D. and Sies, H., Eds., Springer-Verlag, New York, 1984, 278.
71a. **Zielke, C. L.,** unpublished results.
72. **Dennis, S. C., Padma, A., DeBrysere, M. S., and Olson, M. S.,** Studies on the regulation of pyruvate dehydrogenase in the isolated perfused rat heart, *J. Biol. Chem.*, 254, 1252, 1979.
73. **Tsai, C. S., Burgett, M. W., and Reed, L. J.,** Alpha-keto acid dehydrogenase complexes, *J. Biol. Chem.*, 248, 2848, 1973.
74. **Tildon, J. T.,** Glutamine: a possible energy source for the brain, in *Glutamine, Glutamate and GABA in the Central Nervous System*, Hertz, L., Kvamme, E., McGeer, E. G., and Schousboe, A., Eds., Alan R. Liss, New York, 1983, 415.
75. **Yu, A. C. H., Fisher, T. E., Hertz, E., Tildon, J. T., Schousboe, A., and Hertz, L.,** Metabolic fate of ^{14}C-glutamine in mouse cerebral neurons in primary culture, *J. Neurosci.*, 11, 351, 1984.
76. **Schwerin, P., Bessman, S. P., and Waelsch, H.,** The uptake of glutamic acid and glutamine by brain and other tissues of the rat and mouse, *J. Biol. Chem.*, 184, 37, 1948.
77. **Oldendorf, W. H.,** Brain uptake of radiolabeled amino acids, amines and hexoses after arterial injection, *Am. J. Physiol.*, 221, 1629, 1971.
78. **Thanki, C. M., Sugden, D., Thomas, A. J., and Bradford, H. F.,** In vivo release from cerebral cortex of (^{14}C)-glutamate synthesized from (^{14}C)-glutamine, *J. Neurochem.*, 41, 611, 1983.
79. **Abdul-Ghani, A. S., Marton, M., and Dobkin, J.,** Studies on the transport of glutamine in vivo between the brain and blood in resting state and during afferent electrical stimulation, *J. Neurochem.*, 31, 541, 1978.
80. **Balazs, R. and Cremer, J. E., Eds.,** *Metabolic Compartmentation in the Brain*, Macmillan, London, 1973.
81. **Berl, S., Clarke, D. D., and Schneider, E., Eds.,** *Metabolic Compartmentation and Neurotransmission: Relation to Brain Structure and Function*, Plenum Press, New York, 1975.
82. **Kvamme, E., Svenneby, G., Hertz, L., and Schousboe, A.,** Properties of phosphate activated glutaminase in astrocytes cultured from mouse brain, *Neurochem. Res.*, 7, 761, 1982.
83. **Ward, H. K., Thanki, G. M., and Bradford, H. F.,** Glutamine and glucose as precursors of transmitter amino acids: ex vivo studies, *J. Neurochem.*, 50, 855, 1983.
84. **Ardawi, M. S. M. and Newsholme, E. A.,** Glutamine metabolism in lymphocytes of the rat, *Biochem. J.*, 212, 835, 1983.
85. **Ardawi, M. S. M. and Newsholme, E. A.,** Glutamine metabolism in lymphoid tissues, in *Glutamine Metabolism in Mammalian Tissues*, Häussinger, D. and Sies, H., Eds., Springer-Verlag, New York, 1984, 235.
86. **Brand, K.,** Glutamine and glucose metabolism during thymocyte proliferation, *Biochem. J.*, 228, 353, 1985.
87. **Crawford, J. and Cohen, H. J.,** The essential role of L-glutamine in lymphocyte differentiation in vitro, *J. Cell. Physiol.*, 124, 275, 1985.

88. **Kafkewitz, D. and Bendich, A.,** Enzyme-induced asparagine and glutamine depletion and immune system function, *Am. J. Clin. Nutr.,* 37, 1025, 1983.

89. **Rapoport, S., Rost, J., and Schultze, M.,** Glutamine and glutamate as respiratory substrates of rabbit reticulocytes, *Eur. J. Biochem.,* 23, 166, 1971.

90. **Rost, J. and Rapoport, S. M.,** The pathway of glutamate oxidation in rabbit reticulocytes, *Eur. J. Biochem.,* 26, 106, 1972.

91. **Ishikawa, Y., Chin, J. E., Hubbard, H. L., and Wuthier, R. E.,** Utilization and formation of amino acids by chicken epiphyseal chondrocytes: comparative studies with cultured cells and native cartilage tissue, *J. Cell. Physiol.,* 123, 79, 1985.

92. **Trayhurn, P. and Van Heyningen, R.,** The metabolism of glutamine in the bovine lens: glutamine as a source of glutamate, *Exp. Eye Res.,* 17, 148, 1973.

93. **Vinay, P., Lemieux, G., and Gougoux, A.,** Characteristics of glutamine metabolism by rat kidney tubules: a carbon and nitrogen balance, *Can. J. Biochem.,* 57, 346, 1979.

94. **Dass, P. D. and Wu, M.-C.,** Uptake and metabolism of glutamine in cultured kidney cells, *Biochim. Biophys. Acta,* 845, 94, 1985.

95. **Stanisz, J., Wire, B. M., and Kennell, D. E.,** Comparative energy metabolism in cultured heart muscle and HeLa cells, *J. Cell. Physiol.,* 115, 320, 1983.

96. **Bae, I.-H. and Foote, R. H.,** Utilization of glutamine for energy and protein synthesis by cultured rabbit follicular oocytes, *Exp. Cell Res.,* 90, 432, 1975.

97. **Dass, P. D., Murdock, F. E., and Wu, M-C.,** Glutamine promotes colony formation in bone marrow and HL-60 cells; accelerates myeloid differentiation in induced HL-60 cells, *In Vitro,* 20, 869, 1984.

98. **Leonard, E. and Orloff, J.,** Regulation of ammonia excretion in the rat, *Am. J. Physiol.,* 182, 131, 1955.

99. **Curthoys, N. P., Shapiro, R. A., and Haser, W. G.,** Enzymes of renal glutamine metabolism, in *Glutamine Metabolism in Mammalian Tissues,* Häussinger, D. and Sies, H., Eds., Springer-Verlag, New York, 1984, 16.

100. **Raina, P. N. and Rosen, F.,** Induction of glutamine synthetase by cortisol, *Biochim. Biophys. Acta,* 165, 470, 1968.

101. **Wu, C.,** Glutamine synthetase. III. Factors controlling its activity in the developing rat, *Arch. Biochem. Biophys.,* 106, 394, 1964.

102. **Wu, C. and Morris, H. T.,** Responsiveness of glutamine-metabolizing enzymes in Morris hepatomas to metabolic modulations, *Cancer Res.,* 30, 2675, 1970.

103. **Gebhardt, R. and Mecke, D.,** The role of growth hormone, dexamethasone and triiodothyronine in the regulation of glutamine synthetase in primary cultures of rat hepatocytes, *Eur. J. Biochem.,* 100, 519, 1979.

104. **Baverel, G., Michoudet, C., and Martin, G.,** Role of fatty acids in simultaneous regulation of flux through glutaminase and glutamine synthetase in rat kidney cortex, in *Glutamine Metabolism in Mammalian Tissues,* Häussinger, D. and Sies, H., Eds., Springer-Verlag, New York, 1984, 187.

105. **Knox, W. E., Kupchik, H. Z., and Liu, L. P.,** Glutamine and glutamine synthetase in fetal, adult, and neoplastic rat tissues, *Enzyme,* 12, 88, 1971.

106. **Tildon, J. T., Ozand, P. T., and Cornblath, M.,** The effects of hyperketonemia on neonatal brain metabolism, in *Normal and Pathological Development of Energy Metabolism,* Hommes, F. and Van Den Berg, C. J., Eds., Academic Press, New York, 1975, 143.

107. **Hotta, S. S. and Levinson, B. S.,** The effects of aminooxyacetate on the metabolism of glucose and glutamate by homogenates of guinea pig cerebral hemispheres, *Toxicol. Appl. Pharmacol.,* 16, 154, 1970.

108. **Ozand, P. T., Stevenson, J. H., Tildon, J. T., and Cornblath, M.,** Effects of hyperketonemia on glutamate and glutamine metabolism in developing rat brain, *J. Neurochem.,* 25, 67, 1975.

109. **Roeder, L. M., Tildon, J. T., and Stevenson, J. H., Jr.,** Competition among oxidizable substrates in brains of young and adult rats. Whole homogenates, *Biochem. J.,* 219, 125, 1984.

110. **Roeder, L. M., Tildon, J. T., and Holman, D. C.,** Competition among oxidizable substrates in brains of young and adult rats. Dissociated cells, *Biochem. J.,* 219, 131, 1984.

111. **Kvamme, E.,** Enzymes of cerebral glutamine metabolism, in *Glutamine Metabolism in Mammalian Tissues,* Häussinger, D. and Sies, H., Eds., Springer-Verlag, New York, 1984, 32.

112. **Zielke, C. L., Zielke, H. R., and Ozand, P. T.,** A radioisotope assay for L-glutaminase: the measurement of tritiated water formation from the reaction of L-2-^{3}H glutamine with the L-glutaminase and glutamate oxalacetate transaminase couple, *Anal. Biochem.,* 127, 134, 1982.

113. **Zielke, H. R., Sumbilla, C. M., and Ozand, P. T.,** Effect of glucose on aspartate and glutamate synthesis by human diploid fibroblasts, *J. Cell. Physiol.,* 107, 251, 1981.

Chapter 11

METABOLISM OF GLUTAMINE AND GLUTAMATE IN THE LIVER — REGULATION AND PHYSIOLOGICAL SIGNIFICANCE

J. D. McGivan

TABLE OF CONTENTS

I. INTRODUCTION

The liver contains considerable activities of the enzymes glutaminase and glutamine synthetase[1] and has the capacity for either the net synthesis or net degradation of glutamine. However, as recently as 1976, little was known about the mechanisms involved in the regulation of glutamine metabolism. In a review published in that year,[2] it was reported that the rate at which glutamine was synthesized in isolated hepatocytes was very low compared to the maximum activity of glutamine synthetase. Further, while glutamine at high concentrations was a good substrate for gluconeogenesis and urea synthesis, glutamine at physiological concentrations was not metabolized. These findings demonstrated clearly that glutamine metabolism in the liver must be subject to metabolic regulation. In the past 10 years, considerable advances have been made in understanding the detailed mechanisms by which glutamine metabolism is controlled. Even so, it is only very recently that the role of liver glutamine metabolism in ammonia detoxification and in physiological pH regulation has been fully appreciated.

This review will concentrate on three particular aspects of glutamine metabolism in the rat liver. The transport of glutamine across the liver cell membrane will be discussed, and this will be followed by a consideration of the properties and regulation of phosphate-dependent, phosphate-activated glutaminase. Research in this area was greatly assisted by the availability of methods for the preparation of isolated hepatocytes[3] and much information has also been obtained from work on isolated liver mitochondria and work at the submitochondrial level. The third aspect which will be discussed is recent work on the isolated perfused liver which has led to a greatly increased understanding of the control and metabolic significance of glutamine metabolism at the level of the intact organ.

Research in this area has been very active and for this reason, a number of recent reviews of various aspects of glutamine metabolism are already available. General aspects have been reviewed by Krebs[4] and by Lund,[5] while mitochondrial aspects were reviewed by Kovacevic and McGivan.[6] The reader is particularly referred to recent reviews by Seis and Häussinger[7] on liver glutamine and ammonia metabolism and by McGivan et al.[8] on liver glutaminase.

II. PATHWAYS OF GLUTAMINE AND GLUTAMATE METABOLISM IN THE LIVER

The liver obtains glutamine from the portal circulation as a result of absorption from the gut. A second source of glutamine is that produced as an end-product of amino acid metabolism by the muscle and other extrahepatic tissues. In the perfused liver and isolated liver cells, added glutamine is converted quantitatively to glucose and urea; each glutamine molecule metabolized produces one molecule of urea and half a molecule of glucose.

Glutamine is transported across the cell plasma membrane into the cytosol and is then transported into the mitochondria where it undergoes deamidation via a reaction catalyzed by liver phosphate-dependent glutaminase (E.C. 3.5.1.2). This enzyme represents 90% of the glutamine-hydrolyzing activity of the liver.[9] Other pathways of glutamine metabolism such as the aminotransferase (transamination) pathway[10] are not of primary importance in glutamine degradation in the absence of exogenously added ketoacids. The glutamate produced from glutamine hydrolysis is transaminated with endogenous oxaloacetate via glutamate-oxaloacetate aminotransferase to form aspartate plus 2-oxoglutarate. The aspartate together with the ammonia formed in the glutaminase reaction enter the urea cycle and contribute the two nitrogen atoms of the urea molecule; the carbon skeleton of fumarate is then converted to oxaloacetate for transamination with further glutamate molecules. The 2-oxoglutarate produced by transamination is metabolized via oxoglutarate dehydrogenase to succinyl-CoA and this is metabolized eventually to oxaloacetate which then enters the pathway of gluconeogenesis. In the liver, very little glutamine is totally oxidized to CO_2. Glutamine is also an important precursor of a number of complex molecules, in particular of pyrimidines and purines. These pathways will not be discussed further in the present context.

Glutamate is a poor primary substrate for gluconeogenesis in the liver,[11] and has been assumed to penetrate the liver membrane relatively slowly (but see Section V). Glutamate is formed from the transamination of a number of amino acids with 2-oxoglutarate, and also by the metabolism of histidine, ornithine, and proline, as well as glutamine. Glutamate is also formed by the reductive amination of 2-oxoglutarate via glutamate dehydrogenase, and this reaction is of importance in urea synthesis from exogenous ammonia. Glutamate degradation proceeds either via the aminotransferase pathway as described above, or via the glutamate dehydrogenase reaction, producing ammonia and 2-oxoglutarate. A feature of glutamine and glutamate metabolism in the liver is the important role of mitochondrial enzymes in these pathways.[6] Thus, glutaminase, glutamate dehydrogenase, 2-oxoglutarate dehydrogenase, glutamate-oxoaloacetate aminotransferase, ornithine transcarbamylase, proline dehydrogenase, and carbamoyl phosphate synthetase are all located in the mitochondrial matrix. A reaction of particular importance in liver mitochondria is the conversion of glutamate to *N*-acetylglutamate via the enzyme *N*-acetylglutamate synthetase. *N*-Acetylglutamate is the essential activator of carbamoyl phosphate synthetase, an enzyme which is important in the regulation of urea synthesis.

There is considerable literature on the metabolism of glutamate in isolated liver mitochondria,[6,12] and the importance of these investigations in relation to the metabolism of glutamate in the intact cell has been discussed.[6,12,13] It is now generally accepted that in the intact liver cell, the mitochondrial enzymes glutamate dehydrogenase and glutamate oxaloacetate aminotransferase are very active and catalyze "near-equilibrium" reactions. Therefore, these enzymes are not of primary importance in the regulation of glutamate metabolism. In this review, glutamate metabolism will be considered mainly in the context of the synthesis of glutamine via the glutamine synthetase reaction. Other aspects of glutamate metabolism have been reviewed elsewhere.[6] The important subject of the synthesis of *N*-acetylglutamate and its role in the regulation of urea synthesis have been reviewed[14] and will not be discussed in detail here.

III. LIVER-SPECIFIC REACTIONS IN GLUTAMINE METABOLISM

The first two steps in glutamine metabolism in the liver involve glutamine transport across the cell membrane and glutamine hydrolysis via phosphate-dependent glutaminase. Both the cell membrane glutamine-transport system and the glutaminase enzyme appear to be different from their counterparts in other tissues. Since these reactions are of importance in the regulation of liver glutamine metabolism, they will now be considered in some detail.

A. Glutamine Transport Across the Liver Cell Membrane

The transport of neutral amino acids into isolated hepatocyte cells has been widely studied (see References 15 and 16 for recent reviews). Isolated hepatocytes contain transport systems similar to the so-called A, ASC, and L systems originally identified in Ehrlich Ascites cells. The A system in isolated hepatocytes is Na-dependent and is characterized by its sensitivity to inhibition by *N*-methylaminoisobutyrate. L-Cysteine serves as an ASC system-specific substrate,[17] while the transport of L-leucine is Na-independent and proceeds via the L-system.[18] These various transport systems show widely overlapping specificities for their amino acid substrates. The existence of further transport systems has also been postulated.[19] In many cell types, glutamine is transported mainly by System A or System ASC.[20]

Joseph et al.[21] originally reported that glutamine was accumulated across the liver cell membrane by a Na-dependent transport system, and proposed on kinetic grounds that this system differed from that responsible for alanine transport. It was shown by Kilberg et al.[22] that a *N*-methylaminoisobutyrate-insensitive transport system specific for the transport of glutamine, arginine, and histidine exists in the liver cell. This transport system was termed system N, and has so far not been identified in any other tissue. Glutamine transport via system N was not stimulated by insulin or glucagon over a period of hours but was slightly induced on culturing liver cells in the absence of amino acids.[22] Glutamine transport in liver cells from starved rats was not stimulated compared to that in cells from fed rats while the transport of alanine in starved rats was significantly stimulated.[23] These results confirm the existence of separate transporting systems for alanine and glutamine in the liver. The glutamine transporting system is much less inducible than that for alanine. Recent experiments have shown that both glucagon and cyclic AMP (cAMP) exert a short-term transitory stimulation of glutamine transport in isolated hepatocytes.[24] Alanine transport is subjected to a similar short-term regulation by glucagon and this has been ascribed to an increase in cell membrane potential by this hormone.[25]

Fafarnoux et al.[26] have presented evidence for the existence of both an Na-dependent and an Na-independent glutamine transport system in hepatocytes. Both systems were inhibited by histidine. It was suggested that the Na-dependent system serves to catalyze accumulation of glutamine while the Na-independent system allows the hepatocytes to release glutamine when the intracellular concentration is high.

The existence of a transport system for glutamine in the liver different from that in other tissues cannot yet be rationalized in metabolic terms. The possibility that the glutamine transporting system is a rate-controlling step in glutamine metabolism has been considered. Work on isolated hepatocytes has indicated that (1) the kinetics of the glutamine transport are such that at physiological concentrations the transport is fast enough to account for the observed rates of metabolism,[8] (2) the steady-state concentration of glutamine in the cell is much higher than that in the medium even when glutamine metabolism is stimulated[27] and the same situation applies in vivo,[28,29] (3) glucagon stimulates the glutamine transport by only 10%[24] but has a much greater effect on glutamine metabolism,[27] and (4) vasopressin, which stimulates glutamine metabolism more than glucagon[30] does not stimulate the glutamine transport.[24] These results suggest that the regulation of glutamine degradation does not occur primarily at the level of the transport, but rather at the level of intracellular enzyme activity.

The role of the transport in the regulation of glutamine metabolism was further explored by Häussinger et al.[29] by measurement of glutamine uptake and release by the perfused liver and determination of intracellular glutamine concentrations. Glutamine uptake and release was inhibited by histidine, an inhibitor of system N, and this inhibition was not due to inhibition of glutamine-metabolizing enzymes. Stimulation of glutamine metabolism either by stimulating glutaminase flux or by providing substrates for glutamine transamination decreased the intracellular glutamine concentration; such a decrease was also previously observed in isolated hepatocytes.[27] It was concluded that the glutamine transport is a potential regulatory site in glutamine metabolism, especially in the presence of physiological concentrations of histidine.

The conclusions to be drawn from these studies do not appear to be contradictory. Glutamine transport is able to exert a regulatory influence on glutamine metabolism. The transport may be the major rate-controlling factor when glutaminase activity is stimulated, especially when inhibitors of the transport such as histidine are present. Nevertheless, the stimulation of glutamine metabolism occurs by the activation of intracellular enzymes rather than by activation of the transport.

The transport of glutamate into the liver is less well characterized. A transport system for the uptake of aspartate and glutamate has been identified in liver plasma membrane vesicles,[31] and a hormonally induced Na-dependent glutamate transport in cultured liver cells has been reported.[32]

The transport of glutamine into liver mitochondria was studied by Joseph and Meijer.[33] Glutamine equilibrated across the mitochondrial membrane within 10 sec at 30°C. The transport of glutamine was inhibited by mersalyl but not by *N*-ethylmaleimide or 5,5′-dithiobis(2-nitrobenzoic acid) DTNB, and L-glutamine was transported much faster than D-glutamine. From these findings it was assumed that a specific transport system for glutamine exists in the mitochondrial membrane. Glutamate transport across the liver mitochondrial membrane has been extensively investigated and this work has been reviewed.[6] It is not now believed that the rate of transport of either glutamate or glutamine into mitochondria is a limiting factor for the metabolism of these amino acids.

B. Glutaminase
1. Purification and Properties of Liver Glutaminase

Phosphate-dependent glutaminase in liver mitochondrial extracts does not crossreact with antibodies prepared to the purified kidney enzyme,[34] and is, thus, a different protein. Unlike the kidney enzyme, liver glutaminase does not polymerize in a phosphate-borate buffer[35] and polymerization cannot, therefore, be used as a convenient method for the isolation of the enzyme.

So far, attempts to purify liver glutaminase have proven unsuccessful due to the high lability of this enzyme and in particular to its sensitivity to dilution. Using ammonium sulfate fractionation and Sepharose® chromatography, Huang and Knox[35] achieved a fourfold purification starting from a freeze-dried mitochondrial preparation. The molecular weight was 170,000 as judged by sucrose density gradient centrifugation. Patel and McGivan[36] achieved a 50-fold increase in specific activity over that of a liver homogenate using diethylaminoethyl (DEAE) cellulose chromatography of a mitochondrial sonicate. The molecular weight by Sepharose® chromatography was reported to be approximately 290,000. A correlation of activity as eluted from a Sepharose® column with sodium dodecyl sulfate (SDS)-polyacrylamide gels of the various fractions led to a tentative identification of glutaminase subunits with a peptide of 73,500 mol wt. A major problem in this study was the inability of the authors to separate glutaminase from glutamate dehydrogenase which was a very similar charge and molecular weight. Recently, Smith and Watford[37] have achieved a 663-fold purification of glutaminase using ammonium sulfate fractionation and hydroxyapatite chromatography to remove glutamate dehydrogenase contamination, and it is hoped that this procedure will lead to an unambiguous identification of the enzyme protein.

It was shown by Charles[38] in 1968 that glutamine hydrolysis in mitochondria was stimulated by ammonia, and this finding was subsequently confirmed in the perfused liver[39] and in isolated hepatocytes.[27] However, it was shown only recently that in mitochondria glutaminase requires ammonia as an obligatory activator.[40] Only when this fact was realized was it possible to understand the kinetics of this enzyme. With a preparation of sonicated mitochondria or with the partially purified enzyme in the presence of excess glutamine plus phosphate the rate of glutamate production was not linear but increased with time[41] (Figure 1). Preincubation of the enzyme with excess ammonium chloride led to a linear rate on addition of glutamine. This unusual phenomenon of product activation was not recognized in earlier studies due to the presence of ammonia in commercially available preparations of glutamine. Further analysis of glutaminase activity in mitochondrial sonicates showed that the activation by added ammonium chloride was highly pH-dependent and less ammonium chloride was required for activation as the pH increased (Table 1). It was calculated that half-maximum activity was obtained at NH_3 concentrations of 8 μM and that this value was independent of pH. Therefore, it was concluded that the activating species is NH_3 rather than NH_4^+. Deviations from this behavior were observed in intact mitochondria below pH

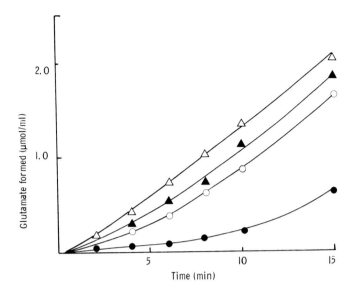

FIGURE 1.   Effect of added ammonia on the time course of the glutaminase reaction. Sonicated mitochondria were incubated with excess glutamine and phosphate at pH 7.2 together with the following concentrations of NH₄Cl: ● = none, ○ = 0.25 mM, ▲ = 0.5 mM, and △ = 2 mM. (From McGivan, J. D. and Bradford, N. M., *Biochim. Biophys. Acta,* 759, 241, 1983. With permission.)

Table 1
ACTIVATION OF GLUTAMINASE BY AMMONIA IN SONICATED MITOCHONDRIA

pH	Concentration of total (NH₄⁺ + NH₃) required for half-maximal velocity (μM)	Corresponding [NH₃](μM)
7.05	1340 ± 67 (5)	8.21 ± 0.41
7.2	959 ± 72 (11)	8.28 ± 0.62
7.4	537 ± 52 (8)	7.31 ± 0.71
7.7	304 ± 44 (5)	8.14 ± 1.17

Note: Sonicated mitochondria were incubated with saturating concentrations of phosphate and glutamine. Numbers of observations are represented in parentheses.

From McGivan, J. D. and Bradford, N. M., *Biochim. Biophys. Acta,* 759, 241, 1983. With permission.

7,[40] and the alternative possibility that the interaction of NH₄⁺ with the enzyme is in fact pH-dependent cannot be excluded.

In the presence of excess ammonia, the activity of partially purified glutaminase was completely dependent on the presence of phosphate, with a half-maximum activation at 5 mM phosphate.[36] The glutamine dependence was highly sigmoidal with half-maximum velocity at 22 mM glutamine. Unlike the kidney enzyme, liver glutaminase is insensitive to inhibition by glutamate.[1,36,42] Apart from phosphate and ammonia, the enzyme appears to have no other effectors of physiological significance. Phosphate-dependent glutaminase from

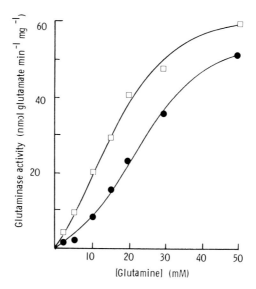

FIGURE 2. Effect of a mitochondrial membrane fraction on the kinetics of glutaminase. A partially purified preparation of glutaminase was incubated at pH 8.0 with saturating concentrations of ammonium chloride and phosphate together with glutamine as shown in the absence (●) or the presence (□) of a mitochondrial membrane fraction. (From McGivan, J. D., Vadher, M., Lacey, J. H., and Bradford, N. M., *Eur. J. Biochem.*, 148, 323, 1985. With permission.)

the human liver has been shown to resemble the rat liver enzyme in terms of ammonia activation and sigmoidicity of glutamine dependence.[43]

2. Interaction of Glutaminase with the Mitochondrial Membranes

After freezing and thawing of liver mitochondria, glutaminase was recovered in the membrane fraction, while matrix enzymes were released. On sonication of mitochondria, however, glutaminase appeared in the soluble fraction.[44] These results were taken to indicate that glutaminase in the liver is loosely associated with the inner mitochondrial membrane. Following the initial finding that the activity of solubilized glutaminase is modified by the addition of phospholipids,[45] reconstitution studies were carried out using partially purified glutaminase and preparations of mitochondrial membranes.[46] Incubation of glutaminase with membranes had a considerable effect on glutaminase kinetics (Figure 2). The glutamine dependence became less sigmoidal with half-maximum activation at about 8 mM glutamine, while the maximum velocity was unchanged. The phosphate dependence was also altered, with a reduction in the requirement for added phosphate for half-maximum activity from 5 mM to <2 mM. These effects were reversed by high concentrations of Mg^{2+}. It was suggested that reversible association with the mitochondrial membrane may change the kinetics of glutaminase leading to a marked activation at low glutamine concentrations. It is possible that Mg^{2+} ions interfere with the binding of glutaminase to the membrane, but there is yet no direct evidence on this point.

3. Glutamine Hydrolysis in Isolated Mitochondria

Since glutaminase is a mitochondrial enzyme, a consideration of its behavior in intact mitochondria is of importance, since in this system the enzyme is present in the same microenvironment as that in the intact cell. Glutaminase activity in intact mitochondria can be measured by following the production of glutamate in the presence of rotenone which inhibits further metabolism of the glutamate formed.

In intact mitochondria, glutamine hydrolysis was found to be enhanced by added ammonia[27,38,40] or by the addition of bicarbonate. The activation by bicarbonate can probably be attributed to alkalization of the medium due to a loss of CO_2 thus increasing the activating effect of endogenous ammonia present either in the mitochondria on isolation or as an impurity in the glutamine added. Bicarbonate did not activate either glutaminase activity in mitochondria[40] or partially purified glutaminase[36] in the absence of ammonia. As for the isolated enzyme, in intact mitochondria glutaminase activity was dependent on phosphate, and half-maximum rates were attained at relatively high glutamine concentrations in the range 15 to 20 mM.[27,47]

Glutamine hydrolysis was activated by energizing the isolated mitochondria by the addition of succinate and was greatly further activated by the addition of valinomycin in the presence of potassium ions. Further, incubation of mitochondria in a hypotonic medium caused activation of glutamine hydrolysis;[48] a difference was observed between incubation in a sucrose medium and in a K^+-containing medium.[8] It is likely that all these effects can be related to swelling of the mitochondria to different extents. Depletion of the mitochondrial magnesium ion concentration by incubation with the ionophore A23187 plus EDTA also activated glutamine hydrolysis.[48] This effect, however, was not considered to be due to swelling. On incubating mitochondria in hypotonic medium or on causing swelling by other means, the glutamine dependence of glutamine hydrolysis became less sigmoidal and the requirement for phosphate decreased. Similar kinetic changes were observed on magnesium depletion. The changes in kinetic parameters observed on swelling were similar to those which occur on reconstitution of glutaminase with a mitochondrial membrane fraction. It was accordingly postulated[46] that swelling (and also possibly magnesium depletion) of mitochondria causes an increased association of glutaminase with the mitochondrial membrane with a consequential change in kinetic properties and that this effect is reversible.

Various hormones activate glutamine metabolism in the perfused liver or intact hepatocytes and this activation is attributable in part to an activation of mitochondrial glutaminase. Mitochondria isolated from glucagon-injected rats exhibited enhanced glutamine-hydrolyzing activity[49] and a similar situation was found in mitochondria isolated from hormone-treated hepatocytes.[50] The activation of glutaminase was lost on disruption of the mitochondria and, therefore, was not due to a stable modification of the enzyme. Analysis of the hormone-induced change in kinetics indicated that the effect of the hormone was to reduce concentrations of both glutamine and phosphate required for half-maximum activation. These effects were quantitatively the same as those produced by incubation of control mitochondria in a hypotonic medium. These results were consistent with the hypothesis that glucagon treatment of rats causes swelling of the mitochondria *in situ* and that the mitochondria persist in a swollen state during isolation.

From the above discussion, it is clear that the regulation of liver glutaminase is complex. Regulation can occur at two different levels of organization. The enzyme itself requires both phosphate and ammonia as obligatory activators and the activation by ammonia is highly pH-dependent. In intact mitochondria, the activity of the enzyme is further determined by the volume of the matrix space, possibly due to an effect of matrix volume change on the degree of association of the enzyme with the membrane. The effect of mitochondrial swelling is likely to be of physiological importance since it is possible that hormonal modulation of glutaminase activity is expressed through this mechanism. These detailed mechanisms of regulation appear to be peculiar to the liver enzyme and may well be essential to its physiological function.

IV. THE REGULATION OF GLUTAMINE METABOLISM IN THE PERFUSED LIVER AND ISOLATED HEPATOCYTES

A. Stimulation of Glutamine Metabolism by Ammonia

It was found in early studies[39] that when the rat liver was perfused with a medium containing 6 mM glutamine, very little glutamine was metabolized. An addition of NH_4Cl increased the rate of glutamine metabolism and this effect was attributed to the activation of glutaminase activity by ammonia. The activation of glutamine degradation in the perfused liver was later studied in considerable detail by Häussinger and Sies,[51] who used glutamine and ammonia concentrations in the physiological range. Glutamine at the physiological concentration of 0.6 mM was not metabolized but metabolism was reversibly stimulated by the addition of ammonium chloride to the perfusion medium; a half-maximum stimulation was obtained at 0.2 to 0.3 mM ammonium ions. A maximum rate of glutamine metabolism occurred at 10 to 12 mM glutamine and this is consistent with the fact that glutaminase has a high K_m for its substrate in isolated mitochondria. Ammonia stimulated the rate of gluconeogenesis from glutamine in isolated hepatocytes.[27] At pH 7.4, a half-maximum effect was observed at 0.5 mM NH_4Cl, and this was consistent with the concentration required to give a half-maximum stimulation of glutaminase activity in intact mitochondria.

A number of other observations are consistent with the activation of glutaminase by ammonia in intact cells. Glutamine degradation in both hepatocytes and the perfused liver exhibited a pronounced lag period before the rate became maximal.[27,52-54] This lag was reduced or abolished on addition of ammonia[27,39,51] and these results are in agreement with the activation of glutaminase by added ammonia in intact mitochondria.[40] When ammonium chloride was administered to rats in vivo, there was a reduction in the liver content of glutamine[55] and this was also consistent with glutaminase activation. Leucine stimulated glutamine degradation in isolated hepatocytes and this effect was originally attributed to an activation of glutaminase by leucine.[56] However, leucine is known to inhibit ornithine transcarbamylase in the urea cycle and, hence, to increase ammonia production by isolated hepatocytes.[13] It is probable that the observed stimulation of glutamine degradation by leucine was secondary to activation of glutaminase by the ammonia accumulating in the cells. Leucine did not activate partially purified glutaminase.[36] Added ornithine overcomes the inhibition of ornithine transcarbamylase and was found to reduce the stimulation of glutamine breakdown by leucine.[57]

The activation of glutamine degradation by ammonia occurs in the range of ammonia concentration which occurs in the portal vein and is therefore likely to be of physiological significance. One physiological role of the activation of glutaminase by ammonia may concern the regulation of carbamoyl phosphate synthetase.[8] Activation of glutaminase by ammonia leads to an increased intramitochondrial concentration of glutamate and this may lead directly to an increased intramitochondrial concentration of N-acetylglutamate, the activator of carbamoyl phosphate synthase.

B. Regulation of Glutamine Metabolism by pH

Lueck and Miller[58] in 1970 observed that a decrease in pH from 7.45 to 7.15 led to a 50% decrease in the rate of glutamine metabolism by the perfused liver, and a similar observation was later made by Saheki and Katunuma.[53] Although the maximum activity of partially purified liver glutaminase decreases sharply below pH 7,[36] it is likely that these findings can be explained primarily by the strong pH dependence of the activation of glutaminase by ammonia observed in intact mitochondria[40] and in submitochondrial preparations.[36,41]

There have been conflicting reports about the effect of bicarbonate on glutamine degradation in intact cells. Häussinger et al.[54] confirmed that a decrease in pH inhibited glutamine metabolism in the perfused liver and showed that the rate of glutamine degradation at constant pH was independent of bicarbonate concentration. These results are consistent with the findings, discussed above, that bicarbonate does not activate partially purified glutaminase. Baverel and Lund[56] have presented results showing that an increase in bicarbonate concentration at constant pH leads to an increased rate of glutamine metabolism in isolated hepatocytes. One factor which, so far, has not been taken into account in this area is that the Na-dependent transport of glutamine (and other amino acids) into isolated hepatocytes is strongly activated by bicarbonate,[21] possibly due to an increase in cell plasma membrane potential.[59] The reason for the discrepancy in results between effects of bicarbonate on glutamine metabolism in the perfused liver and in isolated hepatocytes is not clear at present.

C. Regulation of Glutamine Metabolism by Hormones

The rate of gluconeogenesis from glutamine in isolated hepatocytes was found to be greatly stimulated by glucagon;[27] this stimulation was additive to that produced by ammonia. Similar results have been obtained in the perfused liver.[60] On the basis of the amino acid specificity of the stimulation together with the finding that the increased rate of gluconeogenesis was accompanied by a decrease in the intracellular glutamine concentration, it was concluded that the increase in gluconeogenesis was due to a stimulation of glutaminase.[27] In rats injected with glucagon, the glutaminase activity in subsequently isolated mitochondria was found to be increased compared with that in mitochondria from control livers.[49]

In addition to glucagon, cAMP phenylephrine, vasopressin, and angiotensin II also stimulated gluconeogenesis from glutamine in isolated hepatocytes[30] and stimulation caused by these effectors persisted in mitochondria isolated from hormone-treated hepatocytes.[50] The effects of vasopressin, angiotensin, and adrenergic hormones were absolutely dependent on the presence of Ca^{2+} ions in the external medium, whereas those of glucagon and cAMP were less dependent on Ca^{2+}.[30,50]

The effects of adrenergic hormones and vasopressin on glutamine metabolism in isolated hepatocytes and the perfused liver have been studied in some detail.[42,61-63] The stimulation of glutamine metabolism by norepinephrine[42,61] was associated with a large decrease in the intracellular content of 2-oxoglutarate. Since this decrease was accompanied by an increased flux through 2-oxoglutarate dehydrogenase (a "nonequilibrium enzyme"), these results suggest that 2-oxoglutarate dehydrogenase was stimulated by the hormones. A similar decrease in cell 2-oxoglutarate content was observed during the stimulation of proline metabolism by vasopressin;[63] proline is also metabolized by a pathway involving 2-oxoglutarate dehydrogenase.

2-Oxoglutarate dehydrogenase is activated by calcium ions,[64] and α-adrenergic hormones have been shown to increase cytosolic Ca^{2+} concentrations in hepatocytes.[65-67] It has been proposed that the intramitochondrial free calcium concentration is of the order of micromolar and that stimulation of 2-oxoglutarate dehydrogenase by these hormones involves an increase in intramitochondrial free calcium as a result of the increase in cytosolic Ca^{2+} concentration.[68] It has been shown that 2-oxoglutarate dehydrogenase in isolated liver mitochondria is activated by increases in extramitochondrial Ca^{2+} in the range 0.1 to 10 μM when Na^+ and Mg^+ are present at concentrations which occur in the cytosol.[69,70] Further evidence consistent with this view was provided by a study of the effects of extracellular ATP on glutamine metabolism in isolated hepatocytes.[71] ATP increased the measured cytosolic free Ca^{2+} concentration, and at the same time, increased the flux through 2-oxoglutarate dehydrogenase and reduced the steady-state level of 2-oxoglutarate.

Hormonal stimulation of glutamine metabolism necessarily involves an increase in flux through glutaminase and this enzyme is not significantly inhibited by its products.[42] It follows that the hormones discussed above must act on glutamine metabolism by activating both 2-oxoglutarate dehydrogenase and glutaminase. This was clearly demonstrated recently by

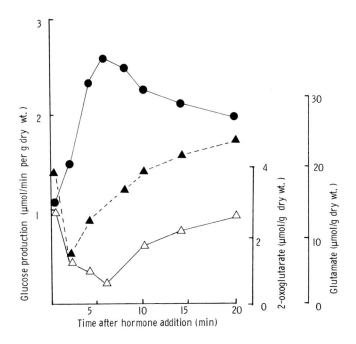

FIGURE 3. Metabolite changes after phenylephrine addition to hepatocytes perfused with glutamine as the substrate. Cells were perfused with 2.5 m*M* glutamine in the presence of 0.25 m*M* NH₄Cl. ● = glucose in perfusate, ▲ = intracellular glutamate, and △ = intracellular 2-oxoglutarate. (Reprinted by permission from *Biochem. J.*, 230, 457, ©1985, The Biochemical Society, London.)

Table 2

EFFECT OF GLUCAGON ON METABOLITE CONCENTRATIONS IN THE RAT LIVER

Time (min)	Glucose (μmol/g)	Glutamine (μmol/g)	Glutamate (μmol/g)	N-Acetylgluta-mate (nmol/g)
0	6.27 ± 0.23 (5)	4.97 ± 0.25 (5)	2.09 ± 0.15 (6)	21.9 ± 1.4 (10)
2	8.90 ± 0.29 (5)***	4.99 ± 0.42 (5)	1.07 ± 0.04 (5)**	25.1 ± 2.5 (6)
5	9.96 ± 0.28 (5)***	5.05 ± 0.45 (5)	0.86 ± 0.08 (5)***	27.1 ± 2.4 (6)
10	11.62 ± 0.33 (5)***	5.20 ± 0.42 (5)	1.27 ± 0.22 (6)*	30.4 ± 2.3 (6)**
15	11.88 ± 0.21 (3)***	3.84 ± 0.41 (3)*	0.98 ± 0.07 (3)**	33.1 ± 6.9 (3)
20	11.25 ± 0.76 (4)***	3.27 ± 0.22 (4)**	1.63 ± 0.34 (4)	31.4 ± 3.9 (5)*

Note: Rats were injected with glucagon at zero time and their livers were freeze-clamped at the times indicated. Numbers of observations are represented in parentheses. Asterisks show level of significance.

Reprinted by permission from *Biochem. J.*, 217, 855, ©1984, The Biochemical Society, London.

Verhoeven et al.[42] In hepatocytes perfused with glutamine, addition of phenylephrine produced a rapid fall in the steady-state intracellular concentration of 2-oxoglutarate and glutamate. The concentrations of these metabolites subsequently increased again while glutamine metabolism was still stimulated (Figure 3). These results were interpreted to indicate a rapid activation of 2-oxoglutarate dehydrogenase followed by an activation of glutaminase which was slower in onset. A relatively slow activation of glutaminase can also be inferred from in vivo experiments[72] (Table 2). Injection of glucagon into rats led to a rapid decrease in the liver glutamate concentration which started to reverse after 10 min. The liver glutamine content remained constant for 10 min and then decreased.

A number of unanswered questions remain about the mechanisms involved in the hormonal control of glutamine degradation. The effects of hormones are additive to those of ammonia and are therefore not mediated simply by an increased ammonia concentration.[27,42,60] The effects of glucagon appear to be different from those of α-adrenergic hormones and vasopressin. Stimulation by glucagon is less in extent and is accompanied by a smaller stimulation of 2-oxoglutarate dehydrogenase.[42,63] It is probable that the effects of the Ca^{2+}-dependent hormones on 2-oxoglutarate dehydrogenase activity can be accounted for by activation of this enzyme via an increased intramitochondrial calcium concentration. The mechanisms of the effects of these hormones on glutaminase activity are still obscure.

Halestrap[73] has shown that addition of α-adrenergic hormones, vasopressin, or glucagon to isolated hepatocytes leads to a light-scattering change interpreted as swelling of mitochondria *in situ*. The swelling obtained with α-adrenergic hormones was rapid and completely Ca^{2+}-dependent while that obtained with glucagon was slower in onset and less dependent on Ca^{2+} ions. A possible hypothesis to explain the hormonal activation of glutaminase is that the activating hormones all cause mitochondrial swelling. The swelling caused by Ca^{2+}-dependent hormones is possibly mediated by an increase in cytoplasmic calcium, while that caused by glucagon is slower and occurs by a different mechanism. Swelling of mitochondria will activate glutaminase, possibly by changing its interaction with the mitochondrial membrane (see Section III above).

The physiological significance of the hormonal regulation of glutamine metabolism is still unclear except for the consideration that a stimulation of glutaminase will lead to an increase in gluconeogenesis from glutamine as the substrate. The hypothesis[6] that a primary function of the glucagon stimulation of glutaminase is to increase mitochondrial glutamate concentration and, hence, increase *N*-acetylglutamate levels is probably no longer tenable. The injection of glucagon in vivo leads to a rapid increase in the liver *N*-acetylglutamate content, but this is accompanied by a decrease, not an increase, in glutamate content[72] (Table 2).

The long-term regulation of liver glutamine metabolism has been relatively little investigated. A recent paper[74] reported that liver glutaminase activity was increased in diabetes and isolated hepatocytes from diabetic rats exhibited an increased rate of glutamine metabolism. Long-term metabolic acidosis had no effect on assayable glutaminase activity in the liver.

D. Glutamine Synthesis in the Liver

Liver homogenates contain high activities of glutamine synthetase. However, the rate of glutamine synthesis in the rat liver perfused with ammonia and lactate or other appropriate carbon sources was only a small fraction of the total activity of the glutamine synthetase present.[75] A similar situation was found in isolated hepatocytes.[2] In retrospect, it can now be seen that the ammonia used as a substrate for glutamine synthesis would simultaneously stimulate glutaminase and, thus, diminish net glutamine production.

The activity of glutamine synthetase in intact cells was first systematically studied using the nonrecirculating perfused liver system. Using u-[14C] glutamine Häussinger and Sies[51] observed a production of $^{14}CO_2$ in the absence of net glutamine metabolism. This was attributed to the simultaneous operation of glutaminase and glutamine synthetase. Under certain conditions net glutamine release was observed in livers perfused with glutamine. This net release was converted into a net uptake by the addition of methionine sulfoxime, an inhibitor of glutamine synthetase.[76] It was further observed that an uptake of oxygen occurred in excess of that accounted for by net urea synthesis and this was also attributed to the existence of a futile cycle between glutamine and glutamine plus ammonia.

This system was further characterized by using [1-14C] glutamine as a substrate.[60] It was shown that flux through glutaminase was accurately represented by $^{14}CO_2$ release from 1-^{14}C glutamine; flux through glutamine synthetase was therefore calculated as the glutaminase flux plus the net glutamine production. Glutamine synthetase flux was increased by ammonia and glucagon in the presence of low concentrations of glutamine, but these effects were abolished or reversed at higher glutamine concentrations. Significantly, flux through glutaminase decreased and flux through glutamine synthetase increased during metabolic acidosis, leading to a higher net glutamine release. In metabolic alkalosis glutamine synthetase flux decreased and that through glutaminase increased, leading to net glutamine uptake.

The metabolic significance of this cycling between glutaminase and glutamine synthetase became apparent when it was shown that these enzymes are located in different cells. This development has been recently reviewed elsewhere[7,77,78] and will be considered relatively briefly here.

V. HEPATOCYTE HETEROGENEITY IN GLUTAMINE METABOLISM

A. Enzyme Localization

The concept of hepatocyte heterogeneity in the liver has been firmly established. This subject has been reviewed by Jungermann and co-workers.[79-81] Cells in the periportal zone receive blood directly from the portal circulation and this is rich in oxygen and substrates. Cells in the perivenous region receive blood which is relatively depleted in substrates and oxygen, but enriched in the metabolic products of cells in the periportal region. The cells in these two regions differ somewhat in their enzymic composition and presumably also in their metabolic capacity. This phenomenon has been studied mainly by determination of enzyme activities following microdissection of lyophilized liver sections, and also in some cases by immunohistochemical detection of various enzymes in preparations of intact tissue. As judged by these techniques, the periportal cells contain relatively higher activities of enzymes specifically involved in gluconeogenesis while the perivenous cells have relatively higher contents of enzymes involved in glucose utilization.

Gebhardt and Mecke[82,83] studied the distribution of glutamine synthetase in liver parenchyma using an immunofluorescence technique. This enzyme was found to be localized exclusively in cells in the perivenous region. In contrast, carbamoyl phosphate synthase is located in the periportal region.[84] These and later related observations[77] of other enzymes indicated heterogeneity in glutamine metabolism with urea synthesis and probably glutamine degradation occurring in the periportal cells and glutamine synthesis occurring in the perivenous region. This picture was also consistent with biochemical findings. Allylformate damages the periportal areas of the liver selectively while carbon tetrachloride destroys mainly the perivenous region. Administration of allylformate decreased the activities of the urea cycle enzymes but had no effect on that of glutamine synthetase while carbon tetrachloride strongly decreased glutamine synthetase but had no effect on enzymes of the urea cycle.[83] In the perfused liver from animals pretreated with carbon tetrachloride, glutamine synthesis from added ammonia was greatly impaired while urea synthesis was unaffected.[85] However, due to the difficulties discussed above in the isolation of liver glutaminase and the failure of antisera to glutaminases from other tissues to crossreact with the liver enzyme, it so far has not been possible to apply immunofluorescence techniques to detect the location of liver glutaminase.

A different approach to this problem was employed by Häussinger[86] using the perfused rat liver. During perfusion in the physiological direction from the portal vein to vena cava ("antegrade perfusion"), substrates in the perfusion medium encounter the periportal region of the parenchyma first. During perfusion in the reverse direction ("retrograde perfusion") substrates are initially presented to the perivenous region. If the distribution of enzymes involved in particular metabolic pathways is not homogeneous throughout the liver, differences in the pattern of metabolism may be expected on reversal of the direction of perfusion.

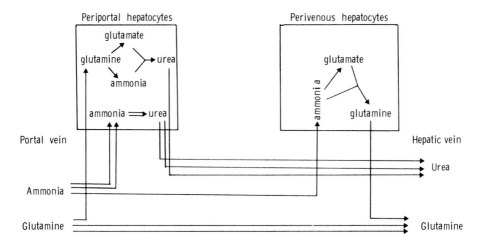

FIGURE 4.   The intercellular glutamine cycle. (From Häussinger, D., *Eur. J. Biochem.*, 133, 269, 1983. With permission.)

Using this technique, it was found that added ammonia was mainly converted to urea in antegrade perfusions, but was preferentially used for glutamine synthesis in retrograde perfusions. Endogenously produced ammonia was mainly converted to urea in antegrade perfusions but was washed out in retrograde perfusions. These results were taken to indicate that glutamine synthesis occurred in the perivenous region while urea synthesis from ammonia was localized in the periportal region. Further, endogenous ammonia was produced by the periportal cells and converted to glutamine by the perivenous cells. The release of $^{14}CO_2$ from 1-^{14}C-glutamine was measured in ante- and retrograde perfusions. $^{14}CO_2$ production was higher in antegrade perfusions and this was attributed to dilution of the specific activity of the isotope in retrograde perfusions by glutamine produced in the perivenous cells. It was concluded from this data that glutamine degradation occurred in the periportal cells.

Further analogous investigations[87] on glutamate uptake and release led to the conclusion that glutamate is taken up from the perfusion medium mainly by the perivenous cells and is then used for glutamine synthesis. The utilization of exogenous glutamate by the periportal cells is restricted by the low permeability of these cells to glutamate; the glutamate-transporting capacity of perivenous cells was estimated to be 20-fold higher than that of periportal cells. However, both perivenous and periportal cells were considered to possess the Na^+-dependent system N for glutamine transport, as judged by the measurement of glutamine uptake and release under various conditions in the perfused liver.[29]

B. The Intercellular Glutamine Cycle

The above investigations[86,87] together with earlier data on glutamine cycling in the perfused liver led to the concept of an intercellular glutamine cycle[7,77,78,86] (Figure 4). Ammonia entering the liver via the portal circulation is mainly converted to urea in the periportal cells and this is also the fate of the ammonia produced in these cells by the deamination of amino acids. The K_m of carbamoyl phosphate synthase for ammonia is in the range 1 to 2 mM.[88] At physiological concentrations of incoming ammonia, some ammonia escapes detoxification via urea synthesis and proceeds to the perivenous region where it is quantitatively converted to glutamine via glutamine synthetase which has a much lower K_m for ammonia (0.3 mM).[89] Glutamine entering the liver is metabolized in the periportal cells and the ammonia produced is mainly converted to urea, but the ammonia which is not used for urea synthesis is reconverted to glutamine in the periportal cells. This intercellular cycle is under regulation by factors which increase glutaminase activity, such as plasma ammonia concentration, plasma pH, and hormones. This mechanism ensures the complete detoxification of ammonia derived either from the portal circulation or from endogenous amino acid metabolism by conversion of the ammonia either into urea or into glutamine.

C. Involvement of Liver Glutamine Metabolism in the Regulation of Blood pH

While the metabolism of fats and carbohydrates in the body produces CO_2 which can be excreted through the lungs, the metabolism of protein produces bicarbonate ions in amounts which are too great to be excreted through the kidneys.[90] Maintenance of pH homeostasis requires continuous removal of this bicarbonate. It has been pointed out[90-93] that synthesis of urea catalyzes the stoichiometric removal of ammonium ions and bicarbonate ions with the production of the excretable products urea and CO_2:

$$2NH_4^+ + HCO_3^- \rightarrow urea + H^+ + 2H_2O$$

$$H^+ + HCO_3^- \rightarrow CO_2 + H_2O$$

$$Net: 2NH_4^+ + 2HCO_3^- \rightarrow urea + CO_2 + 3H_2O$$

Thus, conversion of ammonia to urea consumes bicarbonate ions while the synthesis of glutamine from ammonia does not.

In the context of the intercellular glutamine cycle discussed above, a major influence on the pH modulation of urea synthesis is the strong pH dependence of glutamine degradation as described in an earlier section. During acidosis glutamine hydrolysis is decreased due to the pH dependence of the ammonia activation of glutaminase.[40,41] More ammonia is converted to glutamine and relatively less is converted to urea. Excess nitrogen is then disposed of by an increased hydrolysis of glutamine in the kidney followed by the excretion of the ammonium ions thus formed. According to this view[78,90] the major metabolic function of renal glutamine hydrolysis is the excretion of excess nitrogen rather than pH homeostasis.

There are two further recent developments in this area. In experiments on isolated liver mitochondria, evidence has been obtained for a channeling of ammonia from glutaminase to carbamoyl phosphate synthetase.[94] In this way, it is proposed that activation of glutaminase by ammonia indirectly increases the affinity of urea synthesis for ammonia. In a second report, the pH dependence of urea synthesis from ammonia in the absence of glutamine in the perfused liver has been explained as an effect of pH on the intramitochondrial carbonic-anhydrase dependent supply of bicarbonate ions to carbamoyl phosphate synthetase.[95]

VI. CONCLUDING REMARKS

As will be clear from the above discussion there has been a greatly expanding interest in the study of liver glutamine metabolism in recent years. The elucidation of the properties of liver-specific glutaminase, the discovery of the intercellular glutamine cycle, and the recognition of the importance of the liver in pH homeostasis are all recent developments and progress in this area is now rapid. In addition to its metabolic importance, the study of the hormonal regulation of glutamine degradation has produced results of interest to those concerned with mitochondrial function and with regulation of Ca^{2+} metabolism. The study of glutamine metabolism is also an example of the advantages of the use of a combination of approaches employing submitochondrial extracts, intact mitochondria, isolated hepatocytes, and the isolated perfused liver as experimental material.

The work on hepatocyte heterogeneity and glutamine cycling described above has necessarily been performed on the isolated perfused liver. A number of problems remaining in this area could now be profitably studied using isolated perivenous or periportal hepatocytes; isolated hepatocytes would be particularly suited to the study of glutamine transport and the regulation of glutamine synthetase. Preparations of hepatocytes isolated by conventional collagenase perfusion have not been satisfactorily separated into perivenous and periportal populations. A method involving simultaneous slow antegrade and retrograde liver perfusion with collagenase added only to one inflow has been reported to give populations of cells enriched in either perivenous or periportal hepatocytes, although in very low yield.[96] More recently, a method has been described[97] in which either perivenous or periportal areas of the liver are destroyed selectively by a brief retrograde or antegrade perfusion with digitonin, and hepatocytes are subsequently isolated by conventional collagenase digestion. It is to be hoped that these methods or a development of them will allow investigation of aspects of the regulation of glutamine metabolism in isolated perivenous and/or periportal cells. This is one direction in which research in this interesting area may now be expected to develop.

REFERENCES

1. **Krebs, H. A.,** Metabolism of amino acids. The synthesis of glutamine from glutamic acid and ammonia and the enzymic hydrolysis of glutamine in animal tissues, *Biochem. J.,* 29, 1951, 1935.
2. **Lung, P. and Watford, M.,** Glutamine as a precursor of urea, in *The Urea Cycle,* Grisolia, S., Baguena, R., and Mayor, F., Eds., John Wiley & Sons, New York, 1976, 479.
3. **Berry, M. N. and Friend, D. S.,** High-yield preparation of isolated rat parenchymal cells, *J. Cell Biol.,* 43, 500, 1969.
4. **Krebs, H. A.,** Glutamine metabolism in the animal body, in *Glutamine: Metabolism, Enzymology and Regulation,* Mora, J. and Palacios, R., Eds., Academic Press, New York, 1980, 319.
5. **Lund, P.,** Glutamine metabolism in the rat, *FEBS Lett.,* 117, K86, 1979.
6. **Kovacevic, Z. and McGivan, J. D.,** Mitochondrial metabolism of glutamine and glutamate and its physiological significance, *Physiol. Rev.,* 63, 547, 1983.
7. **Sies, H. and Häussinger, D.,** Hepatic glutamine and ammonia metabolism, in *Glutamine Metabolism in Mammalian Tissues,* Häussinger, D. and Sies, H., Eds., Springer-Verlag, Berlin, 1984, 78.
8. **McGivan, J. D., Bradford, N. M., Verhoeven, A. J., and Meijer, A. J.,** Liver glutaminase, in *Glutamine Metabolism in Mammalian Tissues,* Häussinger, D. and Sies, H., Eds., Springer-Verlag, Berlin, 1984, 122.
9. **Horowitz, M. L. and Knox, W. E.,** A phosphate activated glutaminase in rat liver different from that in kidney and other tissues, *Enzymol. Biol. Clin.,* 9, 241, 1968.
10. **Häussinger, D., Stehle, T., and Gerok, W.,** Glutamine metabolism in isolated perfused liver — the transamination pathway, *Hoppe-Seyler's Biol. Chem.,* 366, 527, 1985.
11. **Ross, B. D., Hems, R., and Krebs, H. A.,** The rate of gluconeogenesis from various precursors in the perfused rat liver, *Biochem. J.,* 102, 942, 1967.
12. **Wanders, R. J. A., Meijer, A. J., Groen, A. K., and Tager, J. M.,** Bicarbonate and the pathway of glutamate oxidation in isolated rat liver mitochondria, *Eur. J. Biochem.,* 133, 245, 1983.
13. **Krebs, H. A., Hems, R., Lund, P., Halliday, D., and Read, W. W. C.,** Sources of ammonia for mammalian urea synthesis, *Biochem. J.,* 176, 733, 1978.
14. **Meijer, A. J. and Hensgens, H. E. S. J.,** Ureagenesis, in *Metabolic Compartmentation,* Sies, H., Ed., Academic Press, New York, 259, 1982.
15. **Kilberg, M. S.,** Amino acid transport in isolated rat hepatocytes, *J. Membr. Biol.,* 69, 1, 1982.
16. **Shotwell, M. A., Kilberg, M. S., and Oxender, D. L.,** The regulation of neutral amino acid transport in mammalian cells, *Biochim. Biophys. Acta,* 737, 267, 1983.
17. **Kilberg, M. S., Handlogten, M. E., and Christensen, H. N.,** Characteristics of system ASC for transport of neutral amino acids in the isolated rat hepatocyte, *J. Biol. Chem.,* 256, 3304, 1981.
18. **McGivan, J. D., Bradford, N. M., and Mendes-Mourao, J. C. P.,** The transport of branched-chain amino acids into isolated rat liver cells, *FEBS Lett.,* 80, 380, 1977.
19. **Weissbach, L., Handlogten, M. E., Christensen, H. N., and Kilberg, M. S.,** Evidence for two Na-independent neutral amino acid transport systems in primary cultures of rat hepatocytes, *J. Biol. Chem.,* 257, 12006, 1982.
20. **Kovacevic, Z. and McGivan, J. D.,** Glutamine transport across biological membranes, in *Glutamine Metabolism in Mammalian Tissues,* Haussinger, D. and Sies, H., Eds., Springer-Verlag, Berlin, 49, 1984.
21. **Joseph, S. K., Bradford, N. M., and McGivan, J. D.,** Characteristics of the transport of alanine, serine and glutamine across the plasma membrane of isolated rat liver cells, *Biochem. J.,* 176, 827, 1978.

22. **Kilberg, M. S., Handlogten, M. E., and Christensen, H. N.,** Characteristics of an amino acid transport system in rat liver for glutamine, asparagine, histidine and closely related analogues, *J. Biol. Chem.,* 255, 4011, 1980.

23. **Hayes, M. R. and McGivan, J. D.,** Differential effects of starvation on alanine and glutamine transport in isolated rat hepatocytes, *Biochem. J.,* 204, 365, 1982.

24. **McGivan, J. D.,** unpublished data.

25. **Edmondson, J. W. and Lumeng, L.,** Biphasic stimulation of amino acid uptake by glucagon in hepatocytes, *Biochim. Biophys. Res. Commun.,* 96, 61, 1980.

26. **Fafarnoux, P., Demigne, C., Remesy, C., and Le Cam, A.,** Bidirectional transport of glutamine across the cell membrane in rat liver, *Biochem. J.,* 216, 401, 1983.

27. **Joseph, S. K. and McGivan, J. D.,** The effects of ammonium chloride and glucagon on the metabolism of glutamine in isolated liver cells from starved rats, *Biochim. Biophys. Acta,* 543, 16, 1978.

28. **Brosnan, J. T. and Williamson, D. H.,** Mechanisms for the formation of alanine and aspartate in rat liver in vivo after administration of ammonium chloride, *Biochem. J.,* 138, 453, 1974.

29. **Häussinger, D., Soboll, S., Meijer, A. J., Gerok, W., Tager, J. M., and Sies, H.,** Role of plasma membrane transport in hepatic glutamine metabolism, *Eur. J. Biochem.,* 152, 597, 1985.

30. **Joseph, S. K., Verhoeven, A. J., and Meijer, A. J.,** Effect of trifluoroperazine on the stimulation by Ca-dependent hormones of gluconeogenesis from glutamine in isolated hepatocytes, *Biochim. Biophys. Acta,* 677, 506, 1981.

31. **Sips, H. J., DeGraaf, P. A., and van Dam, K.,** Transport of L-aspartate and L-glutamate in plasma membrane vesicles from rat liver, *Eur. J. Biochem.,* 122, 259, 1982.

32. **Gebhardt, R. and Mecke, D.,** Glutamate uptake by cultured rat hepatocytes is mediated by hormonally-inducible, sodium-dependent transport systems, *FEBS Lett.,* 161, 275, 1983.

33. **Joseph, S. K. and Meijer, A. J.,** The inhibitory effects of sulphydryl reagents on the transport and hydrolysis of glutamine in rat liver mitochondria, *Eur. J. Biochem.,* 119, 523, 1981.

34. **Curthoys, N. P., Kuhlenschmidt, T., Godfrey, S. S., and Weiss, R. F.,** Phosphate-dependent glutaminase from rat kidney. Cause of increased activity in response to acidosis and identity with glutaminase from other tissues, *Arch. Biochem. Biophys.,* 172, 162, 1976.

35. **Huang, Y. Z. and Knox, W. E.,** A comparative study of glutaminase isoenzymes in rat tissues, *Enzyme,* 21, 408, 1976.

36. **Patel, M. and McGivan, J. D.,** Partial purification and properties of rat liver glutaminase, *Biochem. J.,* 220, 583, 1984.

37. **Smith, E. M. and Watford, M.,** personal communication.

38. **Charles, R.,** Mitochondriale Citrulline Synthese:een Ammonik Fixerend en ATP Verbruikend Proces, Ph.D. thesis, University of Amsterdam, Rototype, Amsterdam, 1968.

39. **Häussinger, D., Weiss, L., and Sies, H.,** Activation of pyruvate dehydrogenase during metabolism of ammonium ions in hemoglobin-free perfused rat liver, *Eur. J. Biochem.,* 52, 421, 1975.

40. **Verhoeven, A. J., Van Iwaarden, J. F., Joseph, S. K., and Meijer, A. J.,** Control of rat liver glutaminase by ammonia and pH, *Eur. J. Biochem.,* 133, 241, 1983.

41. **McGivan, J. D. and Bradford, N. M.,** Characteristics of the activation of glutaminase by ammonia in sonicated rat liver mitochondria, *Biochim. Biophys. Acta,* 759, 241, 1983.

42. **Verhoeven, A. J., Estrela, J. M., and Meijer, A. J.,** Adrenergic stimulation of glutamine metabolism in isolated rat hepatocytes, *Biochem. J.,* 230, 457, 1985.

43. **Snodgrass, P. J. and Lund, P.,** Allosteric properties of human liver glutaminase, *Biochim. Biophys. Acta,* 798, 21, 1984.

44. **McGivan, J. D., Lacey, J. H., and Joseph, S. K.,** Localisation and some properties of phosphate-dependent glutaminase in disrupted liver mitochondria, *Biochem. J.,* 192, 537, 1980.

45. **McGivan, J. D. and Bradford, N. M.,** Influence of phospholipids on the activity of phosphate-dependent glutaminase in extracts of rat liver mitochondria, *Biochem. J.,* 214, 649, 1983.

46. **McGivan, J. D., Vadher, M., Lacey, J. H., and Bradford, N. M.,** Rat liver glutaminase. Regulation by reversible interaction with the mitochondrial membrane, *Eur. J. Biochem.,* 148, 323, 1985.

47. **Joseph, S. K. and McGivan, J. D.,** The effects of ammonium chloride and bicarbonate on the activity of glutaminase in isolated liver mitochondria, *Biochem. J.,* 176, 837, 1978.

48. **Joseph, S. K., McGivan, J. D., and Meijer, A. J.,** The stimulation of glutamine hydrolysis in isolated rat liver mitochondria by Mg^{2+} depletion and hypo-osmotic incubation conditions, *Biochem. J.,* 194, 35, 1981.

49. **Lacey, J. H., Bradford, N. M., Joseph, S. K., and McGivan, J. D.,** Increased activity of phosphate-dependent glutaminase in liver mitochondria as a result of glucagon treatment of rats, *Biochem. J.,* 194, 29, 1981.

50. **Corvera, S. and Garcia-Sainz, J. A.,** Hormonal stimulation of mitochondrial glutaminase. Effects of vasopressin, angiotensin II, adrenaline and glucagon, *Biochem. J.,* 210, 957, 1983.

51. **Häussinger, D. and Sies, H.,** Hepatic glutamine metabolism under the influence of the portal ammonia concentration in the perfused rat liver, *Eur. J. Biochem.,* 101, 179, 1979.

52. **Chamalaun, R. A. F. M. and Tager, J. M.,** Nitrogen metabolism in the perfused rat liver, *Biochim. Biophys. Acta,* 222, 119, 1970.

53. **Saheki, T. and Katunuma, N.,** Analysis of regulatory factors for urea synthesis by isolated perfused rat liver, *J. Biochem.,* 77, 659, 1975.

54. **Häussinger, D., Akerboom, T. P. M., and Sies, H.,** The role of pH and the lack of requirement for hydrogencarbonate in the regulation of hepatic glutamine metabolism, *Hoppe Seyler's Z. Physiol. Chem.,* 361, 995, 1980.

55. **Nordmann, R., Petit, M. A., and Nordmann, J.,** Recherches sur la mecanisme de l'accumulation intra-hepatique d'acides amines dicarboxyliques au cours de l'intoxication ammoniacale, *Biochimie,* 54, 1473, 1972.

56. **Baverel, G. and Lund, P.,** A role for bicarbonate in the regulation of mammalian glutamine metabolism, *Biochem. J.,* 184, 599, 1979.

57. **Meijer, A. J. and van Woerkom, G. M.,** unpublished results, quoted in Reference 8.

58. **Lueck, J. D. and Miller, L. L.,** The effect of perfusate pH on glutamine metabolism in the isolated perfused rat liver, *J. Biol. Chem.,* 245, 5491, 1970.

59. **Bradford, N. M. and McGivan, J. D.,** The use of $^{36}Cl^-$ to measure the membrane in isolated hepatocytes — effects of cAMP and bicarbonate ions, *Biochim. Biophys. Acta,* 845, 10, 1985.

60. **Häussinger, D., Gerok, W., and Sies, H.,** Regulation of flux through glutaminase and glutamine synthetase in isolated perfused rat liver, *Biochim. Biophys. Acta,* 755, 272, 1983.

61. **Ochs, R. S.,** Glutamine metabolism in isolated hepatocytes. Evidence for catecholamine stimulation of α-ketoglutarate dehydrogenase, *J. Biol. Chem.,* 259, 13004, 1984.

62. **Häussinger, D. and Sies, H.,** Effect of phenylephrine on glutamate and glutamine metabolism in isolated perfused rat liver, *Biochem. J.,* 221, 651, 1984.

63. **Staddon, J. M. and McGivan, J. D.,** Distinct effects of glucagon and vasopressin on proline metabolism in isolated hepatocytes, *Biochem. J.,* 217, 477, 1984.

64. **McCormack, J. G. and Denton, R. M.,** The effect of Ca^{2+} ions and adenine nucleotides on the activity of the pig heart 2-oxoglutarate dehydrogenase complex, *Biochem. J.,* 180, 533, 1979.

65. **Charest, R., Blackmore, P. F., Berthon, B., and Exton, J. H.,** Changes in free cytosolic Ca^{2+} in hepatocytes following adrenergic stimulation, *J. Biol. Chem.,* 258, 8769, 1983.

66. **Berthon, B., Binet, A., Mauger, J. P., and Claret, M.,** Cytosolic free Ca^{2+} in isolated rat hepatocytes as measured by quin 2, *FEBS Lett.,* 167, 19, 1984.

67. **Thomas, A. P., Alexander, J., and Williamson, J. R.,** Relationship between inositol polyphosphate production and the increase in cytosolic free Ca^{2+} induced by vasopressin in isolated hepatocytes, *J. Biol. Chem.,* 259, 5574, 1984.

68. **Denton, R. M. and McCormack, J. G.,** On the role of the Ca^{2+} transport cycle in heart and other mammalian mitochondria, *FEBS Lett.,* 119, 1, 1980.

69. **McCormack, J. G.,** Characterisation of the effects of Ca^{2+} on the intramitochondrial Ca^{2+}-sensitive enzymes from rat liver and within intact rat liver mitochondria, *Biochem. J.,* 231, 581, 1985.

70. **McCormack, J. G.,** Studies on the activation of rat liver pyruvate dehydrogenase and 2-oxoglutarate dehydrogenase by adrenaline and glucagon, *Biochem. J.,* 231, 597, 1985.

71. **Staddon, J. M. and McGivan, J. D.,** Effects of ATP and adenosine addition on activity of oxoglutarate dehydrogenase and the concentration of cytoplasmic free Ca^{2+} in rat hepatocytes, *Eur. J. Biochem.,* 151, 567, 1985.

72. **Staddon, J. M., Bradford, N. M., and McGivan, J. D.,** Effects of glucagon in vivo on the N-acetyl-glutamate, glutamate and glutamine contents of rat liver, *Biochem. J.,* 217, 855, 1984.

73. **Halestrap, A. P.,** Hormonal regulation of mitochondrial metabolism, *Biochem. Soc. Trans.,* 13, 655, 1985.

74. **Watford, M. and Smith, E. M.,** Regulation of phosphate-activated glutaminase activity and glutamine metabolism in the streptozocin-diabetic rat, *Biochem. J.,* 224, 207, 1984.

75. **Lund, P.,** Control of glutamine synthesis in rat liver, *Biochem. J.,* 124, 653, 1971.

76. **Meister, A.,** Catalytic mechanism of glutamine synthetase: overview of glutamine metabolism, in *Glutamine: Metabolism, Enzymology and Regulation,* Mora, J. and Palacios, R., Eds., Academic Press, New York, 1980, 1.

77. **Häussinger, D., Sies, H., and Gerok, W.,** Functional hepatocyte heterogeneity in ammonia metabolism. The intercellular glutamine cycle, *J. Hepatol.,* 1, 3, 1984.

78. **Häussinger, D., Gerok, W., and Sies, H.,** Hepatic role in pH regulation: role of the intercellular glutamine cycle, *Trend Biochem. Sci.,* 9, 300, 1984.

79. **Jungermann, K. and Katz, N.,** Functional hepatocyte heterogeneity, *Hepatology,* 2, 385, 1982.

80. **Jungermann, K. and Sasse, D.,** Heterogeneity of liver parenchymal cells, *Trend Biochem. Sci.,* 3, 198, 1978.

81. **Jungermann, K. and Katz, N.,** Metabolic heterogeneity of liver parenchyma, in *Metabolic Compartmentation,* Sies, H., Ed., Academic Press, London, 1982, 411.
82. **Gebhardt, R. and Mecke, D.,** Heterogeneous distribution of glutamine synthetase among rat liver parenchymal cells in situ and in primary culture, *EMBO J.,* 2, 567, 1983.
83. **Gebhardt, R. and Mecke, D.,** Cellular distribution and regulation of glutamine synthetase, in *Glutamine Metabolism in Mammalian Tissues,* Häussinger, D. and Sies, H., Eds., Springer-Verlag, Berlin, 1984, 98.
84. **Gaasbeek-Janzen, J. W., Moorman, A. F. M., Lamers, W. H., Los, J. A., and Charles, R.,** The localization of carbamoyl phosphate synthetase in adult rat liver, *Biochem. Soc. Trans.,* 9, 279, 1981.
85. **Häussinger, D. and Gerok, W.,** Hepatocyte heterogeneity in ammonia metabolism: impairment of glutamine synthesis in CCl_4 induced liver cell necrosis with no effect on urea synthesis, *Chem. Biol. Interact.,* 48, 191, 1984.
86. **Häussinger, D.,** Hepatocyte heterogeneity in glutamine and ammonia metabolism and the role of an intercellular glutamine cycle during ureogenesis in perfused rat liver, *Eur. J. Biochem.,* 133, 269, 1983.
87. **Häussinger, D. and Gerok, W.,** Hepatocyte heterogeneity in glutamate uptake by isolated perfused rat liver, *Eur. J. Biochem.,* 136, 421, 1983.
88. **Lusty, C. J.,** Carbamoyl phosphate synthetase I of rat liver mitochondria, *Eur. J. Biochem.,* 85, 373, 1978.
89. **Deuel, T. F., Louie, M., and Lerner, A.,** Glutamine synthesis from rat liver, *J. Biol. Chem.,* 253, 6111, 1978.
90. **Atkinson, D. E. and Camien, M. N.,** The role of urea synthesis in the removal of metabolic bicarbonate and the regulation of blood pH, *Curr. Top. Cell. Regul.,* 21, 261, 1982.
91. **Bean, E. S. and Atkinson, D. E.,** Regulation of the rate of urea synthesis in liver by extracellular pH, *J. Biol. Chem.,* 259, 1552, 1984.
92. **Oliver, J. and Bourke, E.,** Adaptations in urea and ammonia excretion in metabolic acidosis in the rat: a reinterpretation, *Clin. Sci. Mol. Med.,* 48, 515, 1975.
93. **Oliver, J., Koelz, A. M., Costello, J., and Bourke, E.,** Acid-base induced alterations in glutamine metabolism and ureogenesis in perfused muscle and liver of the rat, *Eur. J. Clin. Invest.,* 7, 445, 1975.
94. **Meijer, A. J.,** Channelling of ammonia from glutaminase to carbamoyl phosphate synthetase in liver mitochondria, *FEBS Lett.,* 190, 249, 1985.
95. **Häussinger, D.,** Hepatic urea synthesis and pH regulation. Role of CO_2, HCO_3^-, pH and the activity of carbonic anhydrase, *Eur. J. Biochem.,* 152, 381, 1985.
96. **Vaananen, H., Lindros, K. O., and Salaspuro, M.,** Selective isolation of intact periportal or perivenous hepatocytes by antero- or retrograde collagenase perfusion, *Liver,* 3, 131, 1983.
97. **Quistorff, B.,** Gluconeogenesis in periportal and perivenous hepatocytes of rat liver, isolated by a new high-yield digitonin/collagenase technique, *Biochem. J.,* 229, 22, 1985.

Chapter 12

RENAL GLUTAMINE METABOLISM

David P. Simpson

TABLE OF CONTENTS

I. INTRODUCTION

The ability of the kidney to adjust ammonium production by regulating the rate of glutamine metabolism is a central process in the regulation of acid-base homeostasis. When net acid production by the body is low, little ammonium needs to be excreted to maintain an acid-base balance and little glutamine is consumed by the kidney. Increased acid production is met by development of metabolic acidosis which causes a gradual increase in renal glutamine extraction; the resulting rise in ammonium production and excretion enables a stable state of acid-base balance to ensue even in the face of large acid loads. The biochemical responses underlying the adaptation of glutamine metabolism to changing requirements for hydrogen ion excretion by the kidney occur principally at the mitochondrial level. Exploration of these responses has revealed special features of mitochondrial glutamine transport and metabolism. In particular, transport of glutamine by its inner membrane carrier has been found to provide a site for the regulation of ammonium formation from glutamine by phosphate-dependent glutaminase (PDG). In this chapter the current state of this knowledge will be reviewed with emphasis on the properties of mitochondrial glutamine metabolism.

II. GLUTAMINE METABOLISM IN VIVO

A. In Normal Man and the Dog Glutamine is the Major Source of Ammonium Produced in the Kidney

In normal man glutamine is removed from the blood entering the kidney in sufficient amount to account for renal ammoniagenesis. Glutamine is present in plasma in a concentration averaging 0.6 mM, making it the most abundant amino acid in the blood. This level plus the very high blood flow to the kidney per gram of tissue causes a large quantity of glutamine, on the order of 600 μmol/min, to be delivered to the kidney each minute.[1,2] Only about 10% of the glutamine entering the kidney is removed in normal man.[1-3] Owen and Robinson[2] studied renal amino acid extraction and ammonium production in normal subjects. Glutamine uptake averaged 47 μmol/min; only small amounts of other amino acids were extracted by the kidney. Ammonium production by the kidney was 75 μmol/min suggesting that some ammonium must come from each nitrogen of glutamine. Similar results have been obtained by Tizianello et al.[3]

The study of glutamine metabolism in dogs has given results quite similar to those in man showing that glutamine is the only amino acid extracted in sufficient amount by the kidney to account for the quantity of ammonium produced.[4] This amount exceeds that which could be derived from the amide nitrogen of glutamine alone but is less than the quantity which could be obtained from both nitrogen containing groups of glutamine.[5] In contrast to man and the dog, glutamine does not appear to be the predominent source of ammonium in the normal, nonacidotic rat kidney. Vinay et al.[5] found total ammonium production by one rat kidney to be 0.72 μmol/min at a time when glutamine extraction was only 0.12 μmol/min. Similarly Yablon and Relman[6] and Parry and Brosnan[7] found that renal extraction of glutamine by control rats was not significantly different from zero.

B. Chronic Metabolic Acidosis is a Powerful Stimulant to Glutamine Extraction by the Kidney

Physiologically, the ability of the kidney to vary ammonium synthesis is a major factor in regulation of the acid-base balance. When an acidifying agent such as ammonium chloride is administered, a gradual increase in ammonium excretion develops. In man and the dog the maximum rate of excretion is achieved in about 6 days;[8-10] in the rat only about 3 days is required for maximum adaptation.[7] Steady-state levels of NH$_4^+$ excretion in chronic metabolic acidosis may be fivefold or more greater than in controls. Increased glutamine extraction accounts for the change in ammonium synthesis and in NH_4^+ excretion in chronic acidosis in man,[2,11,12] the dog,[4,5] and rat[7] (even though in the latter species glutamine is not a major source of ammonium in the nonacidotic animal).

Pitts and colleagues[13] used glutamine labeled with ^{15}N in the amide or amine positions to separate the contribution of these groups to ammonium synthesis in the dog. When ^{15}N-amide-glutamine was infused into one renal artery the contribution to NH_4^+ excretion of ^{15}N was over twice as great as when ^{15}N-amine-glutamine was used. These studies provide direct evidence that the amide-nitrogen of glutamine is the principal source of urinary NH_4^+ with a smaller but important contribution provided by the amine group.

The supply of glutamine to the kidney changes little in chronic acidosis with plasma levels showing little difference from those in controls in the dog and man. The tissue level of glutamine in the renal cortex exceeds that in plasma by up to twofold and this difference does not change appreciably in chronic acidosis[5] or falls slightly.[4,6,7] These findings indicate that during chronic acidosis release of glutamine into the blood by other organs increases to keep pace with increased renal utilization. Also, the transport of glutamine into the cells of renal cortex may be enhanced by chronic acidosis. However, since tissue levels of glutamine do not rise, the transport of glutamine into cells is not the driving mechanism responsible for increased glutamine utilization in acidosis.

The time at which initiation of increased glutamine extraction first occurs in chronic acidosis is uncertain. In the rat ammonium synthesis and glutamine extraction are augmented within minutes after acidosis is produced and after 24 hr ammonium excretion has doubled and the glutamine extraction, initially negligible, is sufficient to account for the increase in NH_4^+ excretion.[7] In man, however, while increased ammoniagenesis develops promptly after acidosis is initiated, no change in glutamine extraction is present after 24 hr.[3] In the dog, in most investigations no immediate increase in glutamine extraction has been found when acute metabolic acidosis is produced by HCl infusion.[5,14] Such studies in the dog are complicated by the reduction in renal blood flow which generally accompanies HCl infusion. This decrease results in the delivery of less glutamine per minute to the kidney. The lack of immediate effect of acidosis on glutamine extraction in the dog could be the result of an increased rate of extraction stimulated by the acidosis but balanced by the decreased extraction arising from the reduction in glutamine delivery. However, in one study of acute acidosis in the dog, no significant change in renal blood flow occurred nor were changes in glutamine extraction observed.[14] In contrast, acute respiratory acidosis does cause a rapid increase in glutamine extraction and ammoniagenesis in the dog.[15]

III. GLUTAMINE METABOLISM IN VITRO BY INTACT CELLS

A. Enhanced Glutamine Utilization and Ammoniagenesis Persist in In Vitro Preparations from Acidotic Animals

Perfused kidneys, tissue slices, and isolated tubule preparations have been used to study glutamine metabolism and its response to acidosis. Such studies provide an important transitional link between glutamine metabolism in the kidney of the intact animal and its characteristics in subcellular systems such as mitochondria. In particular they show that the adaptation of glutamine metabolism to chronic metabolic acidosis is demonstrable under simple in vitro conditions.

In an early study, Goodman et al.[16] incubated tissue slices prepared from the renal cortex of control or 2-day acidotic rats with 10 mM glutamine. The slices from acidotic animals produced 75% more glucose than those from controls. Conversely, glucose production was suppressed in slices from animals made alkalotic by $NaHCO_3$ administration. Subsequently, glutamine metabolism was examined in tissue slices of the dog renal cortex, which does not show an increase in PDG levels in acidosis and which does not contain glutamine synthetase, characteristics of the rat kidney which complicate the interpretation of results in this species. Tissue slices from chronically acidotic dogs were incubated with uniformly labeled ^{14}C-glutamine; ^{14}C-glucose and $^{14}CO_2$ production were measured.[17] The incorporation of labeled glutamine into both end products was stimulated in the acidotic slices. The number of counts in $^{14}CO_2$ was manyfold greater than those in glucose with either acidotic or control slices and acidosis stimulated ^{14}C incorporation into each moiety to about the same extent. These findings indicate that in tissue slices, as in the intact kidney, the major fate of glutamine is oxidation to CO_2. They also show that the stimulus of acidosis lies early in the steps of glutamine metabolism before diversion occurs into separate pathways of CO_2 formation and gluconeogenesis.

Hems[18] compared glutamine metabolism in perfused rat kidney preparations from control and chronically acidotic animals. With 5 mM glutamine as the sole substrate in the perfusion medium, kidneys from rats with 7 to 10 days of acidosis used glutamine at a rate of 387 μmol/hr/g dry weight, a value almost double the consumption by control kidneys. Ammonium production was also twice as great, 721 μmol/hr/g in kidneys from acidotic rats vs. 358 in controls. Glucose production was 101 and 16 μmol/hr/g in the two groups.

The ability to reproduce many of the features of adaptation of glutamine metabolism to chronic acidosis using perfused kidneys or tissue slices shows that this adaptation does not depend on persistence of the internal milieu of chronic acidosis for its expression. The stimulus to glutamine utilization persists in in vitro preparations from acidotic kidneys when the same pH and bicarbonate concentration is present in the incubation medium used for control and acidotic tissue. Also, removal of tissue from exposure to the blood for in vitro studies shows that no immediate hormonal stimulus or change in concentration of some substance in the blood is necessary for enhanced glutamine metabolism to continue in tissue from acidotic animals.

IV. GLUTAMINE METABOLISM IN INTACT MITOCHONDRIA FROM THE KIDNEY

A. Glutamine is Transported Across the Inner Mitochondrial Membrane by a Specific Carrier

Efficient mitochondrial metabolism depends on the ability of specific carriers to transport substrates rapidly in and out of the matrix space.[19,20] Glutamine, an amphoteric compound with balancing positive and negative charges at physiologic pH, is metabolized by PDG located in the interior of mitochondria. For glutamine to reach this enzyme from the cytoplasm it must first be carried across the inner membrane on a specific carrier, strong evidence for which now exists.

Early evidence suggesting the existence of a glutamine carrier was provided by studies of swelling of rat kidney mitochondria.[21,22] When incubated in iso-osmotic L-glutamine, rapid swelling of mitochondria occurs. In contrast, swelling is sluggish when glutamate is substituted for glutamine. When D-glutamine is used, swelling does not occur indicating failure of this isomer to cross the inner membrane.[23]

More definitive evidence for a glutamine carrier has been provided by measurements of L-glutamine distribution in circumstances where the transport and metabolism of glutamine are prevented. A substance which can cross the inner membrane by passive diffusion will accumulate in the matrix space when metabolism is blocked. With no net charge, if glutamine passively entered mitochondria it would reach a concentration equal to that in the incubation medium if no intramitochondrial metabolism occurs. At 0°C no significant formation of glutamate occurs from 1 mM ^{14}C-glutamine in the presence of rotenone (to block conversion of any glutamate formed to other products).[24] Under these conditions, when the distribution of glutamine in dog kidney mitochondria is compared to that of an outer space marker such

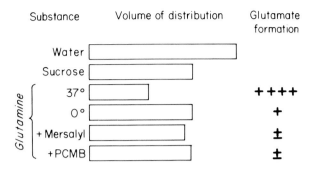

FIGURE 1. Volume of distribution of glutamine compared with that of water or sucrose in dog kidney mitochondria. Except at 37°C, the volume of distribution of glutamine is equal to that of the outer space. When metabolism is rapid at 37°C, glutamine is consumed during the passage of mitochondria through silicone oil, causing the apparent volume of distribution of glutamine to be less than that of the outer space.[24]

as mannitol or sucrose, an identical space of distribution is found (Figure 1); that is, no glutamine is present in the matrix space. However, at a higher temperature rapid accumulation of ^{14}C-glutamate formed from glutamine occurs indicating the presence of a temperature-dependent transport process. Similar results are obtained when glutamine distribution is examined in dog or rat kidney mitochondria in which metabolism is blocked by mersalyl,[24,25] a potent inhibitor of glutamate formation from glutamine in intact mitochondria.

Another property of mitochondrial glutamine metabolism which favors the presence of an active transport mechanism for glutamine entry is energy dependence. When mitochondria are incubated with succinate, or with tetramethyl-*p*-phenylenediamine and ascorbate, in the presence of rotenone, glutamate formation from ^{14}C-glutamine is distinctly increased compared to the amount formed in the absence of these respiratory substrates (Figure 2).[24,26] Not only is the total rate of glutamate formation from glutamine enhanced, but the concentration of labeled glutamate in the matrix space also increases by about twofold. This finding could result either from stimulation of an inner membrane glutamine carrier or by stimulation of PDG. However, the activity of PDG is not known to be affected by an energy source. Since no phosphate was present in the medium, an increase in PDG activity secondary to a rise in matrix phosphate concentration is unlikely. Matrix glutamate levels were higher in the presence of an energy source; if anything, this change would diminish PDG activity since glutamate inhibits the enzyme. The most likely explanation for the influence of an energy source is that it stimulates transport by a glutamine carrier, reflecting a property similar to that possessed by many other inner membrane substrate carriers.

Thus, there is abundant evidence from studies of mitochondrial swelling, from measurements of glutamine distribution, and from characteristics of glutamine metabolism in intact mitochondria that glutamine is transported across the inner membrane by a carrier with properties very similar to those of anionic substrate carriers.

B. The Relationship Between the Glutamine Carrier and Phosphate-Dependent Glutaminase is Unresolved

Several studies have shown that PDG is exclusively a mitochondrial enzyme.[27-29] Curthoys and Weiss[28] studied the distribution of PDG within mitochondria obtaining evidence that it is attached to the inner membrane. Digitonin and Lubrol® were used to fractionate mitochondria and the activity of PDG in different submitochondrial fractions was compared with that of marker enzymes. When the activity of PDG was stabilized with borate, its recovery

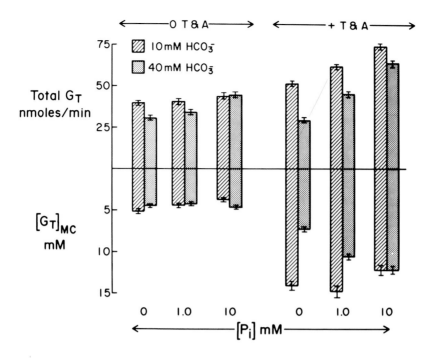

FIGURE 2.   Influence of energy source on glutamine metabolism in dog kidney mitochondria. T and A = tetramethyl-*p*-phenylenediamine plus ascorbate, G_T = glutamate, $[G_T]_{MC}$ = mitochondrial glutamate concentration, and P_i = phosphate concentration. 10 and 40 m*M* HCO_3^- were used in the media. (From Simpson, D. P., *J. Biol. Chem.*, 255, 7123, 1980. With permission.)

in different fractions correlated closely with that of cytochrome oxidase, a component of the inner membrane.

For most mitochondrial substrate carriers, accumulation of the transported compound in the matrix space is readily demonstrated when metabolic degradation of the substrate is blocked with rotenone. In the case of glutamine, however, no convincing demonstration has yet been made of its presence within the matrix space. Yet, glutamate formed from glutamine by PDG accumulates in high concentration in the matrix.

When mitochondria are incubated with ^{14}C-glutamine and then separated from the medium by rapid centrifugation through a silicone oil layer, the volume of distribution of glutamine is less than that of the outer mitochondrial space.[24,26] This peculiarity occurs because during the passage of mitochondria through the silicone oil layer, glutamine continues to be metabolized until the perchloric acid solution beneath the oil is reached. When glutamine metabolism is inhibited in any one of a variety of ways, the discrepancy between the volume of distribution of glutamine and the outer space diminishes until the two are equal. If glutamine were also present in the matrix space, its volume of distribution would exceed the volume of the outer space. No conditions have been found where this occurs: the volume of distribution of glutamine is always less than or equal to that of the outer space.

The failure to detect glutamine in the matrix space may arise from either of two possible relationships between the glutamine carrier and PDG (Figure 3):

1.   The carrier and the enzyme are physically linked so that the carrier transfers transported glutamine directly to the enzyme which deamidates it and releases glutamate into the matrix space. No glutamine is released by the carrier into the matrix space by this mechanism.

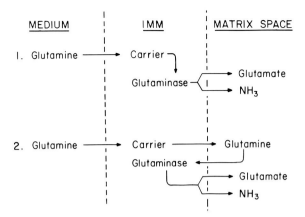

FIGURE 3. Two possible relationships between the glutamine carrier and PDG. In 1, the carrier and the enzyme are linked together in the inner mitochondrial membrane (IMM) so that glutamine is delivered directly to glutaminase without release into the matrix space. In 2, the carrier releases glutamine into the matrix space from which it is removed by glutaminase positioned on the inside of the IMM.

2. After the carrier transports glutamine across the inner membrane, the substrate is released into the matrix space as occurs with other substrates transported by mitochondrial carriers. As soon as glutamine enters the matrix, PDG acts on it, converting it so rapidly to glutamate that free glutamine is present only in unmeasurably low concentrations in the matrix. In this case, the failure to demonstrate glutamine in the matrix when PDG is inhibited by mersalyl or other agent can be accounted for only if the inhibitor also inhibits the carrier as well as PDG.

Regardless of which of the above relationships is correct, the glutamine carrier and not PDG must be the rate-limiting step in converting glutamine to glutamate in intact kidney mitochondria. Otherwise, under some of the conditions tested glutamine would have accumulated in the matrix space.

The conclusion that the carrier is rate limiting has been critized on the basis of results of two other studies. In one, Curthoys and Shapiro[30] purified rat kidney mitochondria using a Ficoll® gradient in order to remove contamination by nonmitochondrial phosphate-independent glutaminase (PIG) activity. After doing this, using conditions similar to those in which no glutamine was found in the matrix space by other investigators, they were able to detect low concentrations of glutamine in the matrix space. They concluded that the failure to detect glutamine in the matrix space in earlier studies was due to the presence of PIG which used up glutamine in the outer space while mitochondria were passing through the silicone oil layer, making the volume of distribution of glutamine less than it actually was. They also found no difference in the concentration of glutamine present in the matrix space of mitrochondria from acidotic or control animals. The mitochondria from acidotic animals formed several times as much glutamate from glutamine as the controls and PDG levels were much higher in mitochondria from chronically acidotic rats (see Section V). The authors argued that if transport was the rate-limiting step, and the enhanced glutamate formation in acidotic mitochondria was due to a stimulation of this step, then a higher concentration of glutamine should have been found in the matrix space of acidotic mitochondria. Since this was not found, they concluded that PDG is the rate-limiting step and enhanced glutamine metabolism in acidosis is due to higher levels of the enzyme present in this condition.

Table 1
VOLUMES OF DISTRIBUTION AND GLUTAMINE METABOLISM IN MITOCHONDRIA FROM THE RAT RENAL CORTEX

Substance	Additions to medium	R^a	$[Glutamate]_M{}^b$ (mM)	Glutamate formation (nmol/min/mg/protein)
^{14}C-Glutamine	0	1.080 ± 0.012	0.317 ± 0.043	1.00 ± 0.033
^{14}C-Glutamine	T + A^c	1.099 ± 0.013	1.15 ± 0.184	1.85 ± 0.043
^{14}C-Ribose	0	1.071 ± 0.004		

^{a}R $= \dfrac{\text{volume of distribution of glutamine or ribose}}{\text{volume of distribution of mannitol}}$

^{b} [Glutamate]$_M$ = concentration of glutamate in matrix.

^{c} T + A = tetramethyl-p-phenylenediamine + ascorbate.

These conflicting findings and conclusions about the presence and significance of glutamine in the matrix space were clarified in a subsequent study. Simpson and Hecker[31] showed that PIG contaminating mitochondrial preparations lies entirely in the loose, fluffy layer above the mitochondrial pellet. This layer was removed by gentle swirling during preparation of mitochondria used in the initial studies in which glutamine could not be detected in the matrix space; consequently, contamination by this enzyme could not account for the distribution of glutamine. The explanation by Curthoys and Shapiro for the apparent presence of glutamine in the matrix space was shown to be due to an underestimation of the outer space volume. In experiments in which the outer space was measured by markers of differing molecular weight, the volume of this space increased with decreasing molecular weight; that is, the smaller molecules penetrated into a slightly larger volume than larger ones. The volume of distribution of ^{14}C-sucrose, used by Curthoys and Shapiro to estimate outer space volume, is smaller than that of ^{14}C-ribose, a compound of molecular size similar to that of glutamine. The volume of distribution of glutamine was reevaluated using several conditions associated with widely different rates of glutamine metabolism. In none of these conditions was the volume of distribution found to exceed that of ^{14}C-ribose (Table 1). The lack of change in the volume of distribution of glutamine in acidosis is thus explained by the fact that all the glutamine is actually in the outer space and not in the matrix.

The second argument against glutamine transport being the rate-limiting step is based on a study of glutamine release from mitochondria loaded with this compound. Kovacević and Bajin[32] developed a technique for loading mitochondria with ^{14}C-glutamine and then studying its rate of release using an inhibitor stop technique. They incubated mitochondria in hypotonic medium containing 40 mM ^{14}C-glutamine. The addition of mersalyl led to the retention of some labeled glutamine in the mitochondrial preparation. The mersalyl block could be removed with thiol reagents and reconstituted with mersalyl and N-ethylmaleimide. The rate of glutamine release was measured by removing the block for timed intervals enabling kinetic measurements to be made. At 0°C the rate of glutamine exit was found to be five to ten times greater than the rate of glutaminase activity. If the rate of exit measured by this technique reflected the activity of the glutamine carrier, these results would suggest that the carrier is not the rate-limiting step in glutamine deamidation. However, subsequent findings by Kovacević and McGivan[33] indicate that the rate of glutamine efflux in this circumstance is determined not by the activity of the carrier but rather by changes in swelling of mitochondria induced by the thiol reagents used to remove the mersalyl block. This finding makes it doubtful that the flux measurements obtained previously with this technique reflected properties of the glutamine carrier.

Thus, no convincing evidence has been obtained for the presence of glutamine within the matrix space. Either of the two associations listed earlier in this chapter between the carrier and PDG remain possible. The bulk of the evidence continues to suggest strongly that transport across the inner membrane is the rate-limiting step in glutamine deamidation.

C. The Properties of Glutaminase Activity in Intact Mitochondria Differ Greatly from Those of Extracted Phosphate-Dependent Glutaminase

PDG has been extracted as a soluble enzyme from kidneys of man,[34] the dog,[27] pig,[35-37] and rat,[38] and its properties have been extensively studied. Characteristics of the solubilized enzyme include:

1. The pH optimum for the reaction is 7.9 to 8.1.[35,37]
2. In the absence of phosphate the enzyme is almost inactive. Half-maximal activation by phosphate occurs at concentrations of 20 to 30 mM.[35,36,39]
3. K_m (at pH 8.1, phosphate 100 mM) is 5 mM.[35,36] The K_m increases markedly as the phosphate concentration declines. Maximum reaction rates are obtained with glutamine concentrations of 25 to 50 mM in 100 mM phosphate buffer.
4. Both L-glutamate and NH_4^+ are potent end-product inhibitors of PDG.[35,37]
5. The enzyme is inhibited by sulfhydryl compounds (*p*-chloromercuribenzoate, mersalyl, and *N*-ethylmaleimide), phthalein dyes (bromcresol green and bromosulfalein),[35] and certain glutamine analogues (6-diazo-5-oxo-L-norleucine).[39] Borate stabilizes the extracted enzyme under some conditions and inhibits its activity under others.[40]
6. Extracts from lyophilized mitochondria contain a monomer of PDG with 160,000 daltons mol wt and a dimer with 330,000.[41] The dimer appears to be the active form of the enzyme.

When glutaminase activity is studied in intact mitochondria incubated with rotenone to prevent metabolism of glutamate, a two-step reaction sequence consisting of transport across the inner membrane followed by enzymatic deamidation is responsible for glutamate and ammonium formation from glutamine. The properties of this two-step process in mitochondria differ in many respects from those of the extracted enzyme outlined above. These differences may be the result of two differences between the reaction in mitochondria and that in extracts. First, the properties of the inner membrane glutamine carrier influence the characteristics of the overall reaction by which extramitochondrial glutamine is converted by mitochondria to glutamate and ammonium. Second, the extraction process by which glutaminase is removed from its inner membrane attachment may alter the properties of the enzyme. The differences between glutamine transport-deamidation in intact mitochondria and deamidation by solubilized glutaminase are sufficiently pronounced that great caution must be exercised in attempting to relate properties of the extracted enzyme to the regulation of glutaminase activity in intact cells.

Major properties in intact mitochondria of glutaminase, representing the combined function of the enzyme and carrier, include the following:

1. In dog kidney mitochondria the pH optimum is 7.8.[24] When bicarbonate buffered medium is used the value falls to 7.1 or below (10 mM bicarbonate, 4% CO_2) (Figure 4).[26] In the presence of bicarbonate-CO_2 buffer, the decreasing pH and bicarbonate concentration stimulate the uptake of many substrates transported by inner membrane carriers.[42] The similarity of this phenomenon to that seen with glutamine suggests that the change in pH optimum observed with bicarbonate buffers is a property of the carrier component of the glutaminase reaction.
2. Phosphate is not required in the medium for effective glutaminase activity in intact mitochondria. A small amount of endogenous phosphate may still be retained in the matrix after isolating mitochondria using phosphate-free solutions. However the con-

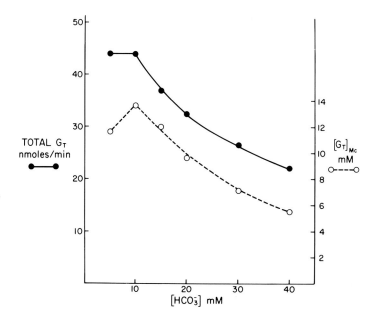

FIGURE 4. Influence of pH and bicarbonate concentration in medium on the formation and accumulation of glutamate formed from 0.5 mM glutamine by dog kidney mitochondria. The media contained an energy source and were gassed with 4% CO_2 and 96% O_2. (From Simpson, D. P., *J. Biol. Chem.*, 255, 7123, 1980. With permission.)

centration in the matrix of retained phosphate is very low compared to the amounts needed for activation of solubilized glutaminase. The presence of bicarbonate-CO_2 buffer also influences the effect of phosphate on intact mitochondrial glutaminase activity.[24,26] The addition of only 0.1 mM phosphate to the medium increases the rate of glutamate formation by almost twofold. However, as phosphate concentration is further increased up to 10 mM, little change occurs in the rate of glutamine conversion to glutamate.

3. Glutamate and NH_4^+ inhibit glutamine deamidation in intact mitochondria as well as in tissue extracts.[24,25] Inhibition of 50% is produced by a glutamate concentration of 6 mM or an NH_4^+ concentration of 1 mM.

4. A striking effect of α-ketoglutarate (2-oxoglutarate) on glutaminase activity in intact rat kidney mitochondria was observed by Goldstein.[43] This effect is present in dog kidney mitochondria in which 50% inhibition occurs with 0.3 mM α-ketoglutarate in the medium.[26] Since the activity of extracted glutaminase is not altered by such low concentrations of α-ketoglutarate, it was suggested that α-ketoglutarate inhibits the glutamine carrier. However, Strzelecki and Schoolwerth[44] found that under the conditions of these experiments, which include rotenone to block glutamate conversion to α-ketoglutarate, considerable amounts of glutamate are formed from α-ketoglutarate by reversal of the glutamate dehydrogenase reaction. Thus the effect of α-ketoglutarate on glutamine deamidation may be secondary to glutamate inhibition of glutaminase activity and not to a direct effect on the glutamine carrier.

5. Sulfhydryl compounds, particularly mersalyl, are potent inhibitors of glutaminase activity in intact mitochondria as well as extracted glutaminase.[24,26] By over 90%, 1 mM mersalyl blocks glutamate formation. *N*-Ethylmaleimide and bromcresol green also inhibit glutamate formation in mitochondria and borate stimulates the reaction.[24] 6-Diazo-5-oxo-L-norleucine, in contrast, has only a small effect on glutamine deam-

idation in a concentration up to 10 mM in intact mitochondria. In part, the failure of this analogue to inhibit glutaminase in intact mitochondria may be due to the lack of penetration of the agent to the enzyme site inside the inner membrane.

6. At low (physiologic) concentrations of glutamine, the reaction in intact mitochondria exhibits a K_m of 0.4 to 0.6. Above 4 mM substrate concentration, a change in the kinetics occurs and a much higher K_m appears to govern the reaction.[24]

V. RESPONSE OF MITOCHONDRIAL GLUTAMINE METABOLISM TO CHRONIC ACIDOSIS

A. The Dog and Rat Kidney Differ in the Adaptation of Phosphate-Dependent Glutaminase (Phosphate-Activated Glutaminase) to Chronic Acidosis

Because of the central role of PDG in ammoniagenesis from glutamine, this enzyme would seem to be a logical site for the regulation of glutamine metabolism to occur. Davies and Yudkin[45] were the first to suggest the possibility that changes in PDG activity occur in acidosis. Shortly thereafter enhanced levels of glutaminase were demonstrated in homogenates of kidneys from chronically acidotic rats.[46,47] In a study of the distribution of PDG in different segments of the rat nephron, Curthoys and Lowry[48] found that PDG activity was highest in the distal portions of the nephron of control animals. However, in chronic acidosis the activity of PDG in distal segments was unchanged but in the proximal convoluted tubules PDG activity increased over 50-fold. These findings and others lent credence to the concept that adaptation of PDG activity accounted for enhanced ammoniagenesis from glutamine.

However, other findings have shown that this attractive hypothesis is untenable. The most compelling of these contrary pieces of evidence comes from study of the adaptation to acidosis in the dog. In this species, as in man, chronic metabolic acidosis is accompanied by increased glutamine extraction and increased ammoniagenesis by the kidney. PDG activity, however, is unaltered in homogenates of the renal cortex from dogs with many days of acidosis.[49,50] The discrepancy in PDG adaptation in the two species has also been demonstrated in mitochondria from chronically acidotic animals. In mitochondria isolated from kidneys of chronically acidotic rats, increased PDG levels are present[25] but in similar preparations from the dog, no change in the enzyme level develops.[24]

In the rat there is also evidence that PDG activity is not an essential component to the adaptation of acidosis. Goldstein[51] showed that treatment of rats with actinomycin prevented the increase in PDG levels in acidotic rats. Yet the rise in NH_4^+ excretion was unaffected. The increase in ammoniagenesis in the rat does not correlate with the time course of change in PDG levels, increased ammonium excretion, or production by tissue slices being evident several hours before detectable alteration in PDG levels develops.[46,52]

Thus in both the dog and rat, chronic acidosis can cause a change in intracellular glutamine metabolism which persists in vitro and results in enhanced ammoniagenesis but is independent of alteration in PDG activity.

B. In Both the Dog and Rat Adaptation of the Glutamine Carrier Develops in Chronic Acidosis

In the rat, increased activity of other enzymes in addition to PDG occurs in chronic metabolic acidosis. Higher levels of phosphoenolpyruvate (PEP) carboxykinase,[52] glutamate dehydrogenase,[49,53] and glutamine ketoacid aminotransferase[54] have been reported. However, as in the case of PDG, changes in the activity of these enzymes are lacking in the acidotic dog kidney.[5,49,50] On the other hand, studies of the mitochondrial glutamine carrier show that alteration in the rate of transport of this carrier can account for enhanced glutamine deamidation in chronic acidosis in both species.

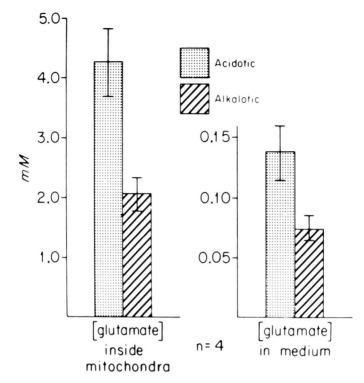

FIGURE 5.   The effect of chronic metabolic acidosis or alkalosis on the accumulation and formation of glutamate from labeled glutamine. Mitochondria were isolated from dogs with acidosis or alkalosis of 10 days or more duration. Incubation medium contained 1 mM [^{14}C]-glutamine and 20 mM KHCO$_3$ and was otherwise identical for the two sets of mitochondria. (From Simpson, D. P., *J. Biol. Chem.*, 250, 8148, 1975. With permission.)

As discussed earlier, incubating mitochondria in the presence of rotenone enables the study of the two-step reaction sequence consisting of the glutamine transport by its inner membrane carrier and conversion of glutamine to glutamate and NH$_3$ by PDG. When this process is examined in mitochondria from the chronically acidotic dog or rat kidney, the rate of glutamate formation is increased severalfold compared to that observed in preparations from the control rat[25] or chronically alkalotic dog (Figure 5).[24] Intramitochondrial glutamate concentration is also markedly increased in the acidotic state so that stimulation of glutamine deamidation occurs despite higher levels of this end-product inhibitor of glutaminase. In neither species is glutamine detectable in the matrix space of mitochondria from acidotic animals. While PDG levels increase in mitochondria from acidotic rats, no such change occurs in the dog. Thus, the stimulation of glutamine metabolism under these conditions must arise either from increased transport by the glutamine carrier in acidosis or from a persistent alteration in PDG activity which occurs without demonstrable change in the tissue levels of the enzyme. No evidence supporting the latter type of process exists so it is reasonable to conclude that the carrier is the site of adaptation leading to enhanced glutamine deamidation in acidosis.

This conclusion is supported by other observations. In the dog kidney the K$_m$ for glutamate formation from glutamine in intact mitochondria is unaltered by chronic acidosis, being 0.4 mM in both control and acidotic preparations (Figure 6).[19] The increase in the rate of glutamine metabolism is attributable to an increase in V$_{max}$ in acidosis. Since it takes several days for the adaptation of glutamine metabolism in acidosis to reach a maximum, the kinetic data suggest that during this time increased activity of the transporter develops due either

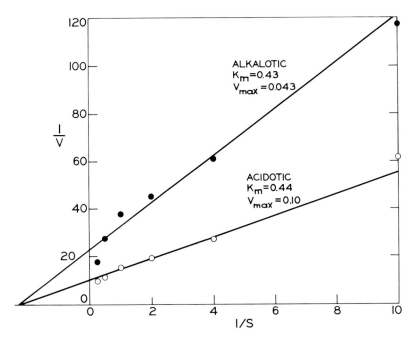

FIGURE 6. Lineweaver-Burk plot of labeled glutamate formation from ^{14}C-glutamine by mitochondria from the renal cortex of chronically acidotic or alkalotic litter-mate dogs. (From Simpson, D. P., *Kidney Int.*, 23, 785, 1983. With permission.)

to development of new carrier units or to gradual unmasking of existing, nonfunctional carrier sites. In the rat kidney, an increase in the rate of glutamate formation in mitochondria is detectable within 3 hr after inducing acidosis, before any change in PDG activity is discernible.[25]

Subsequent studies in rat mitochondria confirmed these observations[23,55-57] and extended them to conditions in which rotenone was not included in the medium so that after glutamate was formed from glutamine subsequent metabolism continued. Tannen and Kunin[56] showed that with or without rotenone, ammoniagenesis was greater in mitochondria from acidotic rats than from controls using both 10 and 0.5 mM concentrations of glutamine in the medium. In a detailed analysis using acidotic rat mitochondria Schoolwerth et al.[57] quantitatively analyzed the contribution of different routes of glutamine metabolism to enhanced ammoniagenesis. Media were used containing either 1 mM glutamine alone or 1 mM glutamine plus 3 mM glutamate, a concentration of the latter substrate approximating that present in the rat kidney cortex. With glutamine as the sole substrate, glutamine utilization by acidotic mitochondria was about 50% greater than in control mitochondria and ammonium production was $2^{1}/_{2}$ times greater. Glutamine deamidation accounted for about half the increase in ammoniagenesis and ammonium formed from the amine group provided the balance. When 3 mM glutamate was also present in the medium, ammonium production was reduced in both control and acidotic mitochondria compared to rates in the absence of glutamate, but was still over threefold greater in the acidotic preparations.

The evidence reviewed above strongly points to the glutamine carrier as the rate-limiting site of adaptation of glutamine metabolism in chronic metabolic acidosis. The limitation to this evidence is the inability as yet to study the transport process in isolation from the deamidation step. However, if the carrier and PDG are physically linked, a possibility entirely compatible with the evidence so far, then separation of the two steps may be almost experimentally impossible. At present, the enhanced transport of glutamine by its inner membrane carrier in chronic acidosis is the only adaptive mechanism which has been demonstrated in both the dog and rat kidney and the only one in which the time course of adaptation parallels changes in ammoniagenesis and NH_4^+ excretion.

C. Mitochondrial Glutamine Metabolism is Influenced by Acid-Base Changes in the Medium

In dog kidney mitochondria incubated with 0.5 mM ^{14}C-glutamine and rotenone in bicarbonate buffered media, decreasing pH and bicarbonate concentration causes marked acceleration of glutamine deamidation (Figure 4).[26] In contrast, in nonbicarbonate buffer the rate of glutamate formation falls off below pH 7.8. The influence of bicarbonate on glutamine metabolism can be attributed to the stimulatory effect of low pH and bicarbonate on the glutamine carrier, an influence similar to that seen with other substrate transporters. Stimulation of glutamine deamidation by a fall in pH and bicarbonate occurs in dog mitochondria even when glutamate, phosphate, and α-ketoglutarate are also present in the medium.

Results of similar studies in rat mitochondria are more complex. With 10 mM glutamine and bicarbonate buffered media, lowering pH and bicarbonate causes a sharp reduction in ammonium formation.[56] This effect, which is opposite to that seen with dog mitochondria, occurs with or without rotenone inhibition of glutamate metabolism. When a more physiologic concentration of glutamine, 0.5 mM, is used, no significant change in ammonia formation from glutamine occurs between pH 7.0 and 7.7. When a nonbicarbonate buffer is used, reducing pH of the medium from 7.4 to 6.8 also diminishes the rate of ammonium formation from glutamine.[58] However, addition of 0.5 mM α-ketoglutarate reverses this effect so that now ammonium production is greater at pH 6.8 than at pH 7.4. This change is found in uninhibited mitochondria and appears due to a greater rate of glutamine deamination by glutamate dehydrogenase; flux through PDG is unaffected under these conditions by a change in pH.

In contrast to the mitochondrial changes in glutamine transport and metabolism induced by chronic metabolic acidosis, the physiologic significance of these in vitro pH-dependent phenomena is unclear. In the intact dog, acute metabolic acidosis has not been shown to result in enhanced glutamine utilization and ammoniagenesis.[5,14,59,60] Thus, the striking in vitro effect of reduced pH and bicarbonate does not have a close parallel in the intact animal. One possible explanation for this discrepancy is that in the intact dog, intracellular bicarbonate is already sufficiently low that further reduction by acute systemic acidosis has little effect on glutamine metabolism. Favoring this explanation is the observation that acute metabolic alkalosis in the dog produced by $NaHCO_3$ infusion does lead to a reduction in renal glutamine extraction,[59] a finding in keeping with the decline in mitochondrial glutamine deamidation when pH and bicarbonate are increased in the medium.

In contrast to the dog, increased glutamine utilization and ammoniagenesis have been demonstrated in response to acute metabolic acidosis in the rat.[5] This response can also be shown in the isolated perfused kidney in which ammonium production is assessed at low or normal pH and bicarbonate concentrations[61] and in similar studies with tubule suspensions.[62,63] Why these findings shown both in vivo and in vitro in intact cells from the rat kidney cannot be reproduced in mitochondria from this species is puzzling. Tannen and Sastrasinh[64] have recently published a detailed review of this subject.

REFERENCES

1. **Tizianello, A., DeFerrari, G., Garibotto, G., Gurreri, G., and Robaudo, C.,** Renal metabolism of amino acids and ammonia in subjects with normal renal function and in patients with chronic renal insufficiency, *J. Clin. Invest.*, 65, 1162, 1980.
2. **Owen, E. E. and Robinson, R. R.,** Amino-acid extraction and ammonia metabolism by the human kidney during the prolonged administration of ammonium chloride, *J. Clin. Invest.*, 42, 263, 1963.
3. **Tizianello, A., Deferrari, G., Garibotto, G., Robaudo, C., Acquarone, N., and Ghiggeri, G. M.,** Renal ammoniagenesis in an early stage of metabolic acidosis in man, *J. Clin. Invest.*, 69, 240, 1982.
4. **Shaloub, R., Webber, W., Glabman, S., Canessa-Fischer, M., Klein, J., deHaas, J., and Pitts, R. F.,** Extraction of amino acids from and their addition to renal blood plasma, *Am. J. Physiol.*, 204, 181, 1963.
5. **Vinay, P., Allignet, E., Pichette, C., Watford, M., Lemieux, G., and Gougoux, A.,** Changes in renal metabolite profile and ammoniagenesis during acute and chronic metabolic acidosis in dog and rat, *Kidney Int.*, 17, 312, 1980.
6. **Yablon, S. B. and Relman, A. S.,** Glutamine as a regulator of renal ammonia production in the rat, *Kidney Int.*, 12, 546, 1977.
7. **Parry, D. M. and Brosnan, J. T.,** Glutamine metabolism in the kidney during induction of, and recovery from, metabolic acidosis in the rat, *Biochem. J.*, 174, 387, 1978.
8. **Sartorius, O. W., Roemmelt, J. C., and Pitts, R. F.,** The renal regulation of acid-base balance in man. IV. The nature of the renal compensations in ammonium chloride acidosis, *J. Clin. Invest.*, 28, 423, 1949.
9. **Simpson, D. P.,** Control of hydrogen ion homeostasis and renal acidosis, *Medicine*, 50, 503, 1971.
10. **Simpson, D. P.,** NH_4^+ excretion by the dog during development of chronic acidosis, *Contr. Nephrol.*, 47, 58, 1985.
11. **Van Slyke, D. D., Phillips, R. A., Hamilton, P. B., Archibald, R. M., Futcher, P. H., and Hiller, A.,** Glutamine as source material of urinary ammonia, *J. Biol. Chem.*, 150, 481, 1943.
12. **Tizianello, A., Defarri, G., Garibotto, G., and Gurreri, G.,** Effects of chronic renal insufficiency and metabolic acidosis on glutamine metabolism in man, *Clin. Sci. Mol. Med.*, 55, 391, 1978.
13. **Pitts, R. F., Pilkington, L. A., and deHaas, J. C. M.,** N^{15} tracer studies on the origin of urinary ammonia in the acidotic dog, with notes on the enzymatic synthesis of labeled glutamic acid and glutamines, *J. Clin. Invest.*, 44, 731, 1965.
14. **Fine, A.,** Effects of acute metabolic acidosis on renal, gut, liver and muscle metabolism of glutamine and ammonia in the dog, *Kidney Int.*, 21, 439, 1982.
15. **Gougoux, A., Vinay, P., Cardoso, M., Duplain, M., and Lemieux, G.,** Immediate adaptation of the dog kidney to acute hypercapnia, *Am. J. Physiol.*, 243, F227, 1982.
16. **Goodman, A. D., Fuisz, R. E., and Cahill, G. F., Jr.,** Renal gluconeogenesis in acidosis, alkalosis and potassium deficiency: its possible role in regulation of renal ammonia production, *J. Clin. Invest.*, 45, 612, 1966.
17. **Simpson, D. P.,** Pathways of glutamine and organic acid metabolism in renal cortex in chronic metabolic acidosis, *J. Clin. Invest.*, 51, 1969, 1972.
18. **Hems, D. A.,** Metabolism of glutamine and glutamic acid by isolated perfused kidneys of normal and acidotic rats, *Biochem. J.*, 130, 671, 1972.
19. **Simpson, D. P.,** Mitochondrial transport functions and renal metabolism, *Kidney Int.*, 23, 785, 1983.
20. **LaNoue, K. F. and Schoolwerth, A. C.,** Metabolite transport in mitochondria, *Annu. Rev. Biochem.*, 48, 871, 1979.
21. **Kovacević, Z., McGivan, J. D., and Chappell, J. B.,** Conditions for activity of glutaminase in kidney mitochondria, *Biochem. J.*, 118, 265, 1970.
22. **Kovacević, Z. and McGivan, J. D.,** Mitochondrial metabolism of glutamine and its physiological significance, *Physiol. Rev.*, 63, 547, 1983.
23. **Brosnan, J. T. and Hall, B.,** The transport and metabolism of glutamine by kidney cortex mitochondria from normal and acidotic rats, *Biochem. J.*, 164, 331, 1977.
24. **Simpson, D. P. and Adam, W.,** Glutamine transport and metabolism by mitochondria from dog renal cortex. General properties and response to acidosis and alkalosis, *J. Biol. Chem.*, 250, 8148, 1975.
25. **Adam, W. and Simpson, D. P.,** Glutamine transport in rat kidney mitochondria in metabolic acidosis, *J. Clin. Invest.*, 54, 165, 1974.
26. **Simpson, D. P.,** Modulation of glutamine transport and metabolism in mitochondria from dog renal cortex. Influence of pH and bicarbonate, *J. Biol. Chem.*, 255, 7123, 1980.
27. **Klingman, J. D. and Handler, P.,** Partial purification and properties of renal glutaminase, *J. Biol. Chem.*, 232, 369, 1958.
28. **Curthoys, N. and Weiss, R. F.,** Regulation of renal ammoniagenesis. Subcellular localization of rat kidney glutaminases, *J. Biol. Chem.*, 249, 3261, 1974.

29. **Kovacević, Z.,** Distribution of glutaminase isoenzymes in kidney cells, *Biochim. Biophys. Acta,* 334, 199, 1974.

30. **Curthoys, N. P. and Shapiro, R. A.,** Effect of metabolic acidosis and phosphate on the presence of glutamine within the matrix space of rat renal mitochondria during glutamine transport, *J. Biol. Chem.,* 253, 63, 1978.

31. **Simpson, D. P. and Hecker, J.,** Glutamine distribution in mitochondria from normal and acidotic rat kidneys, *Kidney Int.,* 21, 774, 1982.

32. **Kovacević, Z. and Bajin, K.,** Kinetics of glutamine efflux from liver mitochondria loaded with ^{14}C-labeled substrate, *Biochim. Biophys. Acta,* 687, 291, 1982.

33. **Kovacević, A. and McGivan, J. D.,** Glutamine transport across biological membranes, in *Glutamine Metabolism in Mammalian Tissues,* Häussinger, D. and Sies, H., Eds., Springer-Verlag, Berlin, 1984, 49.

34. **Kvamme, E., Svenneby, G., Tveter, K. J., and Torgner, R. A.,** Phosphate-activated glutaminase in human kidney, *Contr. Nephrol.,* 47, 145, 1985.

35. **Sayre, F. W. and Roberts, E.,** Preparation and some properties of a phosphate-activated glutaminase from kidneys, *J. Biol. Chem.,* 233, 1128, 1958.

36. **Kvamme, E., Tveit, B., and Svenneby, G.,** Glutaminase from pig renal cortex. I. Purification and general properties, *J. Biol. Chem.,* 245, 1871, 1970.

37. **Svenneby, G., Tveit, B., and Kvamme, E.,** Glutaminase from pig renal cortex. II. Activation by inorganic and organic anions, *J. Biol. Chem.,* 245, 1878, 1970.

38. **Curthoys, N. P., Kuhlenschmidt, T., and Godfrey, S. S.,** Regulation of renal ammoniagenesis. Purification and characterization of phosphate dependent glutaminase from rat kidney, *Arch. Biochem. Biophys.,* 174, 82, 1976.

39. **Shapiro, R. A., Clark, V. M., and Curthoys, N. P.,** Inactivation of rat renal phosphate dependent glutaminase with 6-diazo-5-oxo-L-norleucine. Evidence for interaction at the glutamine binding site, *J. Biol. Chem.,* 254, 2835, 1979.

40. **Roberts, E.,** Glutaminase, in *The Enzymes,* Vol. 4, 2nd ed., Boyer, P. D., Lardy, H., and Myrbäck, K., Eds., Academic Press, New York, 1970, chap. 17.

41. **Godfrey, S. S., Kuhlenschmidt, T., and Curthoys, N. P.,** Correlation between activation and dimer formation of rat renal phosphate-dependent glutaminase, *J. Biol. Chem.,* 252, 1927, 1977.

42. **Simpson, D. P. and Hager, S. R.,** pH and bicarbonate effects on mitochondrial anion accumulation. Proposed mechanism for changes in renal metabolite levels in acute acid-base disturbances, *J. Clin. Invest.,* 63, 704, 1979.

43. **Goldstein, L.,** α-Ketoglutarate regulation of glutamine transport and deamidation by renal mitochondria, *Biochem. Biophys. Res. Commun.,* 70, 1136, 1976.

44. **Strzelecki, T. and Schoolwerth, A. C.,** α-Ketoglutarate modulation of glutamine metabolism by rat renal mitochondria, *Biochem. Biophys. Res. Commun.,* 102, 588, 1981.

45. **Davies, B. M. and Yudkin, J.,** Studies in biochemical adaptation. The origin of urinary ammonia as indicated by the effect of chronic acidosis and alkalosis on some renal enzymes in the rat, *Biochem. J.,* 52, 407, 1952.

46. **Leonard, E. and Orloff, J.,** Regulation of ammonia excretion in the rat, *Am. J. Physiol.,* 182, 131, 1955.

47. **Rector, F. C., Jr., Seldin, D. W., and Copenhaven, J. H.,** The mechanism of ammonia excretion during ammonium chloride acidosis, *J. Clin. Invest.,* 34, 20, 1955.

48. **Curthoys, N. P. and Lowry, O. H.,** The distribution of glutaminase isoenzymes in the various structures of the nephron in normal, acidotic, and alkalotic rat kidney, *J. Biol. Chem.,* 248, 162, 1973.

49. **Rector, F. C., Jr. and Orloff, J.,** The effect of the administration of sodium bicarbonate and ammonium chloride on the excretion and production of ammonia. The absence of alterations in the activity of renal ammonia-producing enzymes in the dog, *J. Clin. Invest.,* 38, 366, 1959.

50. **Pollak, V. E., Mattenheimer, H., DeBruin, H., and Weinman, K. J.,** Experimental metabolic acidosis: the enzymatic basis of ammonia production by the dog kidney, *J. Clin. Invest.,* 44, 169, 1965.

51. **Goldstein, L.,** Actinomycin D inhibition of the adaptation of renal glutamine-deaminating enzymes in the rat, *Nature,* 205, 1330, 1965.

52. **Alleyne, G. A. O. and Scullard, G. H.,** Renal metabolic response to acid-base changes. I. Enzymatic control of ammoniagenesis in the rat, *J. Clin. Invest.,* 48, 364, 1969.

53. **Seyama, S., Sacki, T., and Katunuma, T.,** Comparison of properties and inducibility of glutamate dehydrogenases in rat kidney and liver, *J. Biochem.,* 73, 39, 1973.

54. **Goldstein, L.,** Relation of renal glutaminase-ω-amidase activity to ammonia excretion in the rat, *Nature,* 201, 1229, 1964.

55. **Goldstein, L.,** Glutamine transport by mitochondria isolated from normal and acidotic rats, *Am. J. Physiol.,* 229, 1027, 1975.

56. **Tannen, R. L. and Kunin, A. S.,** Effect of pH on ammonia production by renal mitochondria, *Am. J. Physiol.,* 231, 1631, 1976.

57. **Schoolwerth, A. C., Nazar, B. L., and LaNoue, K. F.,** Glutamate dehydrogenase activation and ammonia formation by rat kidney mitochondria, *J. Biol. Chem.,* 253, 6177, 1978.

58. **Schoolwerth, A. C. and LaNoue, K. F.,** Control of ammoniagenesis by α-ketoglutarate in rat kidney mitochondria, *Am. J. Physiol.,* 244, F399, 1983.

59. **Fine, A., Bennett, F. I., and Alleyne, G. A. O.,** Effects of acute acid-base alterations in glutamine metabolism and renal ammoniagenesis in the dog, *Clin. Sci. Mol. Med.,* 54, 503, 1978.

60. **Silverman, M., Vinay, P., Shinobu, L., Gougoux, A., and Lemieux, G.,** Luminal and antiluminal transport of glutamine in dog kidney: effect of metabolic acidosis, *Kidney Int.,* 20, 359, 1981.

61. **Tannen, R. L. and Ross, B. D.,** Ammoniagenesis by the isolated perfused rat kidney: the critical role of urinary acidification, *Clin. Sci.,* 56, 353, 1979.

62. **Lowry, M. and Ross, B. D.,** Activation of oxoglutarate dehydrogenase in the kidney in response to acute acidosis, *Biochem. J.,* 190, 771, 1980.

63. **Vinay, P., Lemieux, G., Gougoux, A., and Lemieux, C.,** Response of the rat and dog kidney to H$^+$ concentration in vitro — a comparative study with slices and tubules, *Int. J. Biochem.,* 12, 89, 1980.

64. **Tannen, R. L. and Sastrasinh, S.,** Response of ammonium metabolism to acute acidosis, *Kidney Int.,* 25, 1, 1984.

Chapter 13

CYCLIC NUCLEOTIDE REGULATION OF GLUTAMINE METABOLISM IN SKELETAL MUSCLE

C. M. Maillet, A. M. Pujaras Crane, and A. J. Garber

TABLE OF CONTENTS

I. INTRODUCTION

In the intact organism, there is an obligate metabolic requirement for approximately 180 g of glucose per day. This need is met by a combination of hepatic glycogenolysis as well as gluconeogenesis. After an overnight fast glycogen stores are substantially depleted, and glycogenolysis becomes quantitatively less important.[1] Compensatory increases therefore must occur in gluconeogenesis. Glucose production using 3-carbon precursors such as lactate, alanine, and glycerol ensues. Lactate, quantitatively the most important substrate, is derived largely from anaerobic glucolysis in such peripheral tissues as the red blood cell mass. Glycerol is produced by triglyceride hydrolysis during fatty acid mobilization in adipose tissue. Since glucose is required for reesterification of these fatty acids, glycerol may be considered to be, in part, an indirect product of prior glycolysis. Amino acids, principally alanine and glutamine, are the most important sources for *de novo* carbon for the production of glucose. The skeletal muscle is the site of greatest amino acid production and release. Even though alanine and glutamine combined represent only about 10% of the amino acid residues in muscle protein, together they produce more than half of the α-amino nitrogen released from the skeletal muscle.[2-4] In view of these findings, various investigators have demonstrated that the preferential release of glutamine and alanine does not derive from the selective proteolysis of skeletal muscle proteins rich in glutamine and alanine. Instead, both amino acids seem to be produced selectively at the expense of the metabolism of other amino acids, particularly those whose content would lead to the expectation of a higher release rate for each than is found experimentally. Foremost among the precursors of alanine and glutamine are the branched-chain amino acids. However, based on the profile of amino acids released from the skeletal muscle, asparate also appears to make a substantial contribution.

II. AMINO ACID METABOLISM IN THE MUSCLE

In our studies we have used, as an in vitro skeletal muscle preparation, the rat epitrochlaris skeletal muscle preparation, which maintains excellent viability in vitro for periods of at least 6 hr duration. As shown in Figure 1, the release of amino acids from this skeletal muscle preparation parallels to a substantial extent the release of amino acids from most other mammalian skeletal muscle preparations or from in vivo muscle studies reported. Alanine and glutamine are released in the greatest amount; glutamine release exceeds alanine release by 50%. Comparatively, other amino acids are released at a negligible rate. The principal differences between rat skeletal muscle preparations using arteriovenous catheterizations of the human extremity, lie in the release of small quantities of glutamate from rat skeletal muscle preparations, whereas in humans, a small net uptake of glutamate has been observed.[2,3]

Using a variety of inhibitors of alanine aminotransferase, such as aminooxyacetate or cycloserine, inhibition of alanine aminotransferase reduces alanine release from the skeletal muscle by approximately 80%.[5,6] Concomitant with such inhibition of alanine aminotransferase, the release of other, ordinarily poorly released amino acids such as asparate is increased. Similar results have also been obtained for inhibition of glutamine synthetase using methionine sulfoximine.[6] Inhibition of glutamine synthetase resulted in markedly reduced glutamine synthesis and release from the skeletal muscle and a corresponding increase in alanine release.

A number of hypotheses have been advanced to explain the selective synthesis and release of alanine and glutamine from the skeletal muscle. A glucose-alanine cycle has been proposed whereby alanine released from the skeletal muscle is transported to the liver and converted by gluconeogenesis into glucose. This glucose is subsequently released and taken up by the skeletal muscle where it is glycolyzed to pyruvate and transaminated to form alanine. The

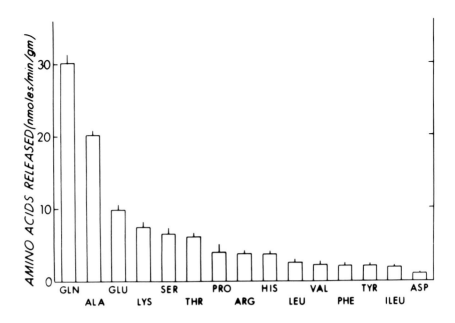

FIGURE 1.   Profile of amino acid release from epitrochlaris preparations of the rat skeletal muscle. Epitrochlaris preparations of rat skeletal muscle were incubated for 1 hr at 37°C in a Krebs-Henseleit bicarbonate buffer (pH 7.4). After incubation muscles were rapidly removed from the media, rinsed, blotted, and frozen in liquid nitrogen. Amino acids in the media were assessed using amino acid analyzer techniques. Values are expressed as the mean ± SEM for at least six experiments and are expressed as nmol/min/g wet weight of muscle.

latter assigns the role to alanine released from the skeletal muscle as primarily that of a nitrogen carrier for urea synthesis. Other investigators[2,5-7] have found that a high proportion of the alanine released from the skeletal muscle does not derive from anaerobic glycolysis of glycose, but derives instead from the net catabolism of other amino acids to form not only the amino group for net alanine synthesis, but also a significant fraction of the carbon skeleton as well. Estimates of the contribution of amino acids to alanine synthesis have suggested that approximately 75% of the alanine released from the skeletal muscle derives from the catabolism of other amino acids and that not more than 20 to 25% of the alanine derived from the muscle reflects a carbon contribution from anaerobic glycolysis.[8] However, a comprehensive basis for an understanding of the metabolic utilization and disposal of glutamine released from the skeletal muscle in the intact organism has not been well defined. Glutamine release from the skeletal muscle accounts for virtually half of the total amino acid output from the skeletal muscle under basal circumstances.[3] During periods of metabolic acidosis, glutamine utilization by the renal mass for ammonia generation with the subsequent formation of other amino acids, such as serine, as well as its utilization of renal gluconeogenesis has been demonstrated.[9] In the nonacidotic state, the metabolic fate of glutamine has not been clearly eludicated. The data of Windmueller and Spaeth[10] demonstrated that substantial oxidation of glutamine in the intestinal mucosa occurs and that in addition metabolized to other 3-carbon precursors, such as alanine and lactate. It is possible that the latter are taken up by the liver and support hepatic gluconeogenesis by an indirect mechanism using glutamine as the substrate. This observation may account for the higher alanine levels found in portal venous blood than have been observed in the arterial blood in man.[11]

III. CONTROL OF AMINO ACID METABOLISM IN THE MUSCLE

Control of the processes of synthesis and release of glutamine and alanine at the cellular

Table 1

**EFFECT OF PYRUVATE, AMMONIUM CHLORIDE, AND
GLUTAMATE ADDITION ON AMINO ACID AND
PYRUVATE RELEASE FROM THE RAT SKELETAL
MUSCLE[a]**

Addition	Glutamine release	Glutamate release	Alanine release	Pyruvate release
Control	29.9 ± 2.0	10.1 ± 1.0	19.8 ± 1.6	20.2 ± 1.8
Pyruvate	20.3 ± 1.8	5.8 ± 0.8	28.8 ± 2.3	
Glutamate	52.1 ± 3.6		29.5 ± 2.1	13.1 ± 2.0
Ammonium chloride	40.1 ± 2.4	15.3 ± 0.8	38.2 ± 2.4	11.9 ± 0.8

[a] Intact rat epitrochlaris preparations were incubated for 1 hr at 37° C in a Krebs-Henseleit buffer, pH 7.4, containing glucose (5 mM), insulin (100 mU/mℓ), and HEPES (5 mM). Neutral solutions of ammonium chloride, glutamate, and pyruvate were added at the concentrations indicated. After incubation, the release of amino acids and pyruvate was determined enzymatically in the media. Values given are mean ± SEM for at least four experiments and are expressed as nmol/min/g muscle, wet weight.

level can occur at a number of points. One such point may be the availability of substrates from outside the cell. However, Goldstein and co-workers[12] have found that in rats in a diabetic ketoacidotic state, where glutamine release is considerably increased, transport across the membrane and membrane permeability were unaltered. Furthermore, it has also been shown that another possible point of control, the synthetic capacity of the glutamine synthetase, the major enzyme responsible for glutamine synthesis in the muscle, was unchanged. Muhlbacher et al.[13] working with an animal model where the stressed state, which leads to increased glutamine synthesis, was mimicked by dexamethasone, found that glutamine synthetase capacity was unaffected. Lemieux and colleagues[14] found similar results in the acidotic rat model.

On the other hand, the control of glutamine synthesis may originate with the control of intracellular mechanisms which preferentially produce glutamate, thereby increasing the production of either glutamine or alanine, depending on the metabolic state of the animal. Direct addition of glutamate to the incubation medium of the epitrochlaris muscle produced an increase in the production of both glutamine and alanine (Table 1). Glutamine synthesis could be decreased by the addition of methinine sulfoxide, an inhibitor of AMP deaminase[3,15] which provides an amino group from AMP in the formation of glutamine from glutamate and NH_3 in the glutamine synthetase reaction. Addition of cysteine, leucine, valine, methionine, isoleucine, tyrosine, lysine, or phenylalanine stimulated glutamine synthesis suggesting that they may contribute either amine groups or carbon in the same reaction.[16] It has also been shown that addition of amine groups, as with ammonium chloride, stimulates glutamine production (Table 1). Therefore, it seems reasonable to conclude that glutamine synthesis is under complex, multifactorial intracellular control.

Two such means of control might be the response of the cyclic nucleotide system to changes in the extracellular environment or the response of the oxidation state to intracellular processes. In our studies we have shown that glutamine release decreases in response to adrenergic[17] and serotoninergic agonists[18] and increases in response to cholinergic agonists.[19] Thus, we feel that it is (at least in part) a cyclic nucleotide-mediated event. Using intact epitrochlaris muscle from the rat forelimb, we found that glutamine release diminished in response to epinephrine, a glucogenolytic hormone in the skeletal muscle, in a dose-related manner (Figure 2). Concomitant increases in lactate and pyruvate release were observed with added epinephrine. Further studies showed that this effect could be mimicked by the

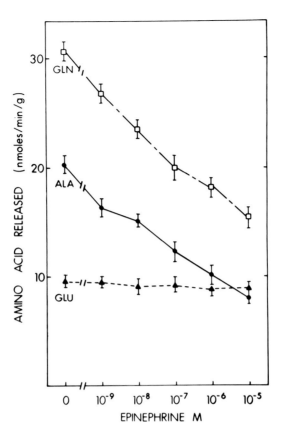

FIGURE 2. Effect of epinephrine on glutamine, alanine, and glutamate release from skeletal muscle preparations in vitro. Epitrochlaris preparations from control animals were obtained and incubated in a Krebs-Henseleit bicarbonate buffer for 1 hr. Varying concentrations of epinephrine were added to the media as indicated. Following incubation, alanine, glutamine, and glutamate released to the media were determined enzymatically. Values shown are the mean ± SEM for at least six experiments and are expressed as nmol/min/g wet weight of muscle.

addition of dibutryl-cAMP and by isoproterenol, but not by α-adrenergic agonists such as phentolamine. This effect could be blocked by β- but not α-adrenergic antagonists.[20] In other incubation systems, such as the hemidiaphragm,[21] either α- or β-adrenergic agonists stimulated glutamine production. cAMP accumulation also increased in response to epinephrine in the intact muscle (Table 2). In rat sarcolemmel membrane, adenylyl cyclase activity, as measured by the conversion of ^{32}P-ATP to ^{32}P-cAMP, was increased in response to epinephrine (Table 3). In a parallel set of experiments using serotonin, a similar effect was found.[20] This series of experiments implicated the cyclic nucleotide-receptor complex in the regulation of glutamine production and/or release. Using the same animal model, the effect of cholinergic agonists was studied. Here it was found that the release of glutamine from an intact muscle was increased in response to carbachol. Studies investigating the accumulation of cGMP indicated that the guanine cyclic nucleotide might also act in a regulatory capacity for glutamine release (Table 4).

An increased synthesis of glutamine from glutamate has been shown in several tissues including diaphragm, although in this tissue an increased synthesis occurs without an in-

Table 2
EFFECT OF EPINEPHRINE AND SEROTONIN ON cAMP LEVELS IN THE SKELETAL MUSCLE OF CONTROL AND UREMIC RATS[a]

| | | cAMP level (pmol/g muscle) | |
Addition	Conc	Control	Uremic
Control		609 ± 39.5	543 ± 30.9
Epinephrine	10^{-8}	726 ± 32.1	595 ± 40.1
	10^{-6}	1710 ± 71.2	794 ± 61.3
	10^{-5}	2246 ± 95.2	1091 ± 84.0
Serotonin	10^{-7}	995 ± 65	649 ± 40
	10^{-5}	1381 ± 45	734 ± 18

[a]   Epitrochlaris preparations from control and uremic rats were incubated with varying concentrations of epinephrine and serotonin as indicated. After a 2 min incubation, the preparations were rapidly removed from their media, rinsed, blotted, and frozen in liquid nitrogen. Levels of cAMP were determined in trichloroacetic acid extracts of the muscle using a sensitive double-antibody radioimmunoassay. Values shown are the mean ± SEM for at least ten experiments.

Table 3
SKELETAL MUSCLE MEMBRANE ADENYLYL CYCLASE ACTIVITY IN CONTROL AND UREMIC RATS[a]

| | Control | | Uremic | |
	Agonist conc (M)	Adenylyl cyclase activity (pmol/mg/min)	Agonist conc (M)	Adenylyl cyclase activity (pmol/mg/min)
Basal		7.56 ± 0.57		6.26 ± 0.24
Epinephrine max	10^{-6}	31.82 ± 1.21	10^{-5}	21.83 ± 0.88
Epinephrine 1/2 max	3×10^{-7}	19.09 ± 0.95	10^{-6}	13.83 ± 1.15

[a]   Membrane preparations were obtained from hindlimb skeletal muscles of control and chronically uremic rats by differential centrifugation of a crude homogenate. An aliquot of the membrane suspension was added to an adenylyl cyclase incubation medium containing [^{32}P]ATP and varying concentrations of epinephrine. [^{32}P]cAMP was isolated. Adenylyl cyclase activity was expressed as μmol cAMP formed/min/mg protein. Values given are the enzymatic activities at the indicated maximal and half-maximal agonist concentration and are the mean ± SEM of six experiments.

creased release.[21,22] Several investigators have proposed a control of the synthetic processes via a combination of (1) branched-chain amino acid anapleurotic reactions which may be altered in metabolically stressed states and (2) a decrease in the availability of oxidizable substrates, as might be modulated by the [NADH]/[NAD] ratio in the cytosol. Palmer et al.[21] theorize that an adrenergic inhibition of branched-chain 2-oxo acid dehydrogenase leads to a decreased availability of those citric acid cycle intermediates which arise from valine and (to a lesser extent) from leucine and isoleucine. The control mechanism for this inhibition seems to be an increase in the [NADH]/[NAD] ratio which may affect the phosphorylation of the enzyme, rendering it inactive. In the hemidiaphragm incubation system used, inhibition

Table 4
EFFECTS OF CARBOMYLCHOLINE ON LEVELS
OF GLUTAMINE RELEASE AND cGMP
ACCUMULATION IN THE RAT SKELETAL MUSCLE[a]

Carbamylcholine conc (M)	Glutamine release (nmol/min/g)	cGMP accumulation (pmol/g muscle)
0	28.8 ± 2.1	12.6 ± 1.6
10^{-10}	31.3 ± 1.8	13.1 ± 1.2
10^{-8}	37.8 ± 2.5	18.4 ± 2.0
10^{-6}	41.6 ± 1.3	33.2 ± 1.9

[a] Effect of carbamylcholine on skeletal muscle synthesis and release of glutamine and on accumulation of cGMP. Epitrochlaris muscles were obtained and incubated in a Krebs-Henseleit bicarbonate buffer containing varying concentrations of carbochol. Following 1 hr incubation, glutamine release to the media was determined enzymatically. Following 10 min incubation, cGMP levels were determined in trichloroacetic acid extracts of each muslce preparation using double-label radioimmunoassay techniques. Values shown are the mean ± SEM of at least eight experiments.

of branched-chain 2-oxo dehydrogenase was produced by the addition of either β- or α-adrenergic agonists to the incubation medium. Buse and colleagues,[22] in their study of control of glutamine formation by reduction-oxidation potential, used the diabetic rat hemidiaphragm as a model. In the diabetic animal, glutamate production in the tissue is significantly increased over that found in normal animals. It was found that when an electron acceptor, methylene blue in this case, was added to the medium the increased appearance of glutamate found in the diabetic animal was returned more nearly to normal. She proposed that the accumulation of NADH in the cytosol acted as a deceleration mechanism on the increased proteolysis found in diabetes by slowing the oxidation of leucine. In the cytosol of diabetic rat diaphragm cells, there is an increased level of aspartate and decreased glutamate levels suggesting a shuttle of reducing equivalents into the mitochondria. Therefore, it seems possible that an increase in the ratio of reductants to oxidants in the cytoplasm may act as a signal to which key enzymes are responsive.

IV. DERANGEMENTS OF GLUTAMINE METABOLISM IN MUSCLE-WASTING STATES

Without any apparent change in membrane permeability, transport, or enzyme synthetic capacity, glutamine release from the skeletal muscle is increased in diabetic and acidotic rats,[12] in animals treated with the synthetic glucocorticoid dexamethasone,[13] in response to somatostatin,[23] in mouse muscular dystrophy,[24] and in chronic uremia.[25]

In the chronic uremic rat model, it was found that muscle wasting was not a result of diminished glutamine or alanine reutilization in terms of muscle protein resynthesis or oxidation to CO_2. Nor was enzyme synthetic capacity altered, since added amino acids produced no further augmentation of the production of glutamine. However, studies using prelabeled [guanido-^{14}C] arginine demonstrated increased proteolysis in uremic animals.[25] Goldstein and co-workers[12] showed that there was no increase in membrane permeability of transport in animals with diabetic ketoacidosis. A lack of insulin did not appear to account for the proteolytic abnormalities; however, it may account for the decreased protein synthesis contributing to a loss of muscle mass.

There is, however, a great deal of evidence for altered glutamine synthesis and for faulty cyclic nucleotide control of glutamine and alanine synthesis and release. Buse[22] found, in her series of studies on the redox potential in the diabetic animal, that the increased glutamate synthesis found in the diabetic rat was ameliorated by the addition of methylene blue to the incubation medium. She proposed that an increase in the level of [NADH] in the cytosol acted as a signal decreasing the production of citric acid cycle intermediates from leucine. Palmer et al.[21] found that in hemidiaphragm preparations in normal animals, branched-chain 2-oxo acid dehydrogenase was inhibited by adrenergic agonists leading to a decrease in the availability of citric acid cycle intermediates formed from leucine and isoleucine, but especially from valine. He implicated the increase in the [NADH]/[NAD] ratio as a control mechanism. In fasting, an increase in free fatty acid levels have been found. In this state [NADH]/[NAD] levels also increase. Although the precise mechanism remains unclear, it appears that the oxidation state of the cytoplasm may act as a controlling mechanism for enzymes involved in proteolysis pathways and, possibly, for the preferential synthesis of glutamate.

In our studies, we have found abnormalities in the cyclic nucleotide control of amino acid synthesis and release. In chronically uremic animals, where glutamine levels of release were elevated in comparison to controls, the inhibiting action of the adrenergic and serotoninergic agonists was not present. Muscles showed a diminished response to the agonists at the level of glutamine release (Figure 3), accumulation of cAMP (Table 2), and the activity of adenylyl cyclase (Table 3). Involvement of the cyclic nucleotide complex is demonstrated by the mimicking in vitro of the "uremic effect" by added parathyroid hormone (PTH), a hormone found in high-circulating concentrations in uremia.[26] Addition of bovine PTH (1-84) or the synthetic fragment (1-34) caused an increased release of glutamine and alanine from the muscle of normal rats, but no increase from the muscle of uremic animals (Figure 4). In the presence of PTH, accumulation of cAMP and cGMP were increased in control but not uremic animals (Table 5). The addition of PTH to the incubation medium in the epitrochlaris muscle system caused a diminution of glutamine release in response to epinephrine (Figure 5). Similarly, when PTH was added to the adenylyl cyclase incubation medium, there was a PTH-dependent decrease in isoproterenol-stimulated adenylyl cyclase activity (Figure 6). The accelerated proteolytic state found in the muscle-wasting diseases appears to be caused, at least in part, by an insensitivity to the control mechanisms found in normal animals. That is, in normal animals the cyclic nucleotide-receptor complex acts as a brake to slow the rate of amino acid release in response to an altered metabolic state, such as fasting, or to stress. In muscle-wasting diseases such as chronic uremia or diabetes this point of control is lost resulting in increased proteolysis. The increased circulating levels of hormones such as the PTH in uremia[27] and epinephrine which are found in diabetes and in the stressed state[28,29] could increase the rate of release of glutamine in these disease states, thereby allowing the animal to meet the challenge of altered gluconeogenesis and of increased ammoniagenesis. In the acidotic state, the derangement of glutamine and alanine synthesis and release occurs without increased proteolysis in the skeletal muscle. There are increased levels of glutamine release,[30,31] decreased alanine release,[14,31] and increased production of urea.[30,31] We have shown that glutamine release from the intact epitrochlaris muscle is increased in the presence of added ammonia. Glutamine is in part extracted by the gut[10] where deamination occurs indirectly producing increased levels of ammonia, or where the carbon skeleton can be converted to alanine or serine. In the kidney, glutamine supports renal gluconeogenesis. The increased production of ammonia in the kidney serves to ameliorate the acid-base imbalance produced by acidosis. It is important to note that increased glutamine production takes place at the expense of alanine production rather than at the expense of muscle mass.

V. SUMMARY

In summary, glutamine production and release appears to be coordinated with alanine

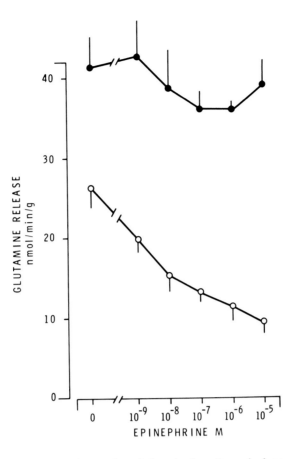

FIGURE 3. Suppression of glutamine formation and release by epinephrine in skeletal muscle preparations of control and uremic rats. Epitrochlaris skeletal muscle preparations from control (O-----O) and chronically uremic rats (●-----●) were obtained and incubated with varying concentrations of epinephrine. Following 1 hr incubation, muscles were rapidly removed from the media, rinsed, blotted, and frozen in liquid nitrogen. Release of glutamine to the incubation media was determined using semimicrofluorometric enzymatic techniques. Values shown are the mean ± SEM for at least ten experiments and are expressed as nmol/min/g wet weight of muscle.

production and release in the skeletal muscle. In an accelerated proteolytic state, increases in cyclic nucleotides, responding to changes in circulating hormone levels, cause a decrease in glutamine release. Precursors of glutamate such as branched-chain amino acids, may be affected by the oxidation state of the cytosol. Increased levels of glutamate may be used in either synthesis of glutamine, which is extracted by the gut and provides indirect substrates for glucose production in the liver and for renal gluconeogenesis, or in the synthesis of alanine, whose carbon skeleton may be used in hepatic and renal gluconeogenesis from alanine. In the nonproteolytic state, increased glutamine release is concurrent with decreased alanine release. Glutamine thus acts as the substrate for both ammoniagenesis and renal gluconeogenesis. The control of skeletal muscle glutamine metabolism appears to be the control of the balance between alanine and glutamine production and release allowing the most efficient response to the metabolically stressed state.

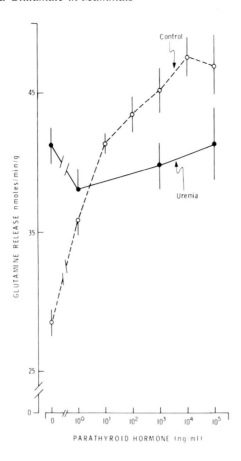

FIGURE 4.   Effect of PTH on glutamine release
from the skeletal muscle. Epitrochlaris preparations
were obtained from control (○) and chronically uremic
(●) rats and incubated at 37°C for 1 hr in a Krebs-
Henseleit bicarbonate buffer (pH 7.4) containing
glucose (5 mM) and varying concentrations of synthetic 1-34 bovine PTH as indicated. After incuba-
tions, the muscles were rapidly removed, rinsed,
blotted, and frozen in liquid nitrogen. Glutamine
released to the media was determined enzymatically
using microfluorometric techniques. Values shown
are the mean ± SEM for at least eight experiments
and are expressed as nmol released/min/g muscle
wet weight.

Table 5
EFFECT OF PTH ON CYCLIC NUCLEOTIDE LEVELS IN THE SKELETAL MUSCLE OF CONTROL AND UREMIC RATS[a]

PTH conc (ng/mℓ)	cAMP level (pmol/g muscle)		cGMP level (pmol/g muscle)	
	Control	Uremic	Control	Uremic
0	631 ± 68	515 ± 15	67 ± 11	86 ± 6
1	1370 ± 123	608 ± 48	94 ± 13	84 ± 13
10	1452 ± 208	705 ± 52	156 ± 37	82 ± 14
100	1573 ± 134	695 ± 33	177 ± 23	76 ± 12
1000	1423 ± 218	618 ± 63	193 ± 17	68 ± 5

[a]   Effect of PTH on cyclic nucleotide levels in the skeletal muscle of control and uremic rats. Epitrochlaris preparations from control and chronically uremic rats were obtained and incubated with varying concentrations of PTH in a Krebs-Henseleit bicarbonate buffer (pH 7.4) containing glucose (5 mM). After the conclusion of the incubation, each muscle was rapidly removed, rinsed, blotted, and frozen in liquid nitrogen. Levels of cAMP and cGMP in trichloroacetic acid extracts of each skeletal muscle preparation were then determined by double antibody radioimmunoassay. Values shown are the mean ± SEM for at least ten experiments.

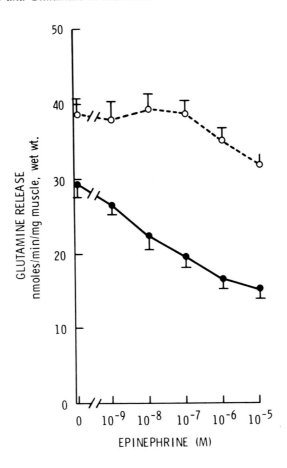

FIGURE 5.   Effect of PTH on the epinephrine-induced inhibition of glutamine release from the skeletal muscle. Epitrochlaris preparations were from normal rats and were
incubated for 1 hr at 37°C under 95% O_2-5% CO_2 in a Krebs-
Henseleit bicarbonate buffer (pH 7.4) containing varying concentrations of epinephrine as indicated either in the presence
(○) or absence (●) of added 1-34 bovine PTH (1000 ng/mℓ).
At the conclusion of the 1 hr incubation, muscles were removed and rapidly rinsed, blotted, and frozen in liquid nitrogen. Glutamine released to the media was determined enzymatically using microfluorometric techniques. Values shown
are the mean ±SEM for at least six experiments and are
expressed as nmol/min/g muscle wet weight.

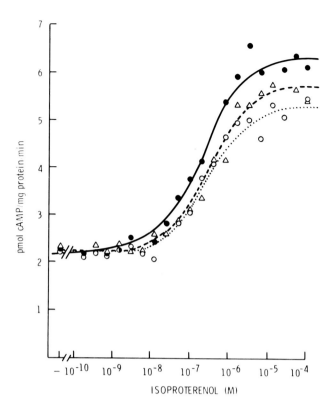

FIGURE 6.   Effect of preincubation with a PTH on isoproterenol-stimulable adenylyl cyclase activity in rat sarcolemma. Skeletal muscle preparations were obtained from control rats and crude preparations of sarcolemma prepared by differential centrifugation. These sarcolemmal omitting [α-^{32}P] ATP but, containing either no added 1-34 bovine PTH (●-----●), 1000 ng/mℓ PTH (△-----△), or 10,000 ng/mℓ of 1-34 PTH (○-----○). After conclusion of the preincubation period, the sarcolemma was used in an adenylyl cyclase activity assay containing varying concentrations of isoproterenol as indicated. Values for adenylyl cyclase activity are the mean ±SEM for at least three experiments and are expressed as pmol of cAMP formed/min/mg protein.

REFERENCES

1. **Garber, A. J., Menzel, P. H., Boden, G., and Owen, O. E.,** Hepatic ketogenesis and gluconeogenesis in humans, *J. Clin. Invest.,* 54, 981, 1974.
2. **Ruderman, N. B. and Lund, P.,** Amino acid metabolism in skeletal muscle: regulation of glutamine and alanine release in the perfused rat hindquarters, *Isr. J. Med. Sci.,* 8, 295, 1972.
3. **Garber, A. J., Karl, I. E., and Kipnis, D. M.,** Alanine and glutamine synthesis and release from skeletal muscle. I. Glycolysis and amino acid release from skeletal muscle, *J. Biol. Chem.,* 251, 826, 1976.
4. **Kominz, D. R., Hugh, A., Symond, P., Laki, K.,** The amino acid composition of actin, myosin, tropomyosin, and the meromyosins, *Arch. Biochem. Biophys.,* 50, 148, 1954.
5. **Goldstein, L. and Newsholme, E. A.,** The formation of alanine from amino acids in diaphragm muscle of the rat, *Biochem. J.,* 154, 555, 1976.
6. **Garber, A. J., Karl, I. E., and Kipnis, D. M.,** Alanine and glutamine synthesis and release from skeletal muscle. II. The precursor role of amino acids in alanine and glutamine synthesis, *J. Biol. Chem.,* 251, 836, 1976.

7. **Snell, K. and Duff, D. A.,** The release of alanine by rat diaphragm muscle in vitro, *Biochem. J.,* 162, 399, 1977.

8. **Snell, K.,** Alanine as a gluconeogenic carrier, *Trends Biochem. Sci.,* 4, 124, 1979.

9. **Owen, O. E., Felig, P., Morgan, A. P., Wahren, J., and Cahill, G. F., Jr.,** Liver and kidney metabolism during prolonged starvation, *J. Clin. Invest.,* 48, 574, 1969.

10. **Windmueller, H. G. and Spaeth, A. E.,** Uptake and metabolism of plasma glutamine by the small intestine, *J. Biol. Chem.,* 249, 5070, 1974.

11. **Felig, P., Wahren, J., Karl, I., Cerasi, E., Luft, R., and Kipnis, D. M.,** Glutamine and glutamate metabolism in normal and diabetic subjects, *Diabetes,* 22, 573, 1973.

12. **Goldstein, L., Perlman, D. F., McLaughlin, P. M., King, P. A., and Cha, C.-J.,** Muscle glutamine production in diabetic ketoacidotic rats, *Biochem. J.,* 214, 757, 1983.

13. **Muhlbacher, F., Kapadia, C. R., Colpoys, M. F., Smith, R. J., and Wilmore, D. W.,** Effects of glucocorticoids on glutamine metabolism in skeletal muscle, *Am. J. Physiol.,* 247, E75, 1984.

14. **Lemieux, G., Watford, M., Vinay, P., and Gougoux, A.,** Metabolic changes in skeletal muscle during chronic metabolic acidosis, *J. Biochem.,* 12, 75, 1980.

15. **Ruderman, N. B. and Berger, M.,** The formation of glutamine and alanine in skeletal muscle, *J. Biol. Chem.,* 249, 5500, 1974.

16. **Karl, I. E., Garber, A. J., and Kipnis, D. M.,** Alanine and glutamine formation and release in skeletal muscle. III. Dietary and hormonal regulation, *J. Biol. Chem.,* 251, 844, 1976.

17. **Garber, A. J., Karl, I. E., and Kipnis, D. M.,** Alanine and glutamine synthesis and release from skeletal muscle. IV. β-Adrenergic inhibition of amino acid release, *J. Biol. Chem.,* 251, 851, 1976.

18. **Garber, A. J.,** Inhibition by serotonin of amino acid release and protein degradation in skeletal muscle, *Mol. Pharmacol.,* 13, 640, 1977.

19. **Garber, A. J., Harari, Y., and Entman, M. L.,** Cholinergic from skeletal muscle, *J. Biol. Chem.,* 253, 7918, 1978.

20. **Ezrailson, E. G., Entman, M. L., and Garber, A. J.,** Adrenergic and serotonergic regulation of skeletal muscle metabolism in the rat. I. The effects of adrenergic and serotonergic antagonists on the regulation of muscle amino acid release, glucogenolysis and cyclic nucleotide levels, *J. Biol. Chem.,* 258, 2494, 1983.

21. **Palmer, T. N., Caldecourt, M. A., and Sugden, M. C.,** Adrenergic inhibition of branched-chain 2-oxo acid dehydrogenase in rat diaphragm muscle in vitro, *Biochem. J.,* 216, 63, 1983.

22. **Buse, M. G., Weigand, D. A., Peeler, D., and Hedden, M. P.,** The effect of diabetes and the redox potential on amino acid content and release by isolated rat hemidiaphragms, *Metabolism,* 29, 605, 1980.

23. **Magno-Sumbilla, C., Collins, R. M., and Ozand, P. T.,** The effects of somatostatin (SRIF) on the release of amino acids from skeletal muscle, *Horm. Metab. Res.,* 12, 439, 1980.

24. **Garber, A. J., Schwartz, R. J., Seidel, C. L., Silvers, A., and Entman, M. L.,** Skeletal muscle protein and amino acid metabolism in hereditary mouse muscular dystrophy: accelerated protein turnover and increased alanine and glutamine formation and release, *J. Biol. Chem.,* 255, 8315, 1980.

25. **Garber, A. J.,** Skeletal muscle protein and amino acid metabolism in experimental chronic uremia in the rat: accelerated alanine and glutamine formation and release, *J. Clin. Invest.,* 62, 623, 1978.

26. **Garber, A. J.,** Effects of parathyroid hormone on skeletal muscle protein and amino acid metabolism in the rat, *J. Clin. Invest.,* 71, 1806, 1983.

27. **Reiss, E. and Canterbury, J.,** A radioimmunoassay for circulating parathyroid hormone in man: preliminary results, *J. Lab. Clin. Med.,* 70, 1012, 1967.

28. **Fushimi, H., Inoue, T., Namikawa, H., Kishino, B., Nunotani, J., Nishikawa, M., Tochino, Y., Funakawa, S., Yamatodani, A., and Wada, H.,** Decreased response of plasma catecholamine to stress in diabetic rats, *Endocrinol. Jpn.,* 29, 593, 1982.

29. **Garber, A. J., Cryer, P. E., Santiago, J. V., Haymond, M. W., Pagiara, A. S., and Kipnis, D. M.,** The role of adrenergic mechanisms in the substrate and hormonal response to insulin-induced hypoglycemia in man, *J. Clin. Invest.,* 58, 7, 1976.

30. **Schroeck, H. and Goldstein, L.,** Interorgan relationships for glutamine metabolism in normal and acidotic rats, *Am. J. Physiol.,* 240, E519, 1981.

31. **Phromphetcharat, V., Jackson, A., Dass, P. D., and Welbourne, T. C.,** Ammonia partitioning between glutamine and urea: interorgan participation in metabolic acidosis, *Kidney Int.,* 20, 598, 1981.

Chapter 14

TRANSPORT AND METABOLISM OF GLUTAMINE AND GLUTAMATE IN THE SMALL INTESTINE

Peter J. Hanson and Dennis S. Parsons

TABLE OF CONTENTS

I. INTRODUCTION

In the late 1940s and early 1950s considerable advances were made in the study of intestinal absorption: these eventually led to an understanding of the principles underlying the processes of intestinal epithelial transport. The advances were based on new methods of studying absorption in vitro and on new analytical techniques. It became realized that to sustain successfully the small intestine in vitro it was necessary that the mucosal surface of the segment was exposed to a well-oxygenated, buffered, balanced saline solution.[1] The improved methods of chemical analysis included enzymic methods and various forms of chromatography. The following introductory survey of these developments together with a description of some general principles of small intestinal biochemistry/physiology will provide a context for this review of the handling of glutamine and glutamate by the small intestine.

A. Intestinal Metabolism During Absorption
1. Carbohydrate
It was early established that segments of rat intestine (e.g., of the jejunum) were capable of translocating some monosaccharides (e.g., D-glucose and D-galactose) from the fluid bathing the mucosal surface across the epithelium into the fluid bathing the serosal surface

of the segment. The movement occurred against a concentration gradient, that is, when the concentration of the hexose in the mucosal fluid was less than that in the fluid bathing the serosa. Because the force driving the movement was not derived from the external concentration gradient, the movement must depend upon some source of energy provided by the epithelium itself ("active transport"). The rate of inward transport (absorption) was determined by the concentration of the hexose in the fluid in the mucosal compartment. The relationship between influx into the epithelium and the concentration in the mucosal compartment was alinear and exhibited saturation at high concentrations, as is the case for enzyme kinetics. There was also some evidence for competition for transport, e.g., between galactose and glucose.

These sorts of findings suggested that there existed somewhere in the epithelium a specific system ("carriers") with which sugars had to combine in order to be transported. Different sugars had different affinities for the carriers and when at high sugar concentrations all the "carriers" were occupied, the transport system was saturated. Naturally there was much speculation as to the nature of the "carriers" and their location in the epithelial cells. It was established at an early stage that the small intestine was an organ with a high rate of metabolism, a relatively high rate of respiration,[2] and a high rate of cellular turnover.[3,4] Balance studies using in vitro preparations, in which the quantities of glucose absorbed and transformed across the epithelium were compared, showed that the influx of glucose into the epithelium from the lumen greatly exceeded the sum of the amounts appearing in the serosal fluid and that retained in the wall of the segment.[5] It was later shown that much of the glucose was converted to lactate secreted largely at the serosal surface.[6,7] In contrast galactose, which was absorbed at similar rates to glucose, was scarcely metabolized. Glucose in the lumen stimulated fluid and salt transport, the nonmetabolized galactose having no such effect. Thus by the mid 1950s, the notion of metabolism by the epithelium of absorbed carbohydrate was well established.

2. Amino Acids

After it was discovered that the L-isomers of some amino acids were absorbed from racemic mixtures more rapidly than the D-isomers[8] attempts were made to discover whether amino acids were transferred from the small intestinal lumen across the epithelium into serosal fluid against a concentration gradient as was the case for glucose and galactose. It was found that such transport did occur with the rat intestine in vitro in the case of the L-isomers of alanine, phenylalanine, methionine, histidine, and isoleucine, but not with glutamic or aspartic acids. In fact, glutamate and aspartate disappeared from the system and it was suggested that these amino acids had been subjected to transamination.[9]

3. Transamination During Absorption

Previous to these experiments Dent and Schilling,[10] studying the absorption of protein, sought the pattern of amino-N in the portal blood; was some of the N transferred as peptide? The amino acid composition of the portal blood was examined by semiquantitative, two-dimensional paper chromatography and also enzymically by manometry and it was concluded that, at the most, only a minor part of the dietary-N was transferred into the portal blood in the form of peptides. Current views largely agree with this conclusion but it is now recognized that substantial amounts of the dietary-N, perhaps as much as 50%, approach the epithelium as oligopeptide to be hydrolyzed either at the brush border surface or after transport into the cell. Dent and Schilling[10] also noted that "it is remarkable that glutamic acid which occurs in casein to the extent of 20% should not increase more in the portal blood during digestion." With the benefit of hindsight it appears from their data for casein that the increase in portal blood alanine is substantial (see their Table 2 in Reference 10).

Having suggested that transamination occurs during the absorption of glutamic and aspartic

B. Transport Across the Basolateral Membrane
1. Glutamate and Alanine
No information seems to be available on the membrane processes underlying the entry or exit of dicarboxylic amino acids across basolateral membranes of mammalian enterocytes, but a system for Na-driven uptake of L-glutamate across the basolateral membrane into renal proximal tubular cells has been reported.[27]

In the frog small intestine, which in many ways resembles that of mammals, it has been found that movement of glutamate across the basolateral membranes is highly asymmetric, the rate constant for the entry into the epithelium from the blood being ten times greater than that for the exit. This asymmetry, which apparently does not depend upon the Na-gradient, favors the trapping of glutamate within the enterocyte thereby favoring transamination. In contrast, the rate constants for the movement of alanine into and out of the epithelium and vascular bed are fast, approximately equal, and of the same order of magnitude as that for the uptake of glutamate from the blood. These findings of Boyd and Perring[28] are in accord with the view that alanine exchanges freely across the plasma membrane of a variety of cells.

2. Glutamine
The basolateral membrane of enterocytes is clearly permeable to glutamine in both directions because during glutamine absorption the amine appears in the blood, while blood-borne glutamine is utilized by the epithelium at very high rates. No work seems to have been reported yet on the transport across vesicles of the intestinal basolateral membrane, but in isolated cells a transport system shared by glutamine and alanine has been detected.[29] The location of this transport system is unknown but it could exchange inwardly moving glutamine for outwardly moving alanine at the basolateral pole of the cell.

3. NH_4^+
The small intestinal epithelium is an important source of blood ammonia; as to its mode of transport across the basolateral membrane, two routes are possible. In the presence of an external gradient of H-ion concentration (acid-cell interior), the outward movement could be as NH_3. On the other hand, it is known that in certain systems NH_4^+ can substitute for K^+ ions, so the possibility of exit through K channels has to be considered.

III. METABOLISM OF GLUTAMINE AND GLUTAMATE

A. Evidence that Glutamine and Glutamate are Metabolized in the Gastrointestinal Tract
1. Experiments In Vivo
a. Metabolism During Absorption
The early work of Dent and Schilling[10] and Neame and Wiseman[12] on metabolism of glutamate during its absorption by the intestine was referred to earlier (see Section I.A.3). Their results were confirmed by Elwyn et al.[30] and by Peraino and Harper.[31] An increased appearance of alanine in the portal blood when glutamine[32] was placed in the intestinal lumen suggested that the intestine also metabolized glutamine during absorption. These initial results have been confirmed and extended by Windmueller and Spaeth[33,34] and by Hanson and Parsons.[35]

b. Metabolism from the Blood
None of these early workers considered the possibility that amino acid metabolism by the small intestine might occur in the absence of the absorption of food. However, metabolism of glutamine by the nonhepatic splanchnic bed does indeed take place when there is no food

in the lumen. Thus, measurement of the difference in the concentration of glutamine between arterial and portal blood demonstrated a net uptake of glutamine by this region in the dog,[30,36] sheep,[37] man,[38] and rat,[39,40] and the cat, hamster, monkey, and rabbit.[40] However, the effect of species differences on glutamine metabolism by the intestine requires further investigation for the guinea pig and chicken intestine did not appear to remove glutamine from the plasma,[41] and apparently no such measurements have been made on other orders of animals.

Glutamate uptake by the GI tract from the plasma has not been observed in any species. Since glutamate is readily metabolized by the intestine when it is absorbed from the lumen it is likely that a low permeability of glutamate across the basolateral membrane prevents its uptake and metabolism from the plasma. Furthermore, in the rat, the arterial concentration of glutamate (0.16 mM) is considerably lower than that of glutamine (0.48 mM).[42]

2. Experiments In Vitro

Although net glutamine removal using slices of small intestine was demonstrated by Finch and Hird,[43] Neptune[44] was the first to demonstrate that [^{14}C]CO$_2$ was produced from [^{14}C]glutamine and that glutamine might therefore be a metabolic fuel. More recently, glutamine metabolism has been observed in isolated small intestinal epithelial cells[45] and vascularly perfused intestine.[35,40,46] The work of Parsons and Volman-Mitchell[13] on glutamate metabolism has been described earlier (see Section I.A.3). Direct measurements of glutamate uptake by isolated epithelial cells were performed by Watford et al.[45]

3. Site of Metabolism of Glutamine and Glutamate

The epithelial cells of the small and large intestine are probably the main sites for metabolism of glutamine in the GI tract. This statement is based mainly on comparisons of enzymic and metabolic activity between various regions of the GI tract. Thus, the activity of the enzyme which initiates glutamine metabolism, phosphate-dependent glutaminase (phosphate-activated glutaminase) (EC 3.5.1.2.), is high in both crypt and villus epithelial cells (enterocytes) in the small intestine, is somewhat lower in the colon, and is comparatively very low in intestinal smooth muscle.[41] Glutamine metabolism is twice as high in enterocytes[45] compared with colonocytes.[47] There may be some variation within the small intestine for metabolism of vascular glutamine by the ileum was 28% lower than in the jejunum.[35]

Metabolism of glutamate during absorption is likely to occur predominantly in the villus epithelial cells of the jejunum and ileum which have a much higher activity of the enzyme which initiates metabolism, alanine aminotransferase (EC 2.6.1.2), than do epithelial cells lower down the GI tract.[48]

B. Products of Metabolism of Glutamine and Glutamate in the Small Intestine

1. Glutamine

a. Fate of Carbon and Nitrogen

In order to understand glutamine metabolism in the intestine it is essential to identify the end products of the process. The first systematic study of the products of glutamine metabolism was performed by Windmueller and Spaeth,[40,49] who used U-[^{14}C]-labeled glutamine to trace the path of the glutamine carbon, which was found predominantly in CO$_2$ (55%) with much smaller proportions in lactate, other organic acids, and alanine. Nitrogenous metabolic products resulting from the addition of glutamine to the lumen in vivo were (percentage of total nitrogen) ammonia (36), alanine (36), ornithine (12), citrulline (10), and proline (7).[34] Hanson and Parsons[35] demonstrated that metabolism of glutamine by vascularly perfused jejunum resulted in the production of alanine, ammonia, and citrulline. Unlike enterocytes, lymphocytes produce much more aspartate than alanine when metabolizing glutamine.[50] The low activity of alanine aminotransferase in the lymphocytes[50] may be partly responsible for this difference from enterocytes. The aspartate/alanine ratio pro-

Table 1
COMPARISON OF THE METABOLISM OF GLUCOSE AND GLUTAMINE BY VASCULARLY PERFUSED RAT JEJUNUM[35] AND BY JEJUNUM IN VIVO[34,49]

Substrate or metabolite	Uptake (−) or release (+) of substrates/metabolites (μmol/hr/g dry weight)			
	Vascularly perfused jejunum		Jejunum in vivo	
	Fed	48-hr fasted	Fed	Overnight-fasted
Glucose	− 171	− 95	− 134	− 69
Glutamine[a]	− 75	− 107	− 140	− 60
Lactate	130	71	101	54
Alanine	30	55	68	44
Glutamate	7	7	5	0.6

[a] Concentration of glutamine in the vascular perfusate was 1.5 mM and in the blood was 0.5 mM.

duced in the presence of glutamine is higher in colonocytes[47] than in enterocytes,[45] and again there is a lower activity of alanine aminotransferase in colonic compared with jejunal epithelium.[48]

b. Metabolism of Glutamine In Vitro and In Vivo

An important point to be considered by workers in this area is that the type of intestinal preparation may influence the products resulting from metabolism of glutamine. Thus, luminally perfused segments of intestine[48a] and intestinal slices[46] convert glutamine to glutamate and produce virtually no alanine. Isolated enterocytes produce glutamate, alanine, and ammonia from glutamine, but citrulline production has not been demonstrated, although this may be for technical reasons.[45] However, little glutamate is produced during metabolism of glutamine by vascularly perfused intestine or in vivo (Table 1). In fact, despite differences in the concentration of glutamine and in the availability of other substrates such as ketone bodies, the results obtained with jejunum in vivo[34,39] are similar to those obtained with vascularly perfused jejunum[35] (Table 1). The major difference seems to be in the effect of fasting on the metabolism of glutamine (see below). Furthermore, contrary to the suggestion of Windmueller and Spaeth,[34] there is little evidence of anoxia in the vascularly perfused preparation. For example, the proportion of glucose converted to lactate is the same, 38% in fed rat jejunum in vitro and in vivo (Table 1).

c. Comparison of Metabolism of Glutamine from the Lumen and the Vascular Bed

There does not seem to be any effect of the route by which glutamine enters the tissue on the metabolism of the carbon atoms in glutamine. Thus, the distribution of ^{14}C among metabolic products was similar whether [14C]glutamine was presented to the tissue from the lumen or the vascular bed.[33] However, alanine-N production expressed as a fraction of the utilization of glutamine-N was 67% if glutamine was presented to the lumen of the vascularly perfused jejunum but only 41% if it was presented from the vascular bed.[35] Calculations from the data of Windmueller and Spaeth[33,34] give values for the same expression of 71% -N (luminal glutamine) and 48% -N (vascular glutamine) in alanine. Thus, if glutamine is provided from the lumen there seems to be a proportionately greater incorporation of the nitrogen into alanine.

2. Glutamate

Metabolism of glutamate carbon is very similar to that of glutamine. Thus, the ^{14}C from [^{14}C]glutamate is found predominantly in carbon dioxide with much smaller amounts of label in lactate, organic acids, and alanine. There are also similarities between glutamine and glutamate in the disposition of glutamate-N among metabolic products although a major difference is the lack of ammonia production from glutamate. The distribution of glutamate nitrogen among metabolic products is (percentage of total nitrogen) ammonia (0), alanine (63), ornithine (17), citrulline (15), and proline (4).[33]

C. Metabolic Routes Involved in the Metabolism of Glutamine and Glutamate

1. Production of Ammonia

The source of ammonia is mainly from degradation of glutamine by phosphate-dependent glutaminase, henceforth referred to as glutaminase. This enzyme has a much higher activity in enterocytes than other enzymes capable of degrading glutamine.[41] The enzyme is localized in mitochondria, has a K_m for glutamine of 2.2 mM at pH 8.1, and is activated by phosphate and NH_4^+. Glutamate dehydrogenase (EC 1.4.1.3) is probably not a major source of ammonia. For example, although luminal glutamate must enter the mitrochondrion to be converted to ornithine and citrulline any ammonia which is produced by glutamate dehydrogenase seems to be incorporated into citrulline.[33] Furthermore, only in enterocytes[51] where ammonia output/ glutamine uptake is greater than one is there clear evidence that activity of glutamate dehydrogenase adds to the net tissue production of ammonia. Production of ammonia from glutamine by the small intestine may have substantial physiological and clinical significance. Thus, 30% of the nitrogen utilized for hepatic ureagenesis may be derived from glutamine breakdown.[52] In the event of hepatic failure this ammonia may escape uptake by the liver with potentially toxic results for tissues like the brain.

2. Production of Alanine

Alanine is produced by transamination of glutamate with pyruvate by alanine aminotransferase and over 90% of the rat enzyme is in the cytosol.[48] Also, Windmueller and Spaeth[49] found very little ^{14}C from [^{14}C]glutamine in alanine. Consequently, Hanson and Parsons[53] proposed that glutamate derived from glutamine left the mitochondrion to be transaminated in the cytosol with a distinct extramitochondrial pool of pyruvate derived from glucose (Figure 1). This proposal requires the transport of glutamate and 2-oxoglutarate across the inner membrane of the mitochondrion and a possible scheme which could account for this is shown in Figure 2. The presence of these carriers has not been established in enterocyte mitochondria and the scheme must therefore be considered speculative. Isolated enterocyte mitochondria produce alanine from glutamine when incubated with 1 mM malate, and it has therefore been suggested that mitochondrial alanine aminotransferase may be involved in alanine production.[54] If this enzyme were an important contributor to overall alanine production, then two mitochondrial pyruvate pools would have to be proposed to explain the virtual absence of ^{14}C derived from [^{14}C]glutamine in alanine.

3. Production of Carbon Dioxide

Oxidation of carbon derived from glutamine and glutamate in the citric acid cycle requires a means of generating pyruvate from citric acid cycle intermediates. The possible alternative pathways involved in this process were discussed by Hanson and Parsons.[53] It was concluded that the mitochondrial NAD(P)-dependent "malic enzyme"[55] was the most likely candidate for this purpose (Figure 1). The enzyme has now been purified.[56] The reasons for believing that this enzyme is involved in glutamine metabolism are (1) the small intestinal mucosa is the most abundant source of the enzyme yet described, (2) its activity is sufficient to account for rates of glutamine oxidation, and (3) the role of the enzyme in energy metabolism is

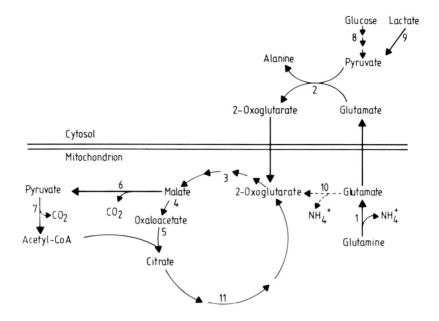

FIGURE 1.   Possible scheme for the metabolism of glutamine in the mucosa of the rat small intestine. The enzymes catalyzing the reactions: 1, glutaminase (EC 3.5.1.2); 2, alanine aminotransferase (EC 2.6.1.2); 3, enzymes of the tricarboxylic acid cycle converting 2-oxoglutarate into malate; 4, malate dehydrogenase (NAD$^+$-dependent) (EC 1.1.1.37); 5, citrate synthase (EC 4.1.3.7); 6, "malic" enzyme [NAD(P)$^+$-dependent]; 7, pyruvate dehydrogenase (EC 1.2.4.1, EC 2.3.1.12, and EC 1.6.4.3); 8, enzymes of glycolytic pathway converting glucose into pyruvate; 9, lactate dehydrogenase (EC 1.1.1.27); 10, glutamate dehydrogenase (EC 1.4.1.3); and 11, enzymes of the tricarboxylic acid cycle converting citrate into 2-oxoglutarate. Broken lines indicate pathways that do not occur at high rates under normal circumstances.

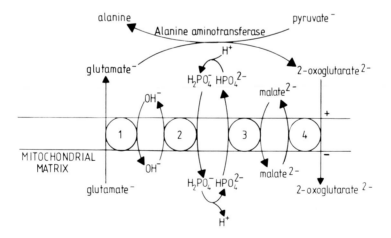

FIGURE 2.   Possible scheme for the movement of glutamate and 2-oxoglutarate across the mitochondrial membrane. The carriers involved: 1, glutamate/hydroxyl antiporter; 2, phosphate carrier; 3, dicarboxylate carrier; and 4, malate/2-oxoglutarate antiporter. The existence of these carriers in enterocyte mitochondria has yet to be established. On the assumption that all the pyruvate for transamination is generated by metabolism in the cytosol then one H$^+$ is transported into the mitochondrion for each molecule of glutamine metabolized.

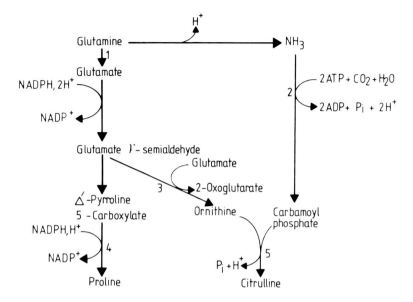

FIGURE 3. Pathways involved in the production of citrulline and proline by enterocytes. The enzymes catalyzing the reactions: 1, glutaminase; 2, carbamoyl-phosphate synthase ammonia (EC 2.7.2.5); 3, ornithine-oxoacid aminotransferase (EC 2.6.1.13); 4, pyrroline 5-carboxylate reductase (EC 1.5.1.2); and 5, ornithine transcarbamoylase (EC 2.1.3.3).

supported by its inhibition by ATP. In isolated rat enterocyte mitochondria oxidation of glutamine is stimulated by malate possibly because oxaloacetate derived from malate transaminates with glutamate to produce aspartate and 2-oxoglutarate.[57]

4. Production of Citrulline

The enzymology of the pathways involved in the production of citrulline and also proline (Figure 3) has been discussed by Windmueller.[52] Two recent findings will be mentioned here. The presence of N-acetylglutamate synthase activity in enterocyte mitochondria[58] suggests that N-acetylglutamate may serve as an activator of carbamoyl-phosphate synthase (EC 6.3.4.16) (Figure 3). Also, enzyme activity promoting the synthesis of pyrroline-5-carboxylate has been found to be associated with a mitochondrial membrane fraction prepared from intestinal mucosa.[59]

5. Purine Biosynthesis

Glutamine probably does not play a part in the *de novo* synthesis of purine nucleotides in the rat small intestine under normal circumstances and the activity of the enzyme glutamine-amidophosphoribosyltransferase (EC 2.4.2.14) in mucosal scrapings is significantly lower than that in the liver and colon. If the diet becomes deficient in purines then small intestinal mucosal cells may be able to perform *de novo* synthesis of purines from glutamine.[60]

6. Unanswered Problems

a. How Much of the Glutamine Carbon Taken Up by the Intestine is Reexported in a Form that can be Used for Gluconeogenesis in the Liver?

Glutamine released from the muscle has conventionally been thought of as ultimately transferring both nitrogen and carbon to the liver so an answer to the above question is important. This importance is emphasized when it is realized that glutamine uptake by the nonhepatic splanchnic bed may exceed the rate of release of glutamine from the total body muscle mass in the rat.[61] There is little doubt that glutamine is oxidized in the intestinal mucosa, but the accurate quantitation of this process from the production of [^{14}C]CO$_2$ from [^{14}C]glutamine is perhaps debatable. The problem results from the operation of the citric acid cycle in such a way that the carbon atoms released during one turn of the cycle are derived from oxaloacetate and not from acetyl-CoA. Thus, the net flux of carbon from [^{14}C]glutamine to [^{14}C]CO$_2$ may be overestimated and the flux to [^{14}C]pyruvate and to subsequent products may be underestimated.[62] To give an example of the problems of using the distribution of label to indicate net metabolic flux, 10% of the carbon from D-3-hydroxy[3-^{14}C]butyrate appears in lactate,[49] yet there cannot be any net flux of carbon from D-3-hydroxybutyrate to lactate. In conclusion, the possibility that the conversion of glutamine carbon to CO$_2$ may have been overestimated and that to alanine may have been underestimated exists.

An alternative, or additional, possibility is that glutamine carbon is indeed substantially oxidized by the small intestine but that pyruvate derived from glucose that would otherwise have been oxidized is saved from oxidation by being transaminated to alanine. The alanine could then be exported to the liver as a gluconeogenic substrate. Thus, oxidation of glutamine by the intestine effectively reduces the oxidation of glucose. This scheme is compatible with a lack of effect of glutamine on the rate of glucose utilization.[35,45]

There is little evidence for any substantial conversion of glutamine carbon to lactate. Thus, no net flux from glutamine to lactate was seen when glucose was absent from the vascular perfusate.[35] Indeed, if glutamine carbon does not appear in alanine there is some difficulty in explaining why it should appear in lactate. It is also unlikely that metabolism of glutamine reduces the oxidation of pyruvate derived from glucose by converting it to lactate because, in the presence of glucose, glutamine did not increase lactate production expressed as a proportion of glucose utilization.[35]

b. Control of Branch Points in the Metabolism of Glutamine and Glutamate

Glutamate derived from glutamine can either be transaminated with alanine or, alternatively, it can be metabolized to form citrulline or proline. It is unclear how this branch point is regulated but the proportionately greater formation of alanine from luminal rather than vascular glutamine mentioned above suggests that some regulation may take place.

D. Adaptation of Glutamine Metabolism to Altered Physiological States

1. Starvation

The activity of glutaminase in rat jejunum expressed per milligram of tissue protein was reduced by about 30% after starvation for 48 hr.[63,64] Glutamine metabolism from the plasma in vivo was reduced to less than 50% after an overnight fast[34,49] (Table 1). However, in the vascularly perfused rat jejunum a slight increase in the rate of metabolism of vascular glutamine was found after a 48 hr fast[35] (Table 1). The reason for this discrepancy seems to be a lower rate of glutamine metabolism in the vascularly perfused intestine than in vivo in fed rats (Table 1). Starvation for 48 hr reduces glutamine metabolism by colonocytes.[47]

In conclusion, it is unclear whether glutamine metabolism falls on fasting, but one way of reconciling the vascular perfusion results with those obtained in vivo is to suggest that some factor present in vivo, but which is absent from the artificial vascular perfusate in vitro, may stimulate the metabolism of glutamine by the intestine of fed rats.

2. Acidosis

Measurements of arterial/portal venous differences suggested an increased uptake of glutamine by the nonhepatic splanchnic bed of acidotic dogs,[36] no change in sheep,[65] and a decrease in rats.[66] Also, the stimulation of enterocyte glutaminase by bicarbonate suggested a means by which acidosis could affect metabolism of glutamine,[51] although the effect was much smaller than that obtained with hepatocytes.

However, isolated enterocytes from normal and acidotic rats exhibited similar metabolic behavior.[67] Schröck and Goldstein,[61] who took account of possible changes in blood flow, found no significant effect of acidosis on the uptake of glutamine by the nonhepatic splanchnic bed of rats in vivo. Also, neither acute nor chronic acidosis altered the activity of glutaminase in the jejunal mucosa,[41,63] and there was no effect of acidosis on the production of ammonia from glutamine by jejunal slices.[63] Finally, Hanson and Parsons[35] found the utilization of glutamine by the vascularly perfused rat jejunum to be slightly increased by chronic acidosis when metabolism was expressed with respect to the tissue dry weight. If account was taken of the decreased weight of jejunal mucosa in acidotic rats then calculations showed that metabolism of glutamine by the whole jejunum was unlikely to have been altered.

In conclusion, it is unlikely that chronic acidosis has a sizable effect on the uptake of glutamine by the rat small intestine.

3. Streptozotocin-Diabetes

The specific activity of glutaminase in enterocytes was not altered 6 days after the induction of streptozotocin-diabetes. There was also no change in the utilization of glutamine by the enterocytes, although the hyperplasia of the intestinal epithelium should have resulted in an increased total capacity to metabolize glutamine.[68] Uptake of glutamine from the blood by the nonhepatic splanchnic bed of streptozotocin-diabetic rats in vivo was unchanged by comparison with controls[61] or was decreased.[68,69] These arteriovenous-difference measurements were all made on fed rats so their interpretation depends on whether there was any glutamine being absorbed from the lumen. This consideration is of particular importance in the present context because long-term streptozotocin-diabetic rats are hyperphagic and therefore perhaps more likely to be absorbing glutamine from the lumen than the controls. In conclusion, the capacity of the small intestine to metabolize glutamine will be increased in medium- to long-term streptozotocin-diabetes, but whether this change in metabolic capacity is actually associated with a change in metabolism in vivo remains an open question.

E. Control and Physiological Significance of Glutamine Metabolism

1. Control

Possible sites for the regulation of metabolism of glutamine are transport into the tissue,[29] entry into mitochondria, and the activity of glutaminase. The concentration of glutamine in enterocytes seems to be below that in the blood[40] and increasing the concentration of glutamine in the vascular perfusate increased the metabolism of glutamine.[35,40] Thus, the transport across the basolateral membrane may be a step with a high flux control coefficient (i.e., its rate will have a major influence on the overall flux through the pathway of glutamine metabolism). This proposal explains the finding of both Windmueller and Spaeth[33] and Hanson and Parsons[35] that the addition of glutamine to the lumen increases the overall rate of glutamine metabolism by the tissue. What happens is that when glutamine enters the tissue by two routes its availability is increased and, therefore, so is its metabolism.

When glutamine (6 mM) is in the lumen some of the amino acid crosses the epithelium unchanged, but 6 mM glutamate is almost completely metabolized by the epithelium.[33] These findings suggest that steps initiating metabolism of glutamine (entry into the mitochondrion and breakdown by glutaminase to glutamate) could also restrict metabolism of glutamine. However, direct information on the importance of these potential control sites is lacking at present.

Metabolism of glutamate from the lumen of the intestine under physiological circumstances is probably controlled largely by the rate at which glutamate can enter the tissue. Thus, as was mentioned earlier (Section I.A.3), when the concentration of glutamate in the lumen is such as might be achieved after a protein meal then the capacity of the transamination system in the rat is sufficient to metabolize all of the glutamate.[13]

2. Physiological Significance

a. Metabolism of Glutamate from the Lumen

Glutamate is poorly taken up by the liver and therefore its metabolism by the small intestine prevents the flooding of the peripheral circulation with glutamate. This detoxifying role for the small intestine may be important for it seems that subjects suffering from "Chinese Restaurant Syndrome" following ingestion of large quantities of monosodium glutamate may have an impaired ability to transaminate glutamate during absorption (see Section IV.A). Oxidation of glutamate carbon will help to provide energy to power absorptive processes (e.g., Na^+ pumping).

b. Metabolism of Glutamine from the Lumen

Probably the most important consequence of the metabolism of luminal glutamine is the provision of energy to aid in the absorption of the products of digestion of food. Indeed, metabolism of luminal glutamine, glutamate, and aspartate can account for 39% of the CO_2 produced by the jejunum in vivo.[34] Furthermore, glutamine increases sodium and fluid transport in everted sacs of rabbit ileum.[70] Some citrulline will also be produced (see below).

c. Metabolism of Glutamine from the Vascular Bed

Metabolism of glutamine may be a characteristic of dividing cells in which changes in division rate can occur quickly (e.g., lymphocytes[50]). The fast turnover of the intestinal epithelium has therefore been used to explain why the intestine metabolizes glutamine from the vascular bed. We are not convinced by this hypothesis. First, neither the chicken nor guinea pig intestine appears to remove glutamine from the plasma[41] and, although plasma glutamine is comparatively low in these species, there is no reason to believe that their intestinal epithelium does not turn over in a similar fashion to other animals. Second, only a fraction of the cells in the crypts and none in the villi can be considered to be dividing rapidly. Villus cells will never be recruited for further division (they move up the villus and are extruded at the tip). However, while enzymes like thymidine kinase (EC 2.7.1.21) which are important in cell replication are of high activity in the crypts, their activity falls as the cells progress up the villi by contrast with glutaminase activity which is similar in the crypt and the villus cells.[41] Thus, some other explanation seems to be required for the retention of a high glutaminase activity in the nondividing villus epithelial cells. Third, the stomach, in which epithelial cells turn over fairly rapidly, extracts little glutamine from the blood[42] and thus glutamine metabolism does not seem to be a prerequisite for turnover of all GI epithelia. In conclusion, although glutamine is indubitably an important substrate for villus enterocytes in many mammals, it seems unlikely that this situation has arisen because of the rapid turnover of the epithelium.

We would speculate that the main significance of glutamine metabolism from the blood by the small intestine of several mammals lies first in the elevation of the portal blood ammonia concentration above the minimum level of 50 μM required for hepatic urea synthesis and, second, in the promotion of the hepatic intercellular glutamine cycle.[71] This system, which may relate the uptake of glutamine by the liver to the regulation of the acid-base balance, requires the presence of both ammonia and glutamine in the portal blood. The use of glutamine as a metabolic fuel would then be a consequence of this need to raise the ammonia concentration in the portal blood, coupled with the undesirability, mentioned above, of adding the glutamate back to the portal blood. Direct evidence in support of this idea is lacking, but in the chicken, where the nitrogenous excretory product is different from mammals, it is interesting to note that the intestine does not remove glutamine from the blood[41] and that enterocytes can both synthesize and catabolize glutamine.[71]

Apart from being used as a source of ammonia and as a metabolic fuel glutamine also is converted to citrulline. Citrulline passes to the kidney where it is converted to arginine.[73] The operation of this pathway explains how some arginine can be synthesized in rats.

IV. CLINICAL ASPECTS

A. Chinese Restaurant Syndrome

Monosodium L-glutamate has been widely used as a food additive (EEC food additive E621:MSG). The amino acid is commonly added in relatively large amounts in Chinese cooking and subjects very fond of this cuisine may ingest several grams of sodium glutamate at a sitting. Some people subsequently suffer burning sensations, feeling of pressure on the face, and very worrying chest pain: the Chinese Restaurant Syndrome.[74] There is no doubt that these symptoms are due to the glutamate and not to other additives because they can be induced by the administration, either orally or intravenously, of the L-amino acid.[75] There is a considerable variation in the threshold of the dose required to produce these effects, but i.v. doses of 200 mg or oral doses of less than 3 g can induce symptoms. Neither D-glutamate or L-aspartate produce effects. Presumably, it is the rate of entry of the amino acid into the mesenteric circulation that is a factor in determining the severity of the symptoms because ingestion of food before consuming the L-glutamate, and hence slowing its absorption, will protect the most susceptible of subjects.[75]

Bazzano et al.[76] administered orally to normal subjects a chemically defined diet containing 16 g N per day in the form of essential amino acids and 137 g of (?D-L) glutamate for periods of up to 42 days without the appearance of symptoms. It would clearly be of value to measure in susceptible subjects the plasma levels of L-glutamate and also to investigate whether transamination reactions are normal in mucosal biopsies; such studies do not seem to have been done.

B. Parenteral Nutrition

1. Adult

The fact that transamination reactions occur during absorption of meals containing the dicarboxylic acids has important implications with respect to the pattern of amino acids that enter the blood of omnivorous and carnivorous animals during absorption. Compared with the pattern present in the mixture undergoing digestion in the intestinal lumen, the amino acids secreted into the blood from the intestine will be relatively deficient in glutamate and aspartate and enriched in alanine. A possible advantage in the use of alanine to ferry amino-N from the intestine to other tissues may be related to the capacity of these tissues to assimilate alanine.[21] These facts, together with the known toxicity of large doses of L-glutamate administered intravenously, are clearly of relevance to the design of mixtures of amino acids used in parenteral nutrition. Evidently, these mixtures ought to be relatively deficient in the L-dicarboxylic acid but enriched with L-alanine.

2. Nutrition of Premature Infants

An important factor in the survival of infants delivered at under 30 weeks gestational age is their nutrition. The intestinal tract is often sufficiently underdeveloped in premature infants to prohibit oral feeding. Because glutamine as well as glucose is a major fuel of the adult intestine and it is known that the rat fetal intestine can metabolize glutamine,[76a] the enrichment with this amino acid of mixtures to be administered parenterally to premature infants ought to be considered at least on the grounds of the nutrition of the developing intestinal tract.

3. Celiac Disease

Wheat proteins and in particular the gliadin of gluten specifically induced relapses in children with celiac disease. A striking feature of gliadin is that no less than 45 amino acid residues out of every hundred consist of glutamine; indeed, it is this composition that makes it so useful in bread making. Naturally, the high glutamine content has been related to its toxic properties in patients suffering from celiac disease, but investigations of γ-glutamyltransferase activity of the mucosa do not throw new light on the condition, neither have studies on peptidases in the mucosa that hydrolyze bonds adjacent to glutamine.[77]

More recently, attention has been directed to the enzyme transglutaminase. Studies by Van der Kamer and Weijers[78] showed that gluten that has been deaminated is no longer toxic, an observation that suggests that there may be an abnormality in the metabolism of glutamine in celiac patients. Transglutaminase[79] in the presence of calcium ions cross-links adjacent polypeptides by forming additional bonds between the γ-carbonyl group of glutamine in one chain with the ε-amino groups of lysine in the other chain. Naturally, gliadin is a very suitable substrate for transglutaminase. The enzyme is present in the intestinal mucosa of normal subjects and is said to be increased in subjects with celiac disease.[77]

The possibility is thus raised of an increased binding by cross-linking of gliadin to cellular proteins including those of the brush borders and basolateral membranes. Such binding could induce cell damage and hence lead to an increase in the turnover of the mucosal epithelial cell population. Clearly, further studies on glutamine metabolism in the intestinal mucosa in health and disease are necessary and likely to be fruitful in throwing light on the biochemical disorders underlying celiac disease.

V. SUMMARY

There is now no doubt that the metabolism of glutamine is of major importance to the small intestinal epithelium. The rate of glutamine utilization is similar to that of glucose,[34,35] and 35% of plasma glutamine is extracted during each passage through jejunal segments.[33] Oxidation of dietary glutamine and glutamate by the intestine during the absorption of nutrients provides energy for the sodium pumping linked with absorption, and prevents overloading of the body tissues with potentially harmful glutamate.

Metabolism of *plasma* glutamine occurs not only during absorption but also in the postabsorptive and fasted states. This continuous removal of glutamine from the plasma by the intestine has major consequences for the body as a whole. Thus, it has been calculated that the rate of glutamine utilization by the GI tract is such that it alone would produce a turnover of the entire plasma pool of the rat every 4.6 min and would account for approximately 15% of the turnover of the entire body glutamine pool.[52] While a high rate of glutamine metabolism in the crypts might be required for the rapid turnover of the epithelium, the retention of this metabolic capacity in the mature villus cells has also to be explained. In this respect, the calculation[52] that the nitrogenous products of intestinal glutamine metabolism could account for 30% of the nitrogen utilized for hepatic ureagenesis seems highly significant.

What remains for the future? The transport of glutamine across brush border, basolateral, and mitochondrial membranes and the regulation of these processes deserve investigation. The role of the intestine in nitrogen metabolism in those animals in which the jejunum apparently does not remove glutamine from the blood also needs clarifying. These are not the only problems (see sections III.C.6, IV.A, and IV.B). Clearly much remains to be done.

ACKNOWLEDGMENT

We are grateful to Dr. P. Lund for comments on the manuscript, to Dr. J. D. McGivan for advice on mitochondrial transport systems, and to Dr. T. J. Peters for providing material that is in press.

REFERENCES

1. **Parsons, D. S.,** Methods for investigation of intestinal absorption, in *Handbook of Physiology, Section 6: The Alimentary Canal,* Vol. 3, Code, C. F., Ed., American Physiological Society, Washington, D.C., 1968, 1164.
2. **Dickens, F. and Weil-Malherbe, H.,** Metabolism of normal and tumour tissue. XIX. The metabolism of intestinal mucous membrane, *Biochem. J.,* 35, 7, 1941.
3. **Leblond, C. P. and Walker, B. E.,** Renewal of cell populations, *Physiol. Rev.,* 36, 255, 1956.
4. **Lipkin, M.,** Proliferation and differentiation in gastrointestinal cells, *Physiol. Rev.,* 53, 891, 1973.
5. **Fisher, R. B. and Parsons, D. S.,** Glucose movements across the wall of the rat small intestine, *J. Physiol.,* 119, 224, 1953.
6. **Wilson, T. H.,** *Intestinal Absorption,* W.B. Saunders, Philadelphia, 1962, chap. 4.
7. **Hanson, P. J. and Parsons, D. S.,** The utilisation of glucose and production of lactate by *in vitro* preparations of rat small intestine: effects of vascular perfusion, *J. Physiol.,* 255, 775, 1976.
8. **Gibson, Q. H. and Wiseman, G.,** Selective absorption of stereoisomers of amino acids from loops of the small intestine of the rat, *Biochem. J.,* 48, 426, 1951.
9. **Wiseman, G.,** Absorption of amino acids using an *in vitro* technique, *J. Physiol.,* 120, 63, 1953.
10. **Dent, C. E. and Schilling, J. A.,** Studies on the absorption of proteins: the amino acid pattern in the portal blood, *Biochem. J.,* 44, 318, 1949.
11. **Matthews, D. M. and Wiseman, G.,** Transamination by the small intestine of the rat, *J. Physiol.,* 120, 55P, 1953.
12. **Neame, K. D. and Wiseman, G.,** The transamination of glutamic and aspartic acids during absorption by the small intestine of the dog *in vivo, J. Physiol.,* 135, 442, 1957.
13. **Parsons, D. S. and Volman-Mitchell, H.,** The transamination of glutamate and aspartate during absorption *in vitro* by small intestine of chicken, guinea-pig and rat, *J. Physiol.,* 239, 677, 1974.
14. **Munck, B. G.,** Intestinal transport of amino acids, in *Physiology of the Gastrointestinal Tract,* Johnson, L. R., Ed., Raven Press, New York, 1981, 1097.
15. **Murer, H. and Burckhardt, G.,** Membrane transport of anions across epithelia of mammalian small intestine and kidney proximal tubule, *Rev. Physiol. Biochem. Pharmacol.,* 96, 1, 1983.
16. **Schultz, S. C., Yu-Tu, I., Alvarez, O. O., and Curran, P. F.,** Dicarboxylic amino acid influx across the brush border of the rabbit ileum, *J. Gen. Physiol.,* 56, 621, 1970.
17. **Lerner, J. and Steinke, D. K.,** Intestinal absorption of glutamic acid in the chicken, *Comp. Biochem. Physiol.,* 57, 11, 1977.
18. **Schneider, E. G., Hammerman, M. R., and Sactor, B.,** Sodium gradient-dependent L-glutamate transport in renal brush border membrane vesicles. Evidence for an electroneutral mechanism, *J. Biol. Chem.,* 255, 7650, 1980.
19. **Silbernagl, S.,** Renal transport of amino acids and oligopeptides, in *Physiology of the Gastrointestinal Tract,* Johnson, L. R., Ed., Raven Press, New York, 1981, 991.
20. **Burston, D., Marrs, T. C., Schleisenger, M. H., Sopanen, T., and Matthews, D. M.,** Mechanisms of peptide transport, in *Peptide Transport and Hydrolysis,* Ciba Foundation Symp., (New Series, Vol. 50,) Elsevier/North-Holland, New York, 1977, 79.
21. **Parsons, D. S.,** Fuels of the small intestinal mucosa, in *Topics in Gastroenterology,* Vol. 3, Truelove, S. C. and Willoughby, C. P., Eds., Blackwell, Oxford, 1979, 253.
22. **Hunjan, M. K. and Evered, D. F.,** Absorption of glutathione from the gastrointestinal tract, *Biochim. Biophys. Acta,* 815, 184, 1985.
23. **Hanes, C. S., Hird, F. J. R., and Isherwood, F. A.,** Enzymic transpeptidisation reactions involving γ-glutamyl peptides and γ-aminoacylpeptides, *Biochem. J.,* 51, 25, 1952.
24. **Meister, A., Tate, S. S., and Ross, L. L.,** Membrane bound γ-glutamyl transpeptidase, in *The Enzymes of Biological Membranes,* Vol. 3, Martinosi, A., Ed., Plenum Press, New York, 1976, 315.
25. **Meister, A. and Tate, S. S.,** Glutathione and related γ-glutamyl compounds: biosynthesis and utilization, *Annu. Rev. Biochem.,* 45, 559, 1976.
26. **Meister, A., Tate, S. S., and Thompson, G. A.,** On the function of the γ-glutamyl cycle in the transport of amino acids and peptides, in *Peptide Transport and Hydrolysis,* Ciba Foundation Symposium, (New Series, Vol. 50,) Elsevier/North-Holland, New York, 1977, 123.
27. **Stevens, B. R., Kaunitz, J. D., and Wright, E. M.,** Intestinal transport of amino acids and sugars: advances using membrane vesicles, *Annu. Rev. Physiol.,* 46, 417, 1984.
28. **Boyd, C. A. R. and Perring, V. S.,** Transamination and asymmetry in glutamate transport across the basolateral membrane of frog small intestine, *Biosci. Rep.,* 1, 851, 1981.
29. **Bradford, N. M. and McGivan, J. D.,** The transport of alanine and glutamine into isolated rat intestinal epithelial cells, *Biochem. Biophys. Acta,* 689, 55, 1982.
30. **Elwyn, D. H., Parikh, H. C., and Shoemaker, W. C.,** Amino acid movements between gut, liver and periphery in unanaesthetised dogs, *Am. J. Physiol.,* 215, 1260, 1968.

31. **Peraino, C. and Harper, A. E.,** Observations on protein digestion *in vivo*. V. Free amino acids in blood plasma of rats force-fed zein, casein, or their respective hydrolysates, *J. Nutr.,* 80, 270, 1963.

32. **Peraino, C. and Harper, A. E.,** Concentrations of free amino acids in blood plasma of rats force-fed L-glutamic acid, L-glutamine, or L-alanine, *Arch. Biochem. Biophys.,* 97, 442, 1962.

33. **Windmueller, H. G. and Spaeth, A. E.,** Intestinal metabolism of glutamine and glutamate from the lumen as compared to glutamine from blood, *Arch. Biochem. Biophys.,* 171, 662, 1975.

34. **Windmueller, H. G. and Spaeth, A. E.,** Respiratory fuels and nitrogen metabolism *in vivo* in small intestine of fed rats, *J. Biol. Chem.,* 255, 107, 1980.

35. **Hanson, P. J. and Parsons, D. S.,** Metabolism and transport of glutamine and glucose in vascularly perfused rat small intestine, *Biochem. J.,* 166, 509, 1977.

36. **Addae, S. K. and Lotspeich, W. D.,** Relation between glutamine utilization and production in metabolic acidosis, *Am. J. Physiol.,* 215, 269, 1968.

37. **Wolff, J. E., Bergman, E. N., and Williams, H. H.,** Net metabolism of plasma amino acids by liver and portal-drained viscera of fed sheep, *Am. J. Physiol.,* 223, 438, 1972.

38. **Felig, P., Wahren, J., and Raf, L.,** Evidence of interorgan amino acid transport by blood cells in humans, *Proc. Natl. Acad. Sci. U.S.A.,* 70, 1775, 1973.

39. **Aikawa, T., Matsutaka, H., Yamamoto, H., Okuda, T., Ishikawa, E., Kawano, T., and Matsumura, E.,** Gluconeogenesis and amino acid metabolism, *J. Biochem.,* 74, 1003, 1973.

40. **Windmueller, H. G. and Spaeth, A. E.,** Uptake and metabolism of plasma glutamine by the small intestine, *J. Biol. Chem.,* 249, 5070, 1974.

41. **Pinkus, L. M. and Windmueller, H. G.,** Phosphate-dependent glutaminase of small intestine: localization and role in intestinal glutamine metabolism, *Arch. Biochem. Biophys.,* 182, 506, 1977.

42. **Anderson, N. G. and Hanson, P. J.,** Arteriovenous differences for amino acids across control and acid-secreting rat stomach *in vivo, Biochem. J.,* 210, 451, 1983.

43. **Finch, L. R. and Hird, F. J. R.,** The uptake of amino acids by isolated segments of rat intestine, *Biochim. Biophys. Acta,* 43, 268, 1960.

44. **Neptune, E. M.,** Respiration and oxidation of various substrates by ileum *in vitro, Am. J. Physiol.,* 209, 329, 1965.

45. **Watford, M., Lund, P., and Krebs, H. A.,** Isolation and metabolic characteristics of rat and chicken enterocytes, *Biochem. J.,* 178, 589, 1979.

46. **Matsutaka, H., Aikawa, T., Yamamoto, H., and Ishikawa, E.,** Gluconeogenesis and amino acid metabolism, *J. Biochem.,* 74, 1019, 1973.

47. **Ardawi, M. S. M. and Newsholme, E. A.,** Fuel utilization in colonocytes of the rat, *Biochem. J.,* 231, 713, 1985.

48. **Volman-Mitchell, H. and Parsons, D. S.,** Distribution and activities of dicarboxylic amino acid transaminases in gastrointestinal mucosa of rat, mouse, hamster, guinea pig, chicken and pigeon, *Biochem. Biophys. Acta,* 334, 316, 1974.

48a. **Parsons, D. S. and Volman-Mitchell, H.,** unpublished work.

49. **Windmueller, H. G. and Spaeth, A. E.,** Identification of ketone bodies and glutamine as the major respiratory fuels *in vivo* for postabsorptive rat small intestine, *J. Biol. Chem.,* 253, 69, 1978.

50. **Newsholme, E. A., Crabtree, B., and Ardawi, M. S. M.,** Glutamine metabolism in lymphocytes: its biochemical, physiological and clinical importance, *Q. J. Exp. Physiol.,* 70, 473, 1985.

51. **Baverel, G. and Lund, P.,** A role for bicarbonate in the regulation of mammalian glutamine metabolism, *Biochem. J.,* 184, 599, 1979.

52. **Windmueller, H. G.,** Glutamine utilization by the small intestine, in *Advances in Enzymology and Related Areas of Molecular Biology,* Vol. 53, Meister, A., Ed., John Wiley & Sons, New York, 1982, 201.

53. **Hanson, P. J. and Parsons, D. S.,** The interrelationship between glutamine and alanine in the intestine, *Biochem. Soc. Trans.,* 8, 506, 1980.

54. **Masola, M., Peters, T. J., and Evered, D. F.,** Transamination pathways influencing L-glutamine and L-glutamate oxidation by rat enterocyte mitochondria and subcellular localization of L-alanine aminotransferase and L-aspartate aminotransferase, *Biochim. Biophys. Acta,* 843, 137, 1985.

55. **Sauer, L. A., Dauchy, R. T., and Nagel, W. O.,** Identification of an NAD(P)$^+$-dependent 'malic' enzyme in small-intestinal-mucosal mitochondria, *Biochem. J.,* 184, 185, 1979.

56. **Nagel, W. O. and Sauer, L. A.,** Mitochondrial malic enzymes, *J. Biol. Chem.,* 257, 12405, 1982.

57. **Evered, D. F. and Masola, B.,** The oxidation of glutamine and glutamate in relation to anion transport in enterocyte mitochondria, *Biochem. J.,* 218, 449, 1984.

58. **Uchiyama, C., Mori, M., and Tatibaba, M.,** Subcellular localization and properties of N-acetylglutamate synthase in rat small intestinal mucosa, *J. Biochem. (Tokyo),* 89, 1777, 1981.

59. **Wakabayashi, Y., Henslee, J. G., and Jones, M. E.,** Pyrroline-5-carboxylate synthesis from glutamate by rat intestinal mucosa. Subcellular localization and temperature stability, *J. Biol. Chem.,* 258, 3873, 1983.

60. **Le Leiko, N. S., Bronstein, A. D., Baliga, B. S., and Munro, H. N.,** De novo purine nucleotide synthesis in rat small and large intestine: effect of dietary protein and purines, *J. Pediatr. Gastroenterol. Nutr.,* 2, 313, 1983.

61. **Schröck, H. and Goldstein, L.,** Interorgan relationships for glutamine metabolism in normal and acidotic rats, *Am. J. Physiol.,* 240, E519, 1981.

62. **Vinay, P., Mapes, J. P., and Krebs, H. A.,** Fate of glutamine carbon in renal metabolism, *Am. J. Physiol.,* 234, F123, 1978.

63. **McFarlane Anderson, N., Bennett, F. I., and Alleyne, G. A. O.,** Ammonia production by the small intestine of the rat, *Biochim. Biophys. Acta,* 437, 238, 1976.

64. **Budohoski, L., Challis, R. J. A., and Newsholme, E. A.,** Effects of starvation on the maximal activities of some glycolytic and citric acid-cycle enzymes and glutaminase in mucosa of the small intestine of the rat, *Biochem. J.,* 206, 169, 1982.

65. **Heitmann, R. N. and Bergman, E. N.,** Glutamine metabolism, interorgan transport and glucogenicity in the sheep, *Am. J. Physiol.,* 234, 197, 1968.

66. **Lund, P. and Watford, M.,** Glutamine at a precursor of urea, in *The Urea Cycle,* Grisolia, S., Baguena, S., and Mayer, F., Eds., John Wiley & Sons, London, 1976, 479.

67. **Lemieux, G., Watford, M., Vinay, P., and Gougoux, A.,** Metabolic changes in skeletal muscle during chronic metabolic acidosis, *Int. J. Biochem.,* 12, 75, 1980.

68. **Watford, M., Smith, E. M., and Erbelding, E. J.,** The regulation of phosphate-activated glutaminase activity and glutamine metabolism in the streptozotocin-diabetic rat, *Biochem. J.,* 224, 207, 1984.

69. **Brosnan, J. T., Man, K-C., Hall, D. E., Colbourne, S. A., and Brosnan, M. E.,** Interorgan metabolism of amino acids in streptozotocin-diabetic ketoacidotic rat, *Am. J. Physiol.,* 244, E151, 1983.

70. **Love, A. H. G., Mitchell, T. G., and Neptune, E. M.,** Transport of sodium and water by rabbit ileum *in vitro* and *in vivo, Nature,* 206, 1158, 1965.

72. **Porteous, J. W.,** Glutamate, glutamine, aspartate, asparagine, glucose and ketone-body metabolism in chick intestinal brush border cells, *Biochem. J.,* 188, 619, 1980.

73. **Windmueller, H. G. and Spaeth, A. E.,** Source and fate of circulating citrulline, *Am. J. Physiol.,* 241, E473, 1981.

74. **Ho Man Kwok, R.,** Chinese restaurant syndrome, *N. Engl. J. Med.,* 278, 796, 1968.

75. **Schaumberg, H. H., Byck, R., Gerstl, R., and Mashman, J. H.,** Monosodium L-glutamate: its pharmacology and role in the Chinese Restaurant Syndrome, *Science,* 163, 826, 1969.

76. **Bazzano, G., D'Elia, J. A., and Olsen, R. E.,** Monosodium glutamate: feeding of large amounts in man and gerbils, *Science,* 169, 1208, 1970.

76a. **Hislop, J. and Parsons, D. S.,** unpublished experiments.

77. **Peters, T. J. and Bjarnason, I.,** Coeliac syndrome: biochemical mechanisms and the missing peptide hypothesis revisited, *Gut,* 25, 913, 1984.

78. **Van de Kamer, J. H. and Weijers, H. A.,** Coeliac disease. V. Some experiments on the cause of the harmful effect of wheat gliadin, *Acta Paediatr.,* 44, 465, 1955.

79. **Folk, J. E.,** Transglutaminases, *Annu. Rev. Biochem.,* 49, 517, 1980.

Index

INDEX